Manual of Temporomandibular Disorders

Manual of Temporomandibular Disorders

Edward F. Wright

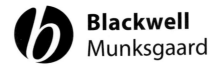
Blackwell
Munksgaard

Edward F. Wright, DDS, MS, MAGD, is an assistant professor at the University of Texas Health Science Center–San Antonio (UTHSCSA). He completed a one-year general dentistry residency and the University of Minnesota's two-year TMJ and Craniofacial Pain Fellowship. He taught TMD diagnosis and treatment to more than 100 U.S. Air Force general dentistry, orthodontic, periodontal, and prosthodontic residents. Upon retiring from the Armed Forces, he completed a two-year research fellowship in TMD diagnosis and treatment at the South Texas Veterans Health Care System and taught TMD diagnosis and treatment to their general dentistry residents. He is now UTHSCSA's Course Director for their undergraduate dentistry students' TMD Course and Dental Anatomy and Occlusion Course, and Module Director for their stabilization appliance rotation. Dr. Wright is the primary author of 23 journal articles and 6 abstracts.

© 2005 by Blackwell Munksgaard,
published by Blackwell Publishing,
a Blackwell Publishing Company

Blackwell Publishing Professional
2121 State Avenue, Ames, Iowa 50014-8300, USA
Tel: +1 515 292 0140
Web site: www.blackwellprofessional.com

Editorial Offices:
9600 Garsington Road, Oxford OX4 2DQ, UK
Tel: 01865 776868

Blackwell Publishing Asia Pty Ltd,
550 Swanston Street, Carlton South,
Victoria 3053, Australia
Tel: +61 (0)3 9347 0300

Blackwell Wissenschafts Verlag, Kurfürstendamm 57,
10707 Berlin, Germany
Tel: +49 (0)30 32 79 060

Library of Congress Cataloging-in-Publication Data

Wright, Edward F.
    Manual of temporomandibular disorders /
        Edward F. Wright.—1st ed.
        p. ; cm. — (Blackwell Munksgaard consult
        library)
    Includes bibliographical references and index.
    ISBN 0-8138-0752-2 (alk. paper)
1. Temporomandibular joint—Diseases—
Handbooks, manuals, etc. 2. Temporomandibular
joint—Diseases—Treatment—Handbooks, manuals,
etc. [DNLM: 1. Temporomandibular Joint
Disorders—therapy. WU 140.5 W948c 2005]
I. Title. II. Series.

RK470.W75 2005
617.5′22—dc22

2004006868

Set in USA by Data Management
Printed and bound in India by Replika

For further information on
Blackwell Publishing's dental publications, visit our
Dentistry Subject Site:
www.dentistry.blackwellmunksgaard.com

The last digit is the print number: 9 8 7 6 5 4 3 2 1

*I dedicate this book to my wife, Barbara,
for her love and understanding
throughout my professional career.*

Contents

Preface

While teaching TMD to postgraduate residents, I commonly heard them complain that there was no concise clinically practical TMD book that (a) was written on the level for the average dentist or dental student, (b) taught evidence-based diagnosis and multidisciplinary treatment for the majority of patients with TMD, (c) taught how to rule out disorders that mimic TMD and identify medical contributing factors for which patients need to be referred, and (d) taught how to identify patients with complex TMD who are beyond the scope of most dentists.

The thrust of this book is to satisfy those complaints; it is the clinical implementation of my assimilated evidence-based TMD knowledge and experience. This book attempts to simplify the complexities of TMD for ease of clinical understanding and application, in addition to integrating the scientific literature, clinical trials, and clinical experiences into an effective strategy. To the degree possible, it provides a systematic guide for how the average dentist can most effectively diagnose and treat the different types of TMD patients.

The book directs how the information obtained from the patient interview and clinical exam can be used to select the most cost-effective evidence-based therapies that have the greatest potential to provide long-term symptom relief for each patient. Whenever possible, the information provided is based on current research findings. When conclusive evidence is not available, I attempt to present a consensus founded on a significant depth of experience and informed thought.

Since this is not a comprehensive textbook on TMD, it periodically warns that certain characteristics are suggestive of an uncommon disorder beyond the book's scope. The book suggests that a practitioner may desire to refer a patient with these specific characteristics to someone with greater expertise in that area.

To speed the practitioner's synthesis of this material, questions that students frequently ask are placed at the beginning of the applicable chapters, and important concepts are highlighted throughout the book. Important terms are in italic or bold, with those listed in the glossary in bold.

Edward Wright

Edward F. Wright

Introduction

Temporomandibular disorder (TMD) is a collective term used for a number of clinical problems that involve the masticatory muscle, *temporomandibular joint* (TMJ), and/or associated structures. It has plagued humanity throughout history, and treatment has been reported even during the time of the ancient Egyptians.[1]

The cardinal signs and symptoms for TMD are pain in the masseter muscle, TMJ, and/or temporalis muscle regions; mouth-opening limitation; and TMJ sounds.[2] TMD pain is by far the most common reason patients seek treatment.[3,4]

◑ FOCAL POINT

The cardinal signs and symptoms for TMD are pain in the masseter muscle, TMJ, and/or temporalis muscle regions; mouth-opening limitation; and TMJ sounds.

TMD is an extremely common disorder that is most often reported in individuals between the ages of 20 and 40. Approximately 33 percent of the population has at least one TMD symptom and 3.6 to 7 percent of the population has TMD with sufficient severity to cause patients to seek treatment.[2,5]

◑ FOCAL POINT

TMD is an extremely common disorder that is most often reported in individuals between the ages of 20 and 40.

Approximately 33 percent of the population has at least one TMD symptom and 3.6 to 7 percent has TMD with sufficient severity that treatment is desired.

TMD symptoms generally fluctuate over time and correlate significantly with masticatory muscle tension, tooth clenching, grinding, and other oral **parafunctional habits**. TMD symptoms are also significantly correlated with an increase in psychosocial factors, e.g., worry, stress, irritation, frustration, and depression.[6-10] It has also been demonstrated that TMD patients with poor psychosocial adaptation have significantly greater symptom improvement when the dentist's therapy is combined with cognitive behavioral intervention.[11]

◉ QUICK CONSULT

Observing TMD Symptom Correlations

TMD symptoms generally fluctuate over time and correlate significantly with masticatory muscle tension, tooth clenching, grinding, and other oral parafunctional habits. TMD symptoms are also significantly correlated with an increase in psychosocial factors, e.g., worry, stress, irritation, frustration, and depression.

Women request treatment more often than do men, providing a female–male patient ratio between 3:1 and 9:1.[2,5] Additionally TMD symptoms are less likely to resolve for women than for men.[6,7,12] Many hypotheses attempt to account for the gender difference, but the underlying reason remains unclear.[3,13]

⊚ **QUICK CONSULT**

Comparing the Response of Men and Women

TMD symptoms are less likely to resolve for women than for men.

Knowledge about TMD has grown throughout the ages. In general, treatment philosophies have moved from a mechanistic dental approach to a biopsychosocial medical model, comparable to the treatment of other joint and muscle conditions in the body.[1,14]

Beneficial occlusal appliance therapy and TMJ disc-recapturing surgery were reported as early as the 1800s.[1,15] During the same period, the understanding of the importance to harmonize the occlusion for the health of the masticatory muscles and TMJs developed as the skills to reconstruct natural teeth advanced. As enthusiasm grew for obtaining optimum health, comfort, and function, the popularity of equilibrating the natural dentition also developed.[1,16]

In the 1930s, Dr. James Costen, an otolaryngologist, brought TMD into the awareness of physicians and dentists, and readers may still find TMD occasionally referred to as *Costen's syndrome*. Dr. Costen reported that TMD pain and secondary otologic symptoms could be reduced with alterations of the occlusion.[17]

Since TMD is a multifactorial disorder (having many etiologic factors), many therapies have a positive impact on any one patient's symptoms. Throughout much of the 1900s, many beneficial therapies were independently identified. Physicians, physical therapists, chiropractors, massage therapists, and others treating the muscles and/or cervical region reported positive responses in treating TMD symptoms. Psychologists working with relaxation, stress management, cognitive-behavioral therapy, and other psychological aspects reported beneficial effects with their therapies. Orthodontists, prosthodontists, and general dentists working with the occlusion also observed the positive impact that occlusal changes provided for TMD symptoms.[1,4,16]

✪ **FOCAL POINT**

Since TMD is a multifactorial disorder (having many etiologic factors), many therapies have a positive impact on any one patient's symptoms.

Surgeons reported positive benefits from many different TMJ surgical approaches. Many forms of occlusal appliance were tried and advocated, from which studies reveal there is similar efficacy for different appliance forms. Medications as well as self-management strategies used for other muscles and joints in the body were also shown to improve TMD symptoms. During this observational period, TMD therapies were primarily based on testimonials and clinical opinions, according to a practitioner's favorite causation hypothesis rather than scientific studies.[1,4,16]

Different philosophies appeared, with enthusiastic nonsurgeons "recapturing" discs through occlusal appliances, whereas surgeons repositioned the discs or replaced discs with autoplastic materials. The eventual breakdown of the autoplastic materials led to heartbreaking sequelae that caused many to step back from their narrowly focused treatment regimens and recognize the multifactorial nature of TMD and the importance of conservative noninvasive evidence-based therapies.[1,4]

In the latter part of the 20th century, much was learned about basic pain mechanisms and the shared neuron pool of the trigeminal spinal nucleus, other cranial nerves, and cervical nerves. This provided a better understanding of the influence that regional and widespread pain may have on TMD, the similarities between chronic TMD pain and other chronic pain disorders, and the need for chronic pain management from a psychosocial and behavioral standpoint.[1,13,18,19]

Today, a large number of potentially reversible conservative therapies are available for our TMD patients. By using the information obtained from the patient interview and clinical exam, practitioners can select cost-effective, evidence-based therapies that have the greatest potential to provide long-term symptom relief. The treatment selected often reduces a patient's contributing factors and facilitates the patient's natural healing capacity. This management is consistent with treatment of other orthopedic and rheumatologic disorders.[2,14,20]

◉ **QUICK CONSULT**

Selecting TMD Therapies

Today, a large number of potentially reversible conservative therapies are available for our TMD patients.

◑ **FOCAL POINT**

By using the information obtained from the patient interview and clinical exam, practitioners can select cost-effective, evidence-based therapies that have the greatest potential to provide long-term symptom relief for patients. The treatment selected often reduces a patient's contributing factors and facilitates the patient's natural healing capacity.

We do not fully understand TMD and the mechanisms causing or sustaining it. Practitioners should bear in mind that not all TMD therapies are equally effective, and no one treatment has been shown to be best for all TMD patients.[4] Most TMD patients can be managed successfully by general practitioners.[6] TMD patients who receive therapy obtain significant symptom relief, whereas patients who do not receive treatment have minimal symptom change.[21]

REFERENCES

1. McNeill C. History and evolution of TMD concepts. Oral Surg Oral Med Oral Pathol Oral Radiol Endod 1997;83:51-60.
2. American Academy of Orofacial Pain, with Okeson JP (ed). Orofacial Pain: Guidelines for Assessment, Diagnosis and Management. Chicago: Quintessence, 1996:116-7.
3. Gremillion HA. The prevalence and etiology of temporomandibular disorders and orofacial pain. Tex Dent J 2000;117(7):30-9.
4. Greene CS. The etiology of temporomandibular disorders: implications for treatment. J Orofac Pain 2001;15(2):93-105.

5. Okeson JP. Management of Temporomandibular Disorders and Occlusion, 5th edition. St Louis: CV Mosby, 2003:153.
6. Egermark I, Carlsson GE, Magnusson T. A 20-year longitudinal study of subjective symptoms of temporomandibular disorders from childhood to adulthood. Acta Odontol Scand 2001;59(1):40-8.
7. Wanman A. Longitudinal course of symptoms of craniomandibular disorders in men and women: a 10-year follow-up study of an epidemiologic sample. Acta Odontol Scand 1996;54(6):337-42.
8. Magnusson T, Egermark I, Carlsson GE. A longitudinal epidemiologic study of signs and symptoms of temporomandibular disorders from 15 to 35 years of age. J Orofac Pain 2000;14(4):310-9.

9. Conti PCR, Ferreira PM, Pegoraro LF, Conti JV, Salvador MCG. A cross-sectional study of prevalence and etiology of signs and symptoms of temporomandibular disorders in high school and university students. J Orofac Pain 1996;10(3):254-62.

10. Vallon D, Milner M, Soderfeldt B. Treatment outcome in patients with craniomandibular disorders of muscular origin: a 7-year follow-up. J Orofac Pain 1998;12(3):210-8.

11. Dworkin SF, Turner JA, Mancl L, Wilson L, Massoth D, Huggins KH, LeResche L, Truelove E. A randomized clinical trial of a tailored comprehensive care treatment program for temporomandibular disorders. J Orofac Pain 2002;16(4):259-76.

12. Garofalo JP, Gatchel RJ, Wesley AL, Ellis III E. Predicting chronicity in acute temporomandibular joint disorders using the Research Diagnostic Criteria. J Am Dent Assoc 1998;129(4):438-47.

13. Gremillion HA. Multidisciplinary diagnosis and management of orofacial pain. Gen Dent 2002;50(2):178-86.

14. McNeill C, Mohl ND, Rugh JD, Tanaka TT. Temporomandibular disorders: diagnosis, management, education, and research. J Am Dent Assoc 1990;120(3):253-63.

15. Goodwillie DH. Arthritis of the temporomaxillary articulation. Arch Med 1881;5:259-63.

16. Dawson PE. Evaluation, Diagnosis and Treatment of Occlusal Problems, 2nd edition. St Louis: CV Mosby, 1989.

17. Costen JB. A syndrome of ear and sinus symptoms dependent upon disturbed function of the temporomandibular joint. Ann Otol Rhinol Laryngol 1934;43:1-15.

18. Raphael KG, Marbach JJ, Klausner J. Myofascial face pain: clinical characteristics of those with regional vs. widespread pain. J Am Dent Assoc 2000;131(2):161-71.

19. Rammelsberg P, LeResche L, Dworkin S, Mancl L. Longitudinal outcome of temporomandibular disorders: a 5-year epidemiologic study of muscle disorders defined by research diagnostic criteria for temporomandibular disorders. J Orofac Pain 2003;17(1):9-20.

20. Fricton JR, Chung SC. Contributing factors: a key to chronic pain. In: Fricton JR, Kroening RJ, Hathaway KM (eds). TMJ and Craniofacial Pain: Diagnosis and Management. St Louis: Ishiyaku EuroAmerica, 1988:27-37.

21. Gaudet EL, Brown DT. Temporomandibular disorder treatment outcomes: first report of a large scale prospective clinical study. Cranio 2000;18(1):9-22.

Part I

Initial Evaluation

The goals of the initial examination are to identify a patient's primary diagnosis; secondary, tertiary, etc., diagnoses; contributing factors; and symptom patterns.

The **primary diagnosis** is the diagnosis for the disorder most responsible for a patient's chief complaint. This diagnosis can be of temporomandibular disorder (TMD) origin [e.g., myofascial pain, TMJ inflammation, or acute temporomandibular joint (TMJ) disc displacement without reduction] or from a different source (e.g., pulpal pathosis, sinusitis, or cervicogenic headache).[1]

Secondary, **tertiary**, etc. **diagnoses** are diagnoses for other disorders that contribute to the primary diagnosis. Typically the primary diagnosis will be of TMD origin (e.g., myofascial pain), and the secondary and tertiary diagnoses will be other TMD diagnoses (e.g., TMJ inflammation and TMJ disc displacement with reduction) that contribute to a patient's chief complaint. When non-TMD disorders (e.g., fibromyalgia) contribute to a TMD primary diagnosis, the non-TMD disorder is designated as a contributing factor to the TMD diagnosis and not as secondary or tertiary diagnosis.[1]

🖲 **FOCAL POINT**

Secondary, tertiary, etc., diagnoses are diagnoses for other disorders that contribute to the primary diagnosis.

Contributing factors are elements that perpetuate the disorder (not allowing it to resolve), e.g., nighttime parafunctional habits, gum chewing, daytime clenching, stress, or poor posture.[1,2] **Symptom patterns** include the period of the day in which the symptoms occur or are most intense (e.g., worse upon awaking) and the location pattern (e.g., begins in the neck and then moves to the jaw).

🖲 **FOCAL POINT**

Contributing factors are elements that perpetuate the disorder (not allowing it to resolve), e.g., nighttime parafunctional habits, gum chewing, daytime clenching, stress, or poor posture.

Symptom patterns include the period of the day in which the symptoms occur or are most intense (e.g., worse upon awaking) and the location pattern (e.g., begins in the neck and then moves to the jaw).

The initial evaluation involves interviewing the patient about his or her symptoms, potential contributing factors, and potential non-temporomandibular disorder (non-TMD). The interview most influences the patient's final treatment approach and generally brings to light concerns that the practitioner will need to evaluate during the clinical examination.

The clinical examination will help to confirm or rule out the structures involved in the patient's complaints and other suspected disorders that may contribute to these complaints. Imaging may be appropriate, but, in my experience, it rarely changes the treatment approach derived by the patient interview and examination.

In the late 1980s, an experience demonstrated that patients with TMD symptoms needed to be evaluated more thoroughly for potential non-TMD. A physician asked if I knew that one of the dentists who worked for me had diagnosed someone with TMD when the patient actually had meningitis. After reviewing the patient's dental record, I found she had been referred by the emergency room physician for possible TMD. The patient told the dentist she had been previously diagnosed with TMD, had an occlusal appliance, and believed she was having a relapse of this disorder. The dentist palpated her masticatory muscles and TMJs and found the muscles were tight and tender to palpation. The dentist confirmed for the patient that she had TMD, gave her TMD self-management instructions, and told her she should see her civilian dentist to have her appliance adjusted (as she was not an active-duty military patient). At the time, it appeared to me the dentist performed an appropriate evaluation and drew a fitting conclusion.

The emergency room record was then reviewed to obtain a better perspective of what had transpired. It was documented that the patient also told the emergency room physician that she had previously been diagnosed with TMD, had an occlusal appliance, and believed she was having a relapse of this disorder. The physician found she had firm masticatory and cervical muscles and a fever, and referred her to the dentist for a TMD evaluation and to a neurologist. When the patient saw the neurologist, he did a spinal tap and found she had meningitis.

This disheartening experience inspired me to research everything I could concerning disorders that mimic TMD. Lists were made of how their symptoms differed from TMD and a fairly brief list of questions was finally formulated that dentists can use to alert a practitioner that a patient may have a non-TMD condition that is mimicking TMD.[3] This questionnaire has been used ever since, adding questions for characteristics that should cause suspicions for referred odontogenic pain and rheumatic disorders.[4,5] This questionnaire is certainly not foolproof, but it helps me identify non-TMD patients, and to the best of my knowledge I have not missed a non-TMD patient since putting this into practice.

REFERENCES

1. Fricton JR. Establishing the problem list: an inclusive conceptual model for chronic illness. In: Fricton JR, Kroening RJ, Hathaway KM (eds). TMJ and Craniofacial Pain: Diagnosis and Management. St Louis: Ishiyaku EuroAmerica, 1988:21-6.
2. McNeill C, Mohl ND, Rugh JD, Tanaka TT. Temporomandibular disorders: diagnosis, management, education, and research. J Am Dent Assoc 1990;120(3):253-63.
3. Wright EF. A simple questionnaire and clinical examination to help identify possible non-craniomandibular disorders that may influence a patient's CMD symptoms. Cranio 1992;10(3):228-34.
4. Wright EF, Gullickson DC. Identifying acute pulpalgia as a factor in TMD pain. J Am Dent Assoc 1996;127:773-80.
5. Wright EF, Des Rosier KE, Clark MK, Bifano SL. Identifying undiagnosed rheumatic disorders among patients with TMD. J Am Dent Assoc 1997;128(6):738-44.

Chapter 1

Patient Interview

FAQs

Q: What should be done if a patient reports having a TMJ Teflon-Proplast implant, or Silastic implant or total TMJ prostheses?
A: A specific protocol has been recommended for TMJ Teflon-Proplast and Silastic implants and total joint prostheses. Follow-up for these is beyond the scope of this book. If the practitioner is unsure of the implant type or management, it is recommended the practitioner refer the patient to, or work in conjunction with, someone who has greater expertise in this area.

Q: What is secondary gain and how common is it for TMD patients?
A: Secondary gain is a situation in which the patient is rewarded for having TMD; e.g., the patient receives disability payments or is excused from undesirable chores or work. Clinically this is not a commonly observed situation, but, if it is present, the patient may not relate improvement from any therapy.

Q: What should be done when a patient appears to have a tooth causing or contributing to the TMD symptoms?
A: A recommended approach to determine whether a tooth is causing or contributing to a patient's TMD symptoms is provided in "Intraoral Examination" in Chapter 3.

A recommended "Initial Patient Questionnaire" is provided (Appendix 1) and may be reproduced for your patients to complete. The questionnaire is designed to efficiently use the time spent interviewing patients. The practitioner's customary medical history form should be used in conjunction with this questionnaire.

◉ QUICK CONSULT
Collecting Symptom History

The "Initial Patient Questionnaire" Is designed to efficiently use the time spent interviewing patients and should be used in conjunction with the practitioner's customary medical history form.

The practitioner may desire to add an additional page to obtain medical and dental insurance information and the name and address of the individual who recommended that the patient come to your office, in addition to the name and address of the patient's physician and dentist. It is comforting to a referring provider to receive a letter acknowledging that the referral was appropriate and providing the practitioner's findings and recommended treatment. This also tends to encourage the referring provider to recommend your office the next time a patient with a similar complaint needs treatment. A copy of this letter is often sent to the patient's physician and dentist (if not the referring doctor); a release statement is included in the "Initial Patient Questionnaire" for this purpose.

The questionnaire appears to keep patients from elaborating in nonproductive discussions or becoming irritated by the number of questions asked, and prevents the practitioner from forgetting to ask relevant information. Clinical experience suggests a patient's responses are not always accurate and the examiner needs to review the answers with the patient. For better patient recall, it appears best if the patient arrives 15 minutes prior to the appointment and completes the questionnaire just prior to the appointment. During the patient interview, the practitioner usually needs to ask the patient to elaborate on some of the answers.

◉ QUICK CONSULT
Confirming Patient Responses

Clinical experience suggests a patient's responses are not always accurate and the examiner needs to review the answers with the patient.

▼ TECHNICAL TIP
Assisting Patient Recall

For better patient recall, it appears best if the patient arrives 15 minutes prior to the appointment and completes the questionnaire just prior to the appointment.

Chapter 2, "Review of Initial Patient Questionnaire," presents the key points for each of the questions and is designed to help a practitioner quickly evaluate a patient's responses. Many of the questions are self-explanatory, but additional discussion for some of the questions as well as supplementary information are provided below:

Question 6 (What treatments have you received?), with additional inquiries, gives an indication of which treatments were previously beneficial for the patient. For example, if the patient found that an occlusal appliance (which the patient no longer has) resolved the symptoms, then fabricating another appliance should be very beneficial. Reinforce to the patient that using the treatments (e.g., application of heat) he or she previously found beneficial can again be beneficial. If the patient has previously received the therapies the practitioner traditionally provides, without satisfactory benefit, the practitioner may desire to refer the patient to someone with greater expertise in this area.

TMJ implants composed of Teflon-Proplast and Silastic have a history of fragmenting, causing a foreign-body response that results in progressive degeneration of the condyle and glenoid fossa. A specific protocol has been recommended for these implants and total joint prostheses.[1] Follow-up for these is beyond the scope of this book. If a practitioner is unsure of the implant type or management, it is recommended the practitioner refer the patient to, or work in conjunction with, someone who has greater expertise in this area.

Question 7 (When are the symptoms the worst?) will often help identify the time when significant contributing factors are present. Patients with nighttime parafunctional habits usually have an increase in pain when they first awake, whereas patients with daytime parafunctional habits have an increase in pain during the day or evening. The examiner may be able to elicit more specific periods, e.g., during or after driving, or when using the computer.

☯ FOCAL POINT

Patients with nighttime parafunctional habits usually have an increase in pain when they first awake, whereas patients with daytime parafunctional habits have an increase in pain during the day or evening.

◉ QUICK CONSULT
Observing for Significant Contributing Factors

When discussing a patient's symptom pattern, an examiner may be able to elicit specific periods when significant contributing factors are present, e.g., during or after driving, or when using the computer.

Question 8 (What docs the pain keep you from doing?) gives the practitioner a sense for how much the pain is affecting the patient's life. This may correlate with how motivated the patient will be to participate in therapy and the level of therapy the patient may be interested in receiving. Occasionally this answer is out of proportion with other features of the examination; e.g., the patient is unable to work, but has only minimal palpation tenderness. Additional questions may reveal the patient continues to participate in other activities, such as yelling at basketball games. This inconsistency may suggest that other factors are involved, commonly referred to as **secondary gain**.[2]

Question 9 (What is the quality of the pain?) helps identify some possible conditions for a patient's pain. Patients most commonly characterize TMD pain as an ache, pressure, or dull pain. If throbbing is one of the components, generally the patient's disorder falls within one or more of the following three situations:

First, some patients report their pain is an ache, pressure, or of dull character and, when it worsens, its character changes to throbbing. The patient may have nausea, photophobia, and/or phonophobia associated with the throbbing pain. Clinically it appears that, if the ache, pressure, or dull pain can be satisfactorily reduced, it can be prevented from escalating to the throbbing level.

◉ QUICK CONSULT
Reducing Throbbing Pain

Clinically it appears that, if a patient relates the ache, pressure, or dull pain worsens to throbbing and can be satisfactorily reduced, this prevents the pain from escalating to the throbbing level.

In a second situation, the patient does not report that an ache, pressure, or dull pain progresses into throbbing pain. This pain is sometimes due to a source that does not respond to TMD therapy. The practitioner may desire to perform an occlusal appliance therapy trial and, if it is not effective, consider a referral to the patient's physician or neurologist for a probable migraine. Studies suggest some migraines respond to TMD therapy, but characteristics for identifying which migraines respond are not well established.[3,4]

For other patients, the throbbing pain may be **referred pain** from an oral problem (most commonly a tooth). Sometimes the perceived painful site (e.g., masseter muscle and/or TMJ) appears as the source to the patient, whereas the actual source (e.g., a tooth) has minimal symptoms. This is similar to how a patient suffering from a heart attack may perceive pain only in the left arm, whereas the pain's source is the heart. Treatment for the pain must be directed toward the source, not the site where it is felt.

⊙ **QUICK CONSULT**

Observing for Throbbing Pain Sources

Throbbing pain may be referred pain from an acute pulpalgia.

A study of patients suspected of having TMD by their dentists, but whose TMD pain upon additional examination was found primarily to be referred odontogenic pain, reported that (a) none of the periapical radiographs revealed apical pathosis and (b) patients related that palpating the perceived painful site often reproduced the patient's pain.[5]

The study found four helpful characteristics for identifying patients who have a tooth causing or contributing to their TMD symptoms: (a) throbbing is a component of the pain, (b) the pain wakes the patient at night, (c) the pain increases when the patient lies down, and (d) the pain increases when the patient drinks hot or cold liquids. Evaluating and treating referred odontogenic pain are discussed further in Question 10 and in "Intraoral Examination" in Chapter 3.

Burning is infrequently reported by TMD patients, whereas most neuropathic pains include a burning quality.[6,7] Sympathetically maintained neuropathic pain occurs from tissue injury and may occur from routine dental procedures, e.g., a simple tooth extraction.[8] Clinical experience has shown that, if burning is combined with the typical TMD pain qualities (ache, pressure, or dull pain), usually the burning correspondingly resolves with the ache, pressure, or dull pain from TMD therapy. If burning has not resolved from initial TMD therapy or is the patient's most prominent pain quality, the

practitioner may desire to refer the patient to someone with greater expertise in this area.

Along with those already discussed, many other pain qualities are possible, e.g., an electrical or stinging sensation. Knowledge of a patient's pain qualities will help a practitioner determine whether treatment for TMD has a high probability of benefiting the patient or whether this treatment may delay the evaluation for another, more probable, disorder.

Question 10 attempts to identify whether the practitioner should be suspicious that sinus congestion or odontogenic pain may be contributing to the patient's complaint. Patients with sinus congestion tend to find an aggravation when they change their head position, i.e., lie down or bend forward. If the patient responds positively to this question, it is recommended that the practitioner further inquire as to whether sinus congestion appears to contribute to the pain; e.g., whether the patient finds decongestants or antibiotics help relieve the pain. If the patient is unaware of the impact decongestants or antibiotics have on the pain and the practitioner suspects sinus congestion involvement, the practitioner may desire to perform a trial treatment with one or both of these medications or to refer to a physician for evaluation and management. Some patients with masticatory muscle pain receive little relief with decongestants, but these symptoms are eliminated completely after administration of antibiotics for a sinus infection.

⊙ **QUICK CONSULT**

Observing for Sinus Congestion Contribution

Patients with sinus congestion tend to find an aggravation when they change their head position, i.e., lie down or bend forward.

Historically patients with odontalgia tend to report their pain wakes them at night, increases when they lie down, and/or increases when they drink hot or cold liquids. If a patient responds positively to one or more of these questions or has throbbing pain, this should raise a suspicion that a tooth may be causing or contributing to the TMD symptoms.[5]

◉ QUICK CONSULT
Observing for Odontalgia Contribution
Historically patients with odontalgia tend to report their pain wakes them at night, increases when they lie down, and/or increases when they drink hot or cold liquids.

Sometimes patients incorrectly answer "Yes" to the question "Does your pain increase when you drink hot or cold liquids?" When these patients elaborate, it becomes apparent that cold only causes tooth discomfort rather than aggravating their facial pain.

When the practitioner suspects that a tooth may be causing or contributing to the TMD symptoms, further evaluation is indicated. A recommended evaluation approach and treatment considerations are provided in "Intraoral Examination" in Chapter 3.

Questions 11, 12, and 13 attempt to quantify the pain, requiring the patient to delineate its intensity, frequency, and duration. The first two questions introduce patients to rating their pain intensity from 0 to 10 and give the practitioner a sense of the patient's pain history. This numerical rating system is the most effective manner we have at this time for rating pain intensity.[9] A concise and commonly used terminology for frequency is *constant* (always present), *daily* (occurs every day, but not constantly), *weekly* (occurs every week, but not daily), etc. Duration may be momentary, the average number of seconds to hours, or constant. The pain may vary greatly and can be difficult to quantify accurately. For brevity, it is often clinically satisfactory to just document the average intensity and frequency in the

patient's record, but in some situations the practitioner may want to include the extremes and/or durations.

Question 14 attempts to identify unusual symptoms, which may be suggestive of other disorders that could mimic or coexist with TMD. For example, a progressively increasing open bite of the anterior teeth may be from the TMJ losing its vertical height, generally due to severe TMJ osteoarthritis. As the condylar height collapses, the most posterior ipsilateral (affected side) tooth becomes the first tooth to contact, acts as a fulcrum, and progressively creates an open bite for the remaining dentition. The open bite generally begins on the contralateral (nonaffected side) anterior teeth and progressively spreads bilaterally until the only tooth that contacts is the most posterior ipsilateral tooth. This disorder and its treatment are complicated and beyond the scope of this book. Practitioners observing this complaint may desire to refer the patient to someone with greater expertise in this area.

It is not uncommon for a patient to relate autonomic changes, which are induced by central excitation produced by the pain. These can include the face becoming red, puffy, or having thermal changes near the area of the pain; the eye becoming bloodshot or tearing; and/or the nose running or becoming congested. These autonomic changes occur when the pain is aggravated and should resolve when it lessens or resolves.[6] They are sometimes reproduced when the practitioner aggravates the pain during the palpation evaluation.

Questions 15, 16, and 17 provide a rapid tool to screen for a non-TMD that may be the cause of the pain or negatively impact it.[10,11] The practitioner can skip each question the patient answers with a "No," but needs to inquire further and consider the comments in a "Review of Initial Patient Questionnaire" (Chapter 2) for each question with a "Yes" answer.

Two disorders that are moderately prevalent among TMD patients often negatively influence TMD symptoms and treatment, and the practitioner must be very observant to identify them. The first is **cervical dysfunction** (cervical pain and/or restricted movement); one study found that 23 percent of TMD patients had cervical dysfunction with a severity that warranted referral.[12] Cervical dysfunction may not only directly affect the masticatory system and its ability to respond to therapy, but it may also cause referred pain to the masticatory structures, which can add to a patient's TMD symptoms or be the sole cause of the TMD symptoms.[11,13]

⊙ **QUICK CONSULT**

Observing Cervical Dysfunction and Fibromyalgia Effects on TMD Therapy

Cervical dysfunction and fibromyalgia often negatively influence TMD symptoms and treatment response.

Recommended cervical palpation techniques to identify referred pain from the cervical region to the head and face are provided in "Palpation" in Chapter 3. The scope of clinical practice for TMD has been determined to include the diagnosis and treatment of disorders affecting the entire head and neck. This is consistent with the historical precedent in dentistry and within the scope of current dental practice.[14]

The other disorder that practitioners must be very astute in identifying is **fibromyalgia**. It is characterized by widespread pain, multiple tender points over the body, poor sleep, stiffness, and generalized fatigue. Only about 2 percent of the general population has fibromyalgia, whereas 18 to 23 percent of TMD patients have it.[11,15]

It has been shown that TMD patients with fibromyalgia, widespread pain, or neck pain do not respond as well to TMD therapies as do those without these comorbid dis-

orders.[16-18] Therefore, it is important to identify patients with these disorders and inform them about the potential negative impact this may have on their treatment. If it appears a patient is not receiving adequate therapy for the coexisting disorder, it is recommended the patient discuss treatment alternatives with their medical provider or be referred to someone who specializes in the area.

It is recommended that patients suspected of having fibromyalgia be referred to a physician for definitive diagnosis and management. There have been instances in which patients diagnosed with fibromyalgia by rheumatologists have had their fibromyalgia advance to other disorders, such as multiple sclerosis.

Questions 18, 19, and 20 ask about TMJ noise and the inability to open or close the mouth. The latter can be of muscle or TMJ origin. A "TMJ Disc Displacements" diagram is provided as Appendix 2 and may be reproduced for your patients. It is helpful for explaining the cause of their TMJ noise and/or inability to open or close.

⊙ **QUICK CONSULT**

Explaining Mechanical Disorder

A "TMJ Disc Displacements" diagram is provided as Appendix 2 and is helpful for explaining the cause of a patient's TMJ noise and/or inability to open or close.

The diagram is broken into four sections, with the top left section providing a view of the skull with the zygomatic arch cut so the entire temporalis muscle can be visualized. This enables the provider to demonstrate how the temporalis muscle functions and how clenching or other oral habits can overuse this muscle, thereby causing pain similar to that caused by overuse of any muscle in the body. The zygomatic arch can be drawn in and the masseter muscle drawn over the ramus, and a similar discussion about muscle-overuse pain can be provided. The lateral pterygoid muscle can also be drawn to explain the symptoms and treatment for lateral pterygoid myospasm (explained in Chapter 9, "Lateral Pterygoid Myospasm"). The articular eminence is also displayed so that condylar dislocation (the condyle catches or locks in front of the eminence) and its treatment may be demonstrated. Conservative therapies for dislocation are also provided in Chapter 11, "TMJ Dislocation."

To orientate the patient for the next section of the diagrams, point to the ear on the skull and then to the ear in the top right section. This drawing provides an avenue to explain the "normal" disc-condyle alignment. If the patient has a TMJ click or pop, the most probable situation is that the elastic ligament (the retrodiscal tissue, in addition to its attachment complex) is stretched and the disc-condyle alignment looks like the top drawing in the bottom left section in which the disc is displaced.[19-21] As the condyle translates forward (e.g., during opening), it moves into the center of the disc (the reduced position), and, as the individual closes, the condyle retrudes off the disc. This is commonly referred to as *TMJ disc displacement with reduction*, which is the terminology that is used in this book.

This section can visually explain the opening and/or closing click. Sometimes patients are also informed about how the tension in the closure muscles (temporalis, masseter, and medial pterygoid) brace the condyle in a superior position, which may promote a greater mechanical interference between the condyle and disc. Clinically patients report this effect by their TMJ click, catch, or lock occurring more frequently or with greater intensity when they are stressed, while eating, or after clenching their teeth.

For patients experiencing limited translation due to the disc blocking their normal opening (*acute TMJ disc displacement without reduction*), the bottom right diagram can help visually explain the mechanical problem and treatment. This is discussed in Chapter 5, "TMD Diagnostic Categories," and in Chapter 10, "Acute TMJ Disc Displacement without Reduction."

Many patients report the presence or history of TMJ noises (*Question 18*), since TMJ clicking or popping is very prevalent among the TMD and general populations.[22] These noises may occur with opening and/or closing, can fluctuate in intensity, and occur sporadically. If a patient has TMJ clicking or popping, the most likely diagnosis is TMJ disc displacement with reduction.[19-21] If the joint noise is course crepitus, then the most likely diagnosis is *chronic TMJ disc displacement without reduction*; see Chapter 5, "TMD Diagnostic Categories," for an explanation of this terminology.[20] A more accurate assessment of the disc-condyle alignment can be obtained by magnetic resonance imaging (MRI) of the TMJ, but the findings rarely change the treatment approach, and MRI is rarely indicated at the initial TMD evaluation.[23] For more information on TMJ imaging, see Chapter 4, "Imaging."

⦿ **QUICK CONSULT**

Requesting MRIs

MRI findings rarely change the treatment approach, and MRI is rarely indicated at the initial TMD evaluation.

The inability to open wide (*Question 19*) is generally due to either a TMJ disorder (e.g., acute disc displacement without reduction) or a muscle disorder. Discussing the onset and its history is often beneficial and may aid in determining the cause. If this limitation is intermittent, patients with an acute disc displacement without reduction are usually aware that the TMJ is blocked at the opening where the TMJ normally clicks or pops. Typically they suddenly have a restricted opening, which just as abruptly releases, allowing them to obtain their normal opening once again. The acute disc displacement without reduction may be persistent, but often has a history of being intermittent. Conversely an intermittent muscle disorder generally develops and resolves slowly for each episode.

If a TMJ disc intermittently blocks a patient from opening wide, the patient is usually aware that the TMJ is blocked at the opening where the TMJ normally clicks or pops, it suddenly occurs, and just as abruptly releases; conversely an intermittent muscle disorder generally develops and resolves slowly for each episode.

If a patient has a restricted opening, the practitioner may be able to determine its origin by stretching the mouth wider. This is usually done by placing the index finger over the incisal edges of the mandibular incisors and the thumb over the incisal edges of the maxillary incisors and pressing the teeth apart by moving the fingers in a scissor-type motion (Figure 1-1). The patient will usually feel tightness or pain at the location of the restriction. From clinical experience, not all patients accurately point to the stretched discomfort location, and it is necessary to palpate the TMJ and musculature to reproduce the discomfort in order to identify its origin.

▼ TECHNICAL TIP
Determining Origin of a Patient's Restricted Opening

The practitioner may be able to determine a patient's restricted opening origin by stretching the mouth wider and determining the location of the created discomfort.

It should be kept in mind that there are other potential, though less common, causes for patients having a restricted opening. Generally these patients complain only about a restricted opening, not pain.[2] Some examples of these are TMJ ankylosis, myofibrotic contracture, and cornoid process im-

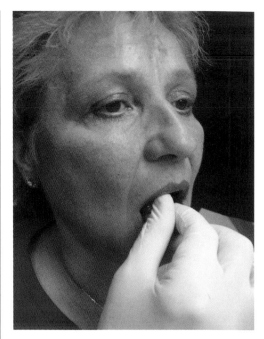

Figure 1-1. Stretching a restricted opening to determine the origin of the restriction.

pedance. These disorders are beyond the scope of this book, and if the practitioner suspects the patient may have one of them, he or she may desire to refer the patient to someone with greater expertise in this area.

Patients may report episodes of being unable to close their mouth (*Question 20*). From clinical experience, there are several common causes for a positive response to this question. If the patient reports the TMJ catches or locks at an opening of 45 mm or wider, the condyle has the potential of being in front of the eminence (TMJ dislocation). Among patients with this complaint, multiple disc-condyle relations have been observed, and investigators have postulated that the catching or locking is due to (a) the articular eminence obstructing the posterior movement of the disc-condyle unit, (b) the disc obstructing the posterior movement of the condyle, or (c) a combination of the two.[24] Traditional TMD therapies have been shown to improve this condition.[25] Conservative treatments for TMJ dislocation are provided in Chapter 11, "TMJ Dislocation."

If the patient's TMJ catches or locks during closure in a range of approximately 10 to 35 mm, the articular eminence should not be involved, and it would most probably be only the disc that is obstructing the posterior movement of the condyle. There is no consistent disc-condyle relationship for this interference, but it is speculated the most common scenario is that the patient has a TMJ disc displacement with reduction. The interference occurs during closure when the condyle is in the reduced position and the condyle has difficulty moving or is temporarily unable to move below the posterior band of the disc; this is the typical location of the closing click. This closing catch or lock occurs similarly to the way in which an opening click's mechanical interference worsens to become an opening catch or lock. The bottom left diagram of the "TMJ Disc Displacements" handout (Appendix 2) may help to explain this mechanical interference visually to patients. From clinical experience, this problem resolves with traditional conservative TMD therapies.

A third common cause of patients reporting an inability to close is a **lateral pterygoid myospasm**. In this situation, the inferior lateral pterygoid muscle is in constant involuntary contraction at a partially shortened position. This is similar to the calf muscle cramp that has awakened many of us in the middle of the night.[26] Upon awaking, the individual notes the calf pain and calf cramp in which he or she has difficulty and increased pain when attempting to move the foot up or down. A patient with a lateral pterygoid myospasm similarly has difficulty and increased pain when attempting to translate the condyle forward or retrude the jaw so the teeth fit into maximum intercuspation. The patient usually complains of the inability to put the ipsilateral posterior teeth together without excruciating pain, the teeth are usually separated by a fraction of a millimeter to a few millimeters, and the first tooth contact is in the area of the contralat-eral canine (if the patient has normal tooth alignment). Since the patient has difficulty translating forward, he or she usually also has a marked limited opening. A diagnostic test and treatments are provided in Chapter 9, "Lateral Pterygoid Myospasm."

Questions 21 through 27 ask about potential contributing factors to a patient's TMD. Some contributing factors are not asked about in this questionnaire, but will become apparent when the provider or staff member reviews the "TMD Self-management Therapies" handout with the patient (e.g., gum chewing, caffeine consumption, or stomach sleeping). This handout is provided as Appendix 3.

Poor sleep may constitute the inability to fall asleep, stay asleep, or awake feeling rested (*Question 21*). Poor sleep has been shown to correlate with increased muscle pain and can be a predictor of patients who will respond poorly to TMD therapy.[27-29] A good system to use to evaluate poor-sleep severity is to ask the patient to rate his or her sleep quality between 0 and 10. Intuitively, when most of us do not get adequate sleep, we tend to feel more aches and pain, be more irritable, etc. The effects of inadequate sleep tend to contribute to a TMD patient's symptoms on both a physical and psychosocial basis.[29] From clinical experience, when a patient relates that poor sleep is primarily due to TMD pain, it has been observed that, when the TMD pain resolves, generally the sleep problem also resolves. To ensure a patient's needs and desires are met, when other causes of poor sleep are involved, the provider may ask the patient to discuss this with his or her physician, refer the patient for relaxation therapy, or refer the patient to someone who specializes in sleep disorders. A book reference is provided in "Sources for Additional TMD Information," Appendix 12, which patients may find helpful for improving their sleep. If the patient has poor sleep and awakes with morning TMD pain, the practitioner may desire to prescribe amitriptyline or nortriptyline; see "Tricyclic Antidepressants" in Chapter 17 for additional information.

Poor sleep has been shown to correlate with an increase in muscle pain and can be a predictor of patients who will respond poorly to TMD therapy.

The usual portion of the day in which a patient feels most tense, aggravated, or frustrated (*Question 22*) is an indicator as to the impact these feelings may have on the TMD symptoms. Patients with TMD tend to hold more tension in their jaws or clench their teeth during these times, and some may be aware of these habits. Some patients may hold their teeth together throughout the day and squeeze them during these times, whereas others may swear they never touch their teeth, but after observing for these habits will later find they clench or tighten their masticatory muscles during such times. It is a challenge to help patients understand their unconscious daytime habits that are contributing to their TMD symptoms. Some dentists train a psychologist or staff member to help patients recognize and break their daytime contributing habits. A diary in which patients hourly record their TMD symptoms and tension levels often helps patients learn about these associations and thereby provides the motivation to change their tension levels.

▼ **TECHNICAL TIP**
Reducing Tension Levels
A diary in which patients hourly record their TMD symptoms and tension levels often helps patients learn about these associations and thereby provides the motivation to change their tension levels and habits.

Clinically it has been observed that TMD patients often deny having stress because they relate the term *stress* to more significant events than they have in their lives. Terms that patients seem to acknowledge having that tend to be associated with these habits are "tension," "aggravations," "frustrations," "concerns," "busyness," "more of life's stuff" or "more of life's situations."

Once patients recognize they have one of these feelings, it is recommended their preferred term be used in future discussions. Discuss the likelihood that this psychosocial contributor is associated with their pain because patients tend to hold more tension in their jaw muscles (also neck and shoulders if they also have pain or tenderness in these areas) during such times.

There are two approaches patients can use to reduce the symptoms related to these psychosocial contributors. They can learn to reduce the psychosocial contributors (using coping strategies, stress management, etc.) and/or become very aware of their propensity to tighten their muscles during such times and break this habit. A combination is generally used when patients are referred for treatment of this problem.

Sometimes a patient's concerns are overwhelming, and the patient desires to discuss them with a trained professional and learn coping skills. Two examples of referrals to a psychologist are provided in Appendix 10.

The portion of the day in which a patient usually feels depressed (*Question 23*) is an indicator as to the impact that depression may have on the TMD symptoms. Clinical experience suggests that patients who are depressed and not open to discussing or receiving treatment for their depression minimize their answer with "Seldom" or "Never." For patients who mark "Always" or "Half the time," it is recommended the practitioner discuss the patient's depression and referral options, i.e., primary medical provider (to discuss treatment options), psychologist (primarily treats through discussions), and/or psychiatrist (a physician who primarily treats with medications). Based on clinical experience, when a patient relates the depression is primarily due to TMD pain, the depression generally resolves when the TMD pain resolves.

⊗ FOCAL POINT

Depression negatively influences TMD symptoms and treatment response.

Suicide was the second leading cause of death among 25- to 34-year-olds in 1997.[30] The propensity that a person will commit suicide increases with the presence of depression and chronic pain.[31,32] If a patient relates he or she has thoughts of hurting himself or herself, or committing suicide (*Question 24*), you must determine lethality. Ask the patient whether he or she has a plan, a time selected, and the means selected of carrying this out (pills, gun, etc.). If the answer is "Yes" to any of these, the patient must immediately be evaluated by someone trained in psychosocial suicide assessment to determine whether suicide is imminent, i.e., a clinical social worker, psychologist, psychiatrist, your local hospital's suicide prevention team, the authority received by calling 911, or the police department's emergency psychiatric evaluation team. Do not allow the patient to leave without an escort (i.e., a staff member, responsible family member, police, or hospital personnel sent to your office) unless he or she has been cleared by an appropriate person.[33] Clearly document your findings, actions, and follow-up on your referral. Your local Suicide Prevention Hotline can provide information about resources available in your community.

A considerable amount of time spent singing or playing a musical instrument (*Question 25*) may also significantly contribute to a patient's TMD symptoms. The impact will vary with the instruments and the amount of time spent in the activity. It has been speculated that wind instruments, some string instruments (violin and viola), and singing have the greatest potential for contributing to TMD symptoms.[34,35] A pa-

tient's symptom time pattern should give an indication of the impact singing or playing the musical instrument has on the symptoms. Sometimes these activities are the patient's sole source of income, so the patient will have to weigh the cost and benefit of limiting or changing the intensity of these activities.

It is recommended the patient never hold his or her teeth together except momentarily when swallowing (*Question 26*). This question nicely leads into discussing the patient's daytime habits and the importance of breaking them. The following analogy is used, demonstrating with my arm, to help the patient understand the impact holding the teeth together may have on his or her pain.

Whenever my fingertips touch the palm of my hand, the muscles in my forearm must flex. If one were to hold this, the muscles would eventually tire and start to hurt. If this were a recurring habit, as the day becomes busy, frustrating, or irritating, the individual would most likely unconsciously squeeze his or her fingertips into the palm and overuse these muscles even more. If the individual were to go to a physician and complain about my forearm pain, he or she would wonder why this muscle is so tender and painful compared to the other muscles in my body. The physician would need to realize this localized pain was caused by that habit and would conclude the best way to treat this muscle disorder is for the individual to break the habit.

If the patient does not have a widespread disorder (e.g., fibromyalgia), I touch his or her biceps and forearm while I say, "Your biceps and forearm are not tender, so there must be something you are doing to overuse your jaw muscles. If your jaw muscles were relaxed, your jaw would drop away from your upper teeth, just as we allow our arms to hang loose and drop (at the same time I allow my arms to go limp and drop). Your jaw should be hanging loose all day with your lips just lightly touching (unless the patient is a mouth breather)."

If patients are aware of clenching, grinding, or any other oral habit (*Questions 27 and 28*), they should be informed of how these negatively affect their TMD symptoms. Sometimes breaking these habits and using the "TMD Self-management Therapies" handout (Appendix 3) will satisfactorily decrease a patient's TMD symptoms.

Question 31 helps a practitioner determine whether a patient might have giant cell arteritis (temporal arteritis).[36] Giant cell arteritis may mimic mild TMD symptoms, has been misdiagnosed as TMD, and may cause blindness within a relatively short time if not treated.[37] It is better to err with an unnecessary referral than allow this disorder to go undiagnosed. If you suspect a patient has giant cell arteritis, it is recommended the patient see a physician within the next few days unless visual symptoms have already developed, in which case the patient should see a physician that day.

◉ **QUICK CONSULT**

Observing for Giant Cell Arteritis

Giant cell arteritis may mimic mild TMD symptoms, has been misdiagnosed as TMD, and may cause blindness within a relatively short time if not treated.

Giant cell arteritis is almost exclusively found in people over the age of 50. It causes a reduction in the blood flow to the structures of the head and neck (including the masticatory muscles and eyes). The decreased masticatory muscle blood flow causes the muscles to tire easily, producing a tired, cramped feeling that resolves within 1 to 2 minutes after use. Some TMD patients without giant cell arteritis may report similar symptoms, and these questions will help to differentiate the two disorders.[36] If a patient has had symptoms suggestive of giant cell arteritis for over a year, it is highly unlikely that he or she has giant cell arteritis.

"Yes" to the first two questions suggests jaw claudication, but a patient with mild TMD symptoms may respond positively to both questions. Consider giant cell arteritis when a patient relates unexplainable scalp tenderness, unexplainable or unintentional weight loss, significant morning stiffness lasting longer than a half-hour, and visual symptoms or visual loss.[36]

A fever (previously asked about in the questionnaire) is also more prevalent among people who have giant cell arteritis.[36] If the fever is not due to a dental condition and has not been evaluated by a physician, it is recommended that the patient be referred for an evaluation. Another sign of giant cell arteritis is an abnormal temporal artery, which is evaluated by comparing the left and right temporal arteries. Relative to the other side, an abnormal vessel would be more visible, have no pulse, or have palpable nodes.

Other symptoms that may occur with giant cell arteritis include fatigue, loss of appetite, mental confusion, depression, diminished taste sensation, tongue numbness or swelling, difficulty swallowing or speaking, and pain with drinking beverages or eating soft foods.[38]

Another clinical presentation that practitioners should be alert to identify is one in which a patient has the worst headache of his or her life, the symptoms started less than 48 hours earlier, and the headache is related to mental impairment (e.g., drowsiness or confusion). It is very unlikely that a patient would come to a dentist's office for treatment of these symptoms, but if this occurs, it is important to realize the symptoms are not suggestive of TMD and that the patient be referred to the emergency room. The patient may have an intracranial hemorrhage, meningitis, encephalitis, etc.

REFERENCES

1. American Association of Oral and Maxillofacial Surgeons. Recommendations for management of

patients with temporomandibular joint implants. Temporomandibular Joint Implant Surgery Workshop. J Oral Maxillofac Surg 1993;51(10):1164–72.

2. Okeson JP. Management of Temporomandibular Disorders and Occlusion, 5th edition. St Louis: CV Mosby, 2003:202–3, 491–8.

3. Quayle AA, Gray RJ, Metcalfe RJ, Guthrie E, Wastell D. Soft occlusal splint therapy in the treatment of migraine and other headaches. J Dent 1990;18(3):123–9.

4. Lamey PJ, Steele JG, Aitchison T. Migraine: the effect of acrylic appliance design on clinical response. Br Dent J 1996;180(4):137–40.

5. Wright EF, Gullickson DC. Identifying acute pulpalgia as a factor in TMD pain. J Am Dent Assoc 1996;127:773–80.

6. Okeson JP. Bell's Orofacial Pains, 5th edition. Carol Stream, IL: Quintessence, 1995:73, 403–56.

7. Jensen TS, Gottrup H, Sindrup SH, Bach FW. The clinical picture of neuropathic pain. Eur J Pharmacol 2001;429(1–3):1–11.

8. Kohjitani A, Miyawaki T, Kasuya K, Shimada M. Sympathetic activity-mediated neuropathic facial pain following simple tooth extraction. Cranio 2002;20(2):135–8.

9. Conti PC, de Azevedo LR, de Souza NV, Ferreira FV. Pain measurement in TMD patients: evaluation of precision and sensitivity of different scales. J Oral Rehabil 2001;28(6):534–9.

10. Wright EF. A simple questionnaire and clinical examination to help identify possible non-craniomandibular disorders that may influence a patient's CMD symptoms. Cranio 1992;10(3):228–34.

11. Wright EF, Des Rosier KE, Clark MK, Bifano SL. Identifying undiagnosed rheumatic disorders among patients with TMD. J Am Dent Assoc 1997;128(6):738–44.

12. Clark GT, Green EM, Dornan MR, Flack VF. Craniocervical dysfunction levels in a patient sample from a temporomandibular joint clinic. J Am Dent Assoc 1987;115(2):251–6.

13. Wright EF. Patterns of referred craniofacial pain in TMD patients. J Am Dent Assoc 2000;131(9):1307–15.

14. Rosenbaum RS, Gross SG, Pertes RA, Ashman LM, Kreisberg MK. The scope of TMD/orofacial pain (head and neck pain management) in contemporary dental practice. Dental Practice Act Committee of the American Academy of Orofacial Pain. J Orofac Pain 1997;11(1):78–83.

15. Plesh O, Wolfe F, Lane N. The relationship between fibromyalgia and temporomandibular disorders: prevalence and symptom severity. J Rheumatol 1996;23:1948–52.

16. Raphael KG, Marbach JJ, Klausner J. Myofascial face pain: clinical characteristics of those with regional vs. widespread pain. J Am Dent Assoc 2000;131(2):161–71.

17. Raphael KG, Marbach JJ. Widespread pain and the effectiveness of oral splints in myofascial face pain. J Am Dent Assoc 2001;132(3):305–16.

18. Rammelsberg P, LeResche L, Dworkin S, Mancl L. Longitudinal outcome of temporomandibular disorders: a 5-year epidemiologic study of muscle disorders defined by research diagnostic criteria for temporomandibular disorders. J Orofac Pain 2003;17(1):9–20.

19. Yatani H, Sonoyama W, Kuboki T, Matsuka Y, Orsini MG, Yamashita A. The validity of clinical examination for diagnosis of anterior disc displacement with reduction. Oral Surg Oral Med Oral Pathol Oral Radiol Endod 1998;85:647–53.

20. Schiffman E, Anderson G, Fricton J, Burton K, Schellhas K. Diagnostic criteria for intraarticular T.M. disorders. Community Dent Oral Epidemiol 1989;17(5):252–7.

21. Eriksson L, Westesson PL, Rohlin M. Temporomandibular joint sounds in patients with disc displacement. Int J Oral Surg 1985;14(5):428–36.

22. Ribeiro RF, Tallents RH, Katzberg RW, Murphy WC, Moss ME, Magalhaes AC, Tavano O. The prevalence of disc displacement in symptomatic and asymptomatic volunteers aged 6 to 25 years. J Orofac Pain 1997;11(1):37–47.

23. Brooks SL, Brand JW, Gibbs SJ, Hollender L, Lurie AG, Omnell K-A, Westesson P-L, White SC. Imaging of the temporomandibular joint: a position paper of the American Academy of Oral and Maxillofacial Radiology. Oral Surg Oral Med Oral Pathol Oral Radiol Endod 1997;83:609–18.

24. Yoda T, Imai H, Shinjyo T, Sakamoto I, Abe M, Enomoto S. Effect of arthrocentesis on TMJ disturbance of mouth closure with loud clicking: a preliminary study. Cranio 2002;20(1):18–22.

25. Kai S, Kai H, Nakayama E, Tabata O, Tashiro H, Miyajima T, Sasaguri M. Clinical symptoms of open lock position of the condyle: relation to anterior dislocation of the temporomandibular joint. Oral Surg Oral Med Oral Pathol 1992;74(2):143–8.

26. Mense S, Simons DG, Russell IJ. Muscle Pain: Understanding Its Nature, Diagnosis, and Treatment. Philadelphia: Lippincott Williams & Wilkins, 2001:112, 122.

27. Ursin R, Endresen IM, Vaeroy H, Hjelmen AM. Relations among muscle pain, sleep variables, and depression. J Musculoske Pain 1999;7(3):59–72.

28. Grossi M, Goldberg MB, Locker D, Tenenbaum HC. Reduced neuropsychologic measures as predictors of treatment outcome in patients with temporomandibular disorders. J Orofac Pain 2001;15(4):329–39.

29. Yatani H, Studts J, Cordova M, Carlson CR, Okeson JP. Comparison of sleep quality and clinical and psychologic characteristics in patients with temporomandibular disorders. J Orofac Pain 2002;16(3):221–8.

30. Grandin LD, Yan LJ, Gray SM, Jamison KR, Sachs GS. Suicide prevention: increasing education and awareness. J Clin Psychiatry 2001;62 Suppl 25:12–6.

31. Fishbain DA. The association of chronic pain and suicide. Semin Clin Neuropsychiatry 1999;4(3):221–7.

32. Paxton R, MacDonald F, Allott R, Mitford P, Proctor S, Smith M. Improving general practitioners' assessment and management of suicide risk. Int J Health Care Qual Assur Inc Leadersh Health Serv 2001;14(2 3):133 8.

33. Reeves II J. The suicidal patient: assessment and management strategies for the orofacial pain specialist. In: 27th Scientific Meeting on Orofacial Pain and Temporomandibular Disorders, April 18–21, 2002, San Antonio. Mt Royal, NJ: American Academy of Orofacial Pain.

34. Yeo DK, Pham TP, Baker J, Porters SA. Specific orofacial problems experienced by musicians. Aust Dent J 2002;47(1):2–11.

35. Taddey JJ. Musicians and temporomandibular disorders: prevalence and occupational etiologic considerations. Cranio 1992;10(3):241–4.

36. Hayreh SS. Masticatory muscle pain: an important indicator of giant cell arteritis. Spec Care Dent 1998;16(2):60–5.

37. Lee AG. Jaw claudication: a sign of giant cell arteritis. J Am Dent Assoc 1995;126:1028–9.

38. Kleinegger CL, Lilly GE. Cranial arteritis: a medical emergency with orofacial manifestations. J Am Dent Assoc 1999;130:1203–9.

Chapter 2

Review of the "Initial Patient Questionnaire"

1. On the diagram, please shade the areas of your pain:

Right   Left

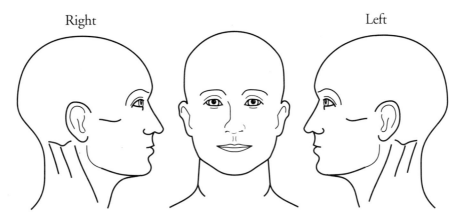

This forces the patient to think of where the pain is located.

2. When did your pain/problem begin? _____

Indicates the chronicity of the disorder. If it is of recent onset, the first occurrence and mild to moderate pain, you may want to prescribe only TMD self-management therapy and ibuprofen, and see whether it resolves.

3. What seemed to cause it to start? _____

This answer may indicate a major contributing factor that can be changed.

---

4. What makes it feel worse? _____

Intuitively, eating, clenching, and stress should aggravate TMD. Listing such problems can help motivate a patient to change these activities. Observe for activities that should not worsen TMD and suggest the patient may have a disorder other than TMD; e.g., symptoms worsen when bearing down for a bowel movement.

5. What makes it feel better? _____

Reinforce the use of these activities. Also, look for activities that suggest the patient may have a disorder other than TMD, e.g., better when taking antibiotics.

6. What treatments have you received? _____

Were these treatments beneficial? These indicate the level of care a patient will need. Did patient receive a TMJ implant that should be followed?

7. When is your pain the worst?
   ○ When first wake up   ○ Later in the day   ○ No daily pattern   ○ Other

Helps identify the significance of nighttime and/or daytime contributing factors and gives a guide to therapy considerations (see "Integration of Conservative Therapies" in Chapter 19).

8. What does the pain keep you from doing? _____

Reflects how much it affects a patient and may correlate with how motivated the patient will be to participate in therapy and the level of therapy the patient may be interested in receiving.

9. Is your pain (check as many as apply):
   ○ Ache   ○ Pressure   ○ Dull   ○ Sharp   ○ Throbbing   ○ Burning   ○ Other

Ache, pressure, or *dull pain* are the usual qualities of TMD pain. *Sharp pain* usually occurs intermittently and is often associated with the TMJ or lateral pterygoid muscle. *Throbbing pain* occurs in one or more of the following three situations:

a. Ache, pressure, or dull is the primary pain character and, when the pain worsens, it changes to throbbing pain. If treatment of the ache, pressure, or dull pain can adequately keep it from escalating into the throbbing pain, the latter will be eliminated.
b. The patient does not report that the ache, pressure, or dull pain progresses into throbbing pain. This pain may be due to a source outside of the dentist's realm of treatment. The practitioner may desire to perform a trial with occlusal appliance therapy and, if it is not effective, consider referring the patient to a physician or neurologist for treatment of a probable migraine. Studies suggest some migraines respond to TMD therapy.

> c. Referred tooth pain; queries suggestive of this are included in Question 10. Burning is sometimes found with TMD pain; if related, it resolves with TMD therapy. Burning may be suggestive of neuropathic pain.

10. Does your pain:
    Wake you up at night? Yes ⭘   No ⭘

> Could be related to nocturnal parafunctional habits, but also to referred tooth pain.

Increase when you lie down? Yes ⭘   No ⭘

> Could be related to gravity's pull on the jaw, but also sinus congestion or referred tooth pain.

Increase when you bend forward? Yes ⭘   No ⭘

> Could be related to gravity's pull on the jaw, but also to sinus congestion.

Increase when you drink hot or cold beverages? Yes ⭘   No ⭘

> TMD pain does not often increase when hot or cold beverages are drunk. What tooth or area does it touch that elicits this response? This response could be due to referred tooth pain (see "Intraoral Examination" in Chapter 3 for more information on referred tooth pain).

11. Please circle the number below to indicate your *present* pain level:
    (No pain) 0 - 1 - 2 - 3 - 4 - 5 - 6 - 7 - 8 - 9 - 10 (The worst pain imaginable)

12. Please circle your *average* pain level during the past 6 months:
    (No pain) 0 - 1 - 2 - 3 - 4 - 5 - 6 - 7 - 8 - 9 - 10 (The worst pain imaginable)

13. Is your pain always present? Yes ⭘   No ⭘ How often do you have it? _____

14. Please describe any symptoms other than pain that you associate with your problem:
    _____
    _____
    _____
    _____

> Look for anything that does not make sense (may be suggestive of non-TMD), e.g., blacking out or decrease in visual field.
>   A progressively increasing open bite of the anterior teeth is suggestive of severe osteoarthritis causing the TMJ to lose vertical height, and is beyond the scope of this book.

Questions 15 through 17 evaluate for non-TMD. Talk to the patient about any "Yes" answer and consider the comments noted after the questions.

15. Have you had:
    Head or neck surgery? Yes ○   No ○

    Is patient's complaint a surgical complication or recurrence from this?

    Whiplash or trauma to your head or neck? Yes ○   No ○

    Is patient's TMD related to this event? If so, was patient adequately evaluated?
        Does the patient have a neck disorder contributing to the TMD?

    Shingles on your head or neck? Yes ○   No ○

    Does the patient have postherpetic neuralgia?

16. Do you have:
    A fever? Yes ○   No ○

    TMD does not cause an elevated temperature. Does the patient have another disorder that may be causing this, e.g., meningitis or sinus infection?
        Consider referring patient to a physician if this has not been evaluated.

    Nasal congestion or stuffiness? Yes ○   No ○

    Is sinus pain the cause for the complaint or contributing to the TMD pain?

    Movement difficulties of your facial muscles, eyes, mouth or tongue? Yes ○   No ○

    Does the patient have a neurological disorder?
        Patients with TMD often report difficulty moving their more painful structures.

    Numbness or tingling? Yes ○   No ○

    Is something more than TMD causing this neurological deficit? Patients with TMD often report small areas of numbness or tingling with a temporal and spatial relationship to their TMD complaint, which correlates with their pain and resolves with their pain. Observe to ensure it resolves with treatment.

    Problems with your teeth? Yes ○   No ○

    Does patient have a tooth problem causing or contributing to the TMD?

Swelling over your jaw joint or in your mouth or throat? Yes ◯   No ◯

Evaluate whether this is causing or contributing to the TMD pain.
    Patients with TMD often report swelling over their painful TMJ or masticatory muscles (see Chapter 1 and Question 14), but this swelling is difficult to discern visually (often only 1 to 2 mm). If it is in a different location or more significant, further evaluation is needed.

A certain spot that triggers your pain? Yes ◯   No ◯

Does the patient have trigeminal neuralgia or some other localized problem? If the patient has only TMD, this is often the source of the primary diagnosis.

Recurrent swelling or tenderness of joints other than in your jaw joint? Yes ◯   No ◯

Does patient have arthritis or some other systemic disorder contributing to the TMD?

Morning stiffness in your body, other than with your jaw? Yes ◯   No ◯

Can be of muscle and/or joint origin and related to systemic disorders.

Muscle tenderness in your body (other than in your head or neck) for more than 50% of the time? Yes ◯   No ◯

Does patient have fibromyalgia, myofascial pain or a systemic disorder?

17. Is your problem worse:
    When swallowing or turning your head? Yes ◯   No ◯

Consider, for example, cervical dysfunction (pain and/or restricted movement), Eagle's syndrome, glossopharyngeal neuralgia, and subacute thyroiditis.

After reading or straining your eyes? Yes ◯   No ◯

The patient may need a new eyeglass prescription or reading glasses, may have a cervical disorder exacerbated by poor posture during the activity, or may clench during this activity.

18. Do your jaw joints make noise? Yes ◯   No ◯ If yes, which: Right ◯   Left ◯

If "Yes," the patient most likely has a disc displacement.

19. Have you ever been unable to open your mouth wide? Yes ○   No ○ If yes, please explain: _____

> Could be due to a TMJ disorder (e.g., acute disc displacement without reduction) or a muscle disorder. The practitioner may need to stretch the patient's mouth to determine the location of restriction.

20. Have you ever been unable to close your mouth? Yes ○   No ○ If yes, please explain:

    _____

    _____

    _____

    _____

> If it occurred at an opening of over 45 mm, the condyle was probably in front of the eminence, and the eminence and/or disc was interfering with the condyle's posterior movement.
>
> If it occurred at an opening of 10 to 35 mm, the condyle was probably unable to get under the posterior band of the disc.
>
> If it occurred at an opening of less than 5 mm, it was probably a lateral pterygoid myospasm.

21. Do you sleep well at night? Yes ○   No ○ Please explain: _____

    _____

    _____

    _____

    _____

> Patients should awake feeling rested. Individuals with fibromyalgia often report they do not sleep well, but there are many other causes for this problem. You may want to consider asking the patient to discuss this with his or her physician, or referring the patient for relaxation therapy or to someone who specializes in sleep disorders. If the patient also awakes with morning TMD pain, you may want to prescribe amitriptyline or nortriptyline.

22. How often are you tense, aggravated or frustrated during a usual day? Always ○ Half the time ○   Seldom ○   Never ○

> If always or half of the time is checked, consider referring the patient for stress management.
>
> Patients tend to hold more tension in their jaws or clench their teeth during these times.

23. How often do you feel depressed during a usual day? Always ○   Half the time ○ Seldom ○   Never ○

> If always or half of the time is checked, consider referring patient for an evaluation.

24. Do you have thoughts of hurting yourself or committing suicide? Yes ○   No ○

If "Yes," determine lethality by asking the patient whether he or she has a plan, a time selected, and the selected means of carrying this out (pills, gun, etc.). If the answer is "Yes" to any of these, the patient must immediately be evaluated by someone trained in this area. A good option is to telephone your local hospital's suicide prevention team and discuss whether immediate referral is necessary. If it is, the patient must be escorted (i.e., by a staff member, responsible family member, or a staff member sent by the hospital). Document your findings and actions, and follow up on your referral.

25. Do you play a musical instrument and/or sing more than 5 hours in a typical week? Yes ○   No ○

This often contributes to the patient's TMD symptoms.

26. What percent of the day are your teeth touching? _____%

As the patient holds his or her teeth together, there is a tendency unconsciously to squeeze as life becomes busy, intense, etc. Encourage the patient to keep his or her teeth apart and relax the jaw.

27. Are you aware of clenching or grinding your teeth: When sleeping? ○
While driving? ○   When using a computer? ○   Other times? ○   Not aware? ○

Encourage the patient to stop clenching or grinding at checked times and become aware of other times he or she may be doing this.

28. Are you aware of oral habits such as: Chewing your cheeks? ○   Chewing objects? ○
Biting your nails or cuticles? ○   Thrusting your jaw? ○   Other habits? ○
Not aware? ○

Encourage the patient to break checked oral habits.

29. What treatment do you think is needed for your problem? _____

Discuss their treatment expectations.

30. Is there anything else you think we should know about your problem? _____
_____
_____

31. If your age is 50 or older, please circle the correct response:
    Docs your pain occur only when you eat? Yes ○ No ○
    Are you pain free when you open wide? Yes ○ No ○
    Do you have unexplainable scalp tenderness? Yes ○ No ○
    Are you experiencing unexplainable or unintentional weight loss? Yes ○ No ○
    Do you have significant morning stiffness lasting more than 1/2 hour? Yes ○ No ○
    Do you have visual symptoms or a visual loss? Yes ○ No ○

These features are more prevalent among people who have **giant cell arteritis** (temporal arteritis), which is almost exclusively found in people over the age of 50 and causes a reduction in the blood flow to the structures of the head and neck. The decreased masticatory muscle blood flow causes the muscles to tire easily, producing a tired, cramped feeling that resolves within 1 to 2 minutes after use. This symptom is also observed among some TMD patients without giant cell arteritis, and these questions are to help differentiate the cause. If the patient has had this symptom for over a year, it is highly unlikely that he or she has giant cell arteritis, which is an important disorder not to miss, because it may progress to cause blindness. It is better to err with an unnecessary referral than allow this disorder to go undiagnosed. If you suspect the patient has giant cell arteritis, he or she should see a physician that day.

A "Yes" response to the first two questions is suggestive of jaw claudication, but a TMD patient with mild TMD symptoms may positively respond to both questions. Consider giant cell arteritis when a patient relates unexplainable scalp tenderness, unexplainable or unintentional weight loss, significant morning stiffness lasting more than 1/2 hour, and visual symptoms or visual loss.

A fever (previously asked in the questionnaire) is also more prevalent among people who have giant cell arteritis. If this is not caused by a dental condition and has not been evaluated by a physician, it is recommended the patient be referred for an evaluation. Another sign of giant cell arteritis is an abnormal temporal artery. This is evaluated by comparing the left and right temporal arteries. Relative to the other side, an abnormal vessel will be more visible, have no pulse, or have palpable nodes.

Chapter 3

Clinical Examination

FAQs

Q: Which should be performed first: measurement of the range of motion or palpation?

A: The range of motion should be measured prior to palpating, because palpation often aggravates the masticatory muscles and/or TMJs, which may cause a decrease in a patient's range of motion.

Q: What is considered to be the minimum of normal range of motion?

A: A general guide for minimum of normal is 40 mm opening (including the overlap), 7 mm right and left lateral, and 6 mm protrusive movements.

Q: Can a dentist write prescriptions or refer a patient for neck pain?

A: Cervical treatment and referrals are within a dentist's scope of clinical practice for TMD.

Q: If odontogenic pain is suspected of contributing to a patient's pain, what are the clinical observations that may aid in locating the offending tooth?

A: Anterior teeth (canine to canine) have been observed referring odontogenic pain bilaterally, whereas the bicuspids and molars have been observed referring pain only to the ipsilateral side.

Substantial information should have been obtained from the patient interview suggesting whether the patient has TMD, other disorders that could contribute to TMD (e.g., odontalgia, sinusitis, neck pain, or cervicogenic headaches), many TMD contributing factors, and the symptom location and time patterns. Consequently prior to performing the clinical examination, the practitioner should have strong suspicions as to which structures are concerns and need further evaluation.

⊙ **QUICK CONSULT**

Obtaining Suspicions of Structures That Are a Concern

From the patient interview, the practitioner should have strong suspicions as to which structures are concerns and need further evaluation.

The primary purpose of the clinical examination is to gather additional information to help confirm or rule out structures involved in a patient's complaints and other suspected disorders that may contribute to these complaints. A potential source can be verified by observing whether stimulating a structure causes the pain to be reproduced (if not present) or exacerbated (if present), or whether anesthetically blocking or alleviating the structure by other means decreases the pain.

⊙ **QUICK CONSULT**

Verifying Potential Sources

A potential source can be verified by observing whether stimulating a structure causes the pain to be reproduced (if not present) or exacerbated (if present), or whether anesthetically blocking or alleviating the structure by other means decreases the pain.

Typically structures are stimulated during the clinical examination to verify their contribution to the pain, and palpation is used to stimulate the masticatory muscles and the TMJs. Generally more than one structure is the source of a TMD patient's pain. Some practitioners grade the palpation tenderness between 0 and 3 for more definitive documentation and to help prioritize a structure's contribution.

Some of the procedures used to anestheti-

cally block or alleviate potential pain sources are (a) a trigger-point anesthetic injection for an individual myofascial trigger point, (b) an anesthetic infiltration or block for a tooth, and (c) a trial of decongestants for the suspected contribution of sinus congestion. Obviously one limiting factor for the anesthetic test is that the pain must be present when the test is performed.

Sometimes structures are both stimulated and injected with anesthetic. For example, a patient with a frontal sinus headache that can be exacerbated by palpating a cervical trigger point (due to referred pain) may desire to have an anesthetic injection of the trigger point to determine the amount the trigger point is contributing to the sinus pain.

RANGE OF MOTION

The patient's range of motion should be measured prior to palpating, because palpation often aggravates the masticatory muscles and/or TMJs, which may cause a decrease in the range of motion. Recording the range of motion enables the practitioner to determine whether the patient has a significant decrease (suggestive of certain disorders) and to follow an objective measure for improvement. (An increase in a restricted range of motion suggests improvement.) Many range-of-motion measures can be performed, e.g., assisted, unassisted, without pain, and despite pain.

The opening measurement routinely obtained is the distance (in millimeters) between the incisal edge of the maxillary central incisors and the incisal edge of the mandibular central incisors when I request of the patient, "Open as wide as you can" (Figure 3-1). Since practitioners may follow a patient's opening measures from appointment to appointment, it is important that practitioners try to be consistent in how the patient is asked to open. Therefore, the phrase and intonation should be consistent at every appointment.

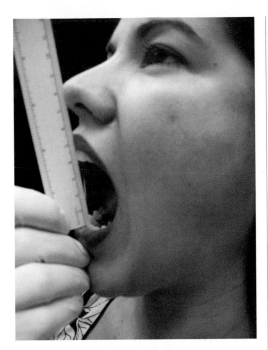

Figure 3-1. Measuring the opening from incisal edge to incisal edge.

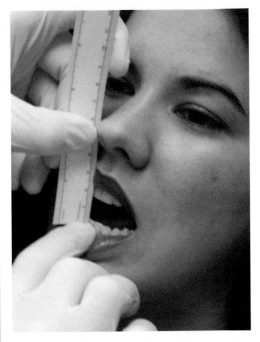

Figure 3-2. Measuring overlap of the central incisors.

▼ TECHNICAL TIP

Opening Consistency

Since a patient's opening may be followed from appointment to appointment, practitioners should try to be consistent in how the patient is asked to open.

The true distance a patient opens includes the overlap of the central incisors. This can easily be determined by asking the patient to close into maximum intercuspation (MI), placing a fingernail on the facial surface of the mandibular central incisor against the maxillary central incisor's incisal edge, asking the patient to open, and measuring the distance from the mandibular central incisor's incisal edge to the fingernail (Figure 3-2). Only the overlap is routinely documented at the initial appointment, and the incisal-to-incisal openings are followed at future appointments. Measuring and adding the overlap at each appointment adds potential for error, and it rarely changes throughout treatment.

A patient who has a significantly limited opening is told about the practitioner's need to look down the patient's throat. Place the head of a mouth mirror against the posterior portion of the tongue, press down on the mirror, and ask the patient to say "Ah" and open as wide as possible. Occasionally a patient who could open only 21 mm may now open 45 mm. There are many potential reasons the patient did not previously open as wide, and these need to be discussed to the practitioner's satisfaction.

Lateral movements can be measured by asking the patient to close into MI and placing a ruler over the maxillary central incisors with the mandibular central incisors' embrasure lined with one of the prominent ruler marks (e.g., the 20-mm mark). The patient is asked to move his or her mandible as far as possible to one side while the practitioner observes the distance the embrasure has moved on the ruler; then the patient is asked to move the mandible in the other direction (Figure 3-3). In general, people do not con-

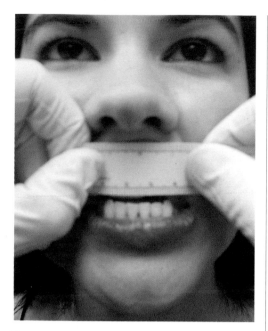

Figure 3-3. Measuring lateral movement.

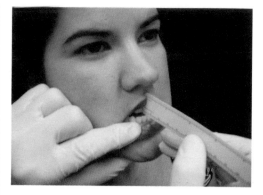

Figure 3-4. Measuring the distance the mandibular incisors are in front of the maxillary incisors.

sciously move their mandible laterally, so some have difficulty when asked to do so. This can usually be resolved by the practitioner demonstrating these movements and asking the patient to practice them in a mirror.

▼ TECHNICAL TIP
Enabling a Patient to Make Excursive Movements
If a patient has trouble making lateral or protrusive movements, asking him or her to practice these by looking into a hand mirror is usually beneficial.

The protrusive movement can be obtained by asking the patient to close in MI and measuring the anterior overjet. The patient is then asked to slide the lower jaw as far forward as possible while the practitioner measures the distance the mandibular incisors are in front of the maxillary incisors and adding the two numbers together (Figure 3-4).

As the patient makes these movements, the practitioner observes for the translation of each condyle. If it is suspected that translation is restricted on one or both condyles, it is recommended he or she feel for the translation. This is performed by placing the palmar surface of the index or middle finger over the condyle and asking the patient to open, close, and move in lateral and protrusive excursions.

▼ TECHNICAL TIP
Observing Restricted TMJ Translation
If the practitioner suspects a patient's TMJ translation is restricted, it is recommended the practitioner feel for the condylar translation.

Slight to moderate restriction in the range of motion is commonly observed among TMD patients. However, range of motion varies with a patient's stature, and the degree of restriction is not always related to severity of TMD symptoms. No minimum of normal ranges has been established, but a general guide for minimum of normal is 40 mm opening (including the overlap), 7 mm right and left lateral, and 6 mm protrusive movements.

TMJ NOISE

TMJ clicks and pops are very prevalent among TMD patients as well as in the general population.[1,2] **Crepitus** is a grating or crackling noise similar to the sound that is created when one walks over gravel. These noises may occur with opening and/or closing, fluctuate in intensity, and occur sporadically.[2,3] It is common for patients to report having a history of TMJ noise, but being unable to reproduce it during the examination.[3]

Practitioners vary in the degree to which they try to verify the TMJ noise. Some palpate for the noise by placing the finger's palmar surface over the TMJ as the patient opens, closes, and moves through lateral and protrusive excursions. Others use a stethoscope to listen for the noise during these movements. The bell-shaped portion of the stethoscope should be used because, when the flat portion of the stethoscope is used, a hair or whisker stub under the flat portion often sounds remarkably similar to TMJ crepitus. Some practitioners use even more sensitive equipment (e.g., Doppler) in an attempt to verify the TMJ noise.

Sometimes the patient and the practitioner have trouble distinguishing which TMJ is generating the click or pop, because the vibration can travel through the mandible and be perceived in the contralateral TMJ. This can usually be differentiated by having the patient start in MI and move the mandible lateral to the one side several times and then lateral to the other side several times. The click or pop is generated during the translation phase, and whichever TMJ was translating when the noise was generated is the source.

Clicking and popping are most commonly related to a disc displacement with reduction,[4-6] course crepitus is most commonly related to a chronic disc displacement without reduction,[5] and fine crepitus does not appear to be highly related to any single articular diagnosis.[5] TMJ inflammation induces osseous changes that may cause rough articular surfaces (Figure 3-5), which can also cause mechanical interferences and TMJ

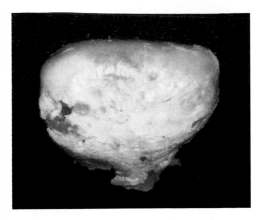

Figure 3-5. Roughness on the condylar surface with a portion of the articular fibrous connective tissue removed to expose the osseous surface.

noises.[7] For additional information on these diagnoses, see "TMJ Articular Disorders" in Chapter 5.

TMJ noise rarely changes my treatment approach, so spending extensive time or specialized equipment to verify the noise is unwarranted. In general, TMJ noise is no more of a concern than is noise in any other joint in the body, and TMJ noise alone does not need to be treated.

⊙ **QUICK CONSULT**

Understanding TMJ Noise Significance

In general, TMJ noise is no more of a concern than is noise in any other joint in the body, and TMJ noise alone does not need to be treated.

TMJ noise generally decreases with TMD therapy, but is less responsive to therapy than are most TMD symptoms.[8] The percentage of patients observing a degree of improvement varies from study to study along with the procedures used to measure the noise. If a patient were to ask for the probability that his or her noise would decrease, as a general conservative guide the patient is informed that from occlusal appliance therapy approximately a third of patients report significant noise reduction or elimination, a third report minor improvement, and a third report no improvement.[8,9] There are no established predictors to suggest a specific individual's results.

PALPATION

The masticatory and cervical muscles and TMJs are generally palpated with the fingertip or palmar surface of the index or middle finger. If applicable, the forces placed on the head are balanced by simultaneously palpating both sides or stabilizing the head by placing the palm of the nonpalpating hand on the contralateral side. It is recommended the practitioner face the patient during the palpation so as to better observe the patient's eyes and facial expressions. The muscles and TMJs are palpated with the muscles relaxed, and healthy muscles do not hurt when palpated.[10]

The muscle and TMJ palpations attempt to stimulate these structures sufficiently so that, if they are contributing to the pain, the palpation will reproduce (if the pain is not present) or exacerbate (if the pain is present) it. The extent to which the practitioner must palpate varies with the ease of reproducing the patient's symptoms; e.g., a patient with exquisite tenderness generally relates light touch reproduces the pain, whereas a muscular man who has not had the pain for a couple of weeks may need forceful palpation to reproduce his pain.

As a point of reference, the TMD Research Diagnostic Criteria[11] recommend using 2 pounds for extraoral muscles and 1 pound on the TMJ and intraoral muscles, but more force may be necessary to generate a patient's chief complaint.[12] It is the author's teaching experience that most practitioners are initially reluctant to use sufficient force to reproduce the TMD symptoms. Conversely, excessive force causes unnecessary palpation and postexamination pain.

Palpation may generate pain within or beyond the structure and/or generate referred pain to a distant location. A variety of palpation techniques provide varying degrees of stimulation to the structure. The degree of stimulation in addition to the sensitivity of the structure govern which of these responses occur. In general, three palpation techniques are used to provide different stimulation intensities: (a) nonspecific palpation in a predetermined location; (b) palpation of a trigger point or nodule of spot tenderness within the muscle (these are localized, firm, hyperirritable nodules that feel like firm knots within the muscle and are more tender than the surrounding muscle); and (c) firm, sustained palpation of these tender nodules.

It is recommended a tiered palpation approach be used. Initially palpate the anterior region of the temporalis muscles, TMJs, and masseter muscles bilaterally in predetermined locations and attempt to generate referred pain from the carotid artery, thyroid, and the muscles just below the occipital protuberance.

Start by palpating the anterior region of the temporalis muscle, TMJs, and masseter muscle; begin with light pressure and slowly increase the force until the patient's eyes or facial expressions convey that the patient is experiencing discomfort. Clinical experience has shown the eyes and face express discomfort prior to patients verbally responding to the discomfort. As the practitioner palpates, the patient is asked whether the palpation is causing discomfort and whether this is his or her pain complaint.

▼ **TECHNICAL TIP**

Reducing Palpation Discomfort

It is recommended the practitioner face the patient during the palpation, so he or she can better observe the patient's eyes and facial expressions; these generally express discomfort prior to patients verbally responding to the discomfort.

After palpating these structures, rule out other specific disorders by palpating the carotid arteries, the thyroid, and the occipital protuberance area of the splenius capitis and trapezius muscles. Additional specific guidance regarding the palpation of this first tier as well as supplementary information are provided below, and a synopsis is provided in Table 3-1, "Recommended Initial Palpations."

The temporalis muscle is often segmented into the anterior, middle, and posterior regions. The muscle fiber direction and the direction the fibers move the mandible vary with each region segment. All three regions

---

Table 3-1. Recommended initial palpations

Anterior region of the temporalis muscle	Bilaterally palpate approximately 1½ inches behind the eye canthus and ½ inch above the zygomatic arch (Figure 3-6).
TMJ	Three areas of the TMJ need to be palpated bilaterally, and any one of these can be tender without tenderness of the others. A common mistake is not having a patient open sufficiently to palpate the TMJ adequately. (a) Ask the patient to open the mouth approximately 20 mm and palpate the condyle's lateral pole. (b) Ask the patient to open as wide as possible and palpate the depth of the depression behind the condyle with the fingertip. (c) With the finger in the depression, pull forward to load the posterior aspect of the condyle (Figure 3-7).
Masseter muscle	Bilaterally palpate the center of the masseter muscle (Figure 3-8). If unsure of the muscle's extent, ask the patient to clench, and its extent can easily be felt.
Carotid artery	Bilaterally palpate the carotid arteries on both sides of the thyroid cartilage (Figure 3-9). This rules out carotidynia for patients who relate this palpation does not reproduce their pain complaint.
Thyroid	Initially touch the suprasternal notch and then bilaterally palpate approximately 1 inch superior and 1 inch lateral to the notch (Figure 3-10). This rules out thyroiditis for patients in whom this palpation does not reproduce their pain complaint.
Splenius capitis muscle	This muscle is located in the depression just posterior to the sternocleidomastoid muscle along the base of the skull. Find the firm nodules within this muscle along the skull base. Palpate approximately 1 inch below the skull so these nodules are compressed up against the skull base. Press to patient tolerance and hold for approximately 5 seconds, attempting to generate referred pain. The head is stabilized during palpation by placing the palm of the other hand above the forehead (Figure 3-11).
Trapezius muscle	Find the firm nodules within this muscle along the base of the skull. Palpate approximately 1 inch below the skull so these nodules are compressed up against the skull base. Press to patient tolerance and hold for approximately 5 seconds, attempting to generate referred pain. The head is stabilized by placing the palm of the other hand above the forehead (Figure 3-12).

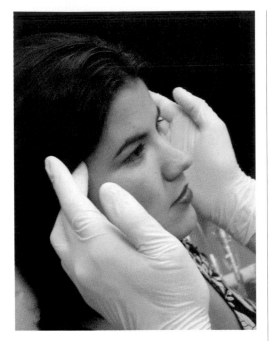

Figure 3-6. Palpation of the anterior region of the temporalis muscle.

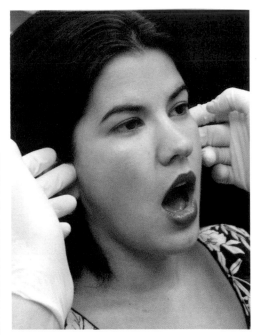

Figure 3-7. Palpation of the TMJ.

may be tender to palpation, have tender nodules, and be a source of the pain. Bilaterally palpate the *anterior region of the temporalis muscle* approximately 1¹/₂ inches behind the eye canthus and ¹/₂ inch above the zygomatic arch (Figure 3-6).

If the anterior region of the temporalis or any other muscle is tender to palpation, the most probable diagnosis is myofascial pain. Ideally the practitioner would identify trigger points to arrive at this diagnosis, but they may be difficult to discern, even for practitioners experienced in palpating muscles.[13] From a clinically practical viewpoint, if the muscle is tender to palpation and no other muscle diagnosis in Chapter 5 ("TMD Diagnostic Categories") better describes the patient's condition, it is recommended the muscle tenderness be diagnosed as myofascial pain. It is estimated that, among the TMD patients I evaluate who have muscle tenderness, more than 95 percent of the time I diagnose the muscle tenderness as myofascial pain.

✪ FOCAL POINT

Muscle palpation tenderness generally provides a clinical diagnosis of myofascial pain, unless another muscle diagnosis in Chapter 5 ("TMD Diagnostic Categories") better describes the patient's condition.

Clinically it has been observed that the *TMJ* needs to be palpated in three locations. Tenderness in one of these locations is not necessarily associated with tenderness in another. Palpate the first location by asking the patient to open approximately 20 mm and palpating the condyle's lateral pole. Then ask the patient to open as wide as possible while you palpate the depth of the depression behind the condyle with your fingertip. Finally with the finger in the depression and the mouth open wide, pull forward to load the posterior aspect of the condyle (Figure 3-7).

Tenderness of the TMJ suggests the patient has capsulitis and/or synovitis, but this cannot be differentiated clinically, so the clinical diagnosis is TMJ inflammation.

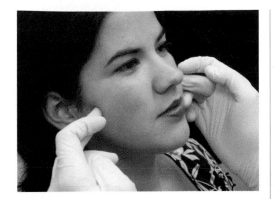

Figure 3-8. Palpation of the masseter muscle.

Clinical training experience has shown that most practitioners do not adequately palpate the TMJ, and the most common mistake is that the patient's mouth is not open wide enough.

✪ FOCAL POINT

TMJ palpation tenderness provides a clinical diagnosis of TMJ inflammation.

The *masseter muscle* is composed of a superficial portion and a deep portion. Bilaterally palpating the center of the masseter muscle will simultaneously stimulate both sections of the muscle (Figure 3-8). If the practitioner is unsure of the muscle's center, it can easily be delineated by asking the patient to clench his or her teeth while the practitioner palpates the extent of the muscle. If the muscle is tender to palpation and no other muscle diagnosis in Chapter 5 ("TMD Diagnostic Categories") better describes the patient's condition, it is recommended the muscle tenderness be diagnosed as myofascial pain.

The *carotid arteries* are palpated on both sides of the thyroid cartilage to determine whether stimulating these structures reproduces a patient's pain (Figure 3-9). This area is tender for most individuals, so, prior to this palpation, it is recommended that the practitioner has palpated this structure on himself or herself to determine the force that

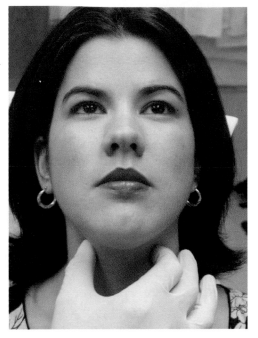

Figure 3-9. Palpation of the carotid arteries.

would not cause undue discomfort. The patient may relate the palpation generates discomfort, but this is different from his or her pain. If this palpation brings on the pain, it suggests carotidynia is causing or contributing to the pain and a referral should be made to the patient's physician.

Bilaterally palpate the *thyroid*. If unsure of its location, first touch the suprasternal notch to establish the landmarks and then bilaterally palpate the thyroid at approximately 1 inch superior and 1 inch lateral to the notch (Figure 3-10). If this palpation reproduces the pain, this suggests thyroiditis is causing or contributing to the pain and a referral should be made to the patient's physician.

It is important to attempt to generate referred pain from the *splenius capitis* (located in the depression just posterior to the sternocleidomastoid muscle along the base of the skull) and *trapezius muscles*, because referred cervicogenic pain is relatively prevalent among TMD patients. A study of 230 TMD patients found palpation of the splenius

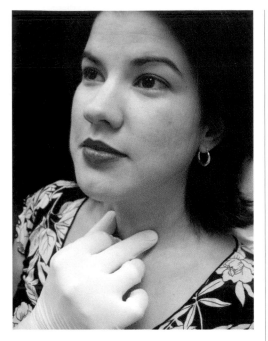

Figure 3-10.   Palpation of the thyroid.

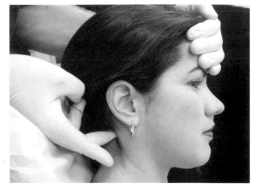

Figure 3-11.   Palpation of the splenius capitis muscle.

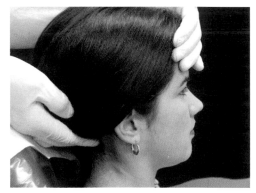

Figure 3-12.   Palpation of the trapezius muscle.

capitis and trapezius muscles generated referred pain to the temporalis muscle region in 18 and 31 patients, respectively. This study observed that palpating these muscles just below the occipital protuberance was one of most common sources for generating referred pain to the forehead, periorbital, vertex, temple, occipital, postauricular, and ear.[14]

◉ **QUICK CONSULT**

Identifying Referred Pain from the Neck

Referred pain from the neck is relatively prevalent among TMD patients. Palpating the neck muscles just below the occipital protuberance most commonly generates referred pain to the forehead, periorbital, vertex, temple, occipital, postauricular, and ear.

Prior to attempting to generate referred pain from either the splenius capitis or trapezius muscles, palpate the muscle to find the most tender nodules within the muscle along the skull base. Then press the fingertip

approximately 1 inch below the skull, up against the skull base, so each nodule is compressed between the fingertip and skull base. Press to patient tolerance (a considerable amount of force may be needed) and hold for approximately 5 seconds. The head is stabilized during the palpation by placing the palm of the other hand above the forehead. See Figure 3-11 for palpation of the splenius capitis muscle and Figure 3-12 for the trapezius muscle. As these muscles are palpated, ask the patient whether pain is being felt in any location other than the palpation site.

The forehead and periorbital (in, behind, or around the eyes) areas are very common sites to which these muscles refer pain. It is believed that practitioners who have not previously palpated these muscles in this manner will be surprised by the frequency with which referred pain is generated from the cervical region.

Clinically it has been observed that the vast majority of TMD patients have their pain reproduced by employing only these initial recommended palpations. If a patient's pain was reproduced by palpating these sites, it is felt that additional masticatory muscle palpation would only cause more discomfort and have little likelihood of changing the diagnoses and treatment plan. Stopping the palpation evaluation for these patients is justified because (a) the initial recommended palpations have demonstrated the pain is from masticatory structures, (b) most conservative TMD therapies treat all the masticatory structures, (c) a muscle and joint contribution comparison can be made with the information obtained, and (d) other structures that commonly refer to the masticatory system or whose source is important to rule out are part of the initial recommended palpations.

If the pain was not reproduced by these initial palpations, more extensive palpation is needed. It is recommended the practitioner next attempt to reproduce the remaining pain complaints by palpating the anterior region of the temporalis muscle, masseter muscle, and/or TMJ more intensely and/or palpating additional structures. The direction the practitioner proceeds typically varies with his or her suspicions and clinical experience.

For practitioners who have not yet developed this clinical experience, Figure 3-13 provides maps of palpation locations that could generate referred pain to the labeled anatomical areas of the head and face.[14] For instance, with a patient complaining of maxillary dentition pain in which no local etiology can be found, the practitioner may desire to test whether it might be due to referred pain from the masticatory or cervical muscles or TMJ. In Figure 3-13, the map for "Maxillary Dentition" has areas of the temporalis muscle, TMJ, and masseter muscle marked on the head, in addition to the lateral pterygoid area and medial pterygoid muscle annotated below. (These are intraoral muscles that could not be drawn on the head.) The masseter muscle is the location marked with the color designated as the more common source, so palpating the masseter muscle more intensely is most likely to generate referred pain to the maxillary dentition. If palpation of this location does not generate the desired referred pain, it is recommended the practitioner similarly palpate the less common sources.

A good technique for more intensely palpating muscles involves finding and loading the trigger points or nodules of spot tenderness within the muscle. These nodules feel like firm knots within the muscle and are more tender than the surrounding muscle.

Once found, apply pressure to each nodule. This will generate more intense pain within that structure, generate pain that may go beyond the structure, and will sometimes refer pain to distant locations. If such a nodule cannot be found, then firmly palpate the desired area of the muscle and, wherever tenderness is noted, hold firm pressure on that area. The TMJ can be similarly stimulated more intensely by palpating its tender locations more vigorously.

The third palpation technique can further stimulate the structure and is typically used when attempting to generate referred pain. This is accomplished by first identifying the tender nodules within the muscle or locations within the TMJ, applying sustained pressure to these sites up to patient tolerance, and holding it for at least 5 seconds or until the desired result occurs. This generates greater local pain that may go beyond the structure and/or referred pain to distant locations. To determine where referred pain is being generated to a distant location, ask the patient whether pain is being felt at a location other than where the practitioner is pressing. Each nodule within a muscle may

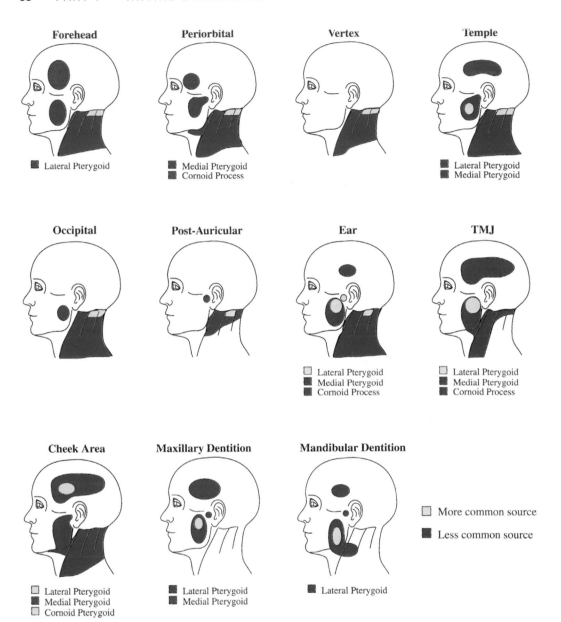

Figure 3-13.   Map of palpation locations that can generate referred pain to the labeled anatomical areas.

refer pain to a different location; therefore, this palpation technique may need to be repeated for each tender nodule.

If a patient's complaint was not reproduced by the recommended initial palpations, and the practitioner believes it is coming from structures not previously palpated, then additional palpations need to be performed. Specific guidance regarding these additional palpations as well as supplementary information are provided below, and a synopsis is provided in Table 3-2, "Additional Palpations."

The sequence for palpating these additional structures varies with a practitioner's suspicions and clinical experience. The prac-

Table 3-2. Additional palpations

Middle temporalis muscle	The temporalis muscle can visibly be divided into its three segments. Bilaterally palpate the central portion of the middle temporalis, approximately 2 inches above the TMJs (Figure 3-15). Referred pain may be generated by locating and applying sustained pressure to the tender nodules within this segment.
Posterior temporalis muscle	Bilaterally palpate the central portion of the posterior temporalis, above and behind the ears (Figure 3-16). Referred pain may also be generated by locating and applying sustained pressure to the tender nodules within this segment.
Anterior digastric muscle	The anterior digastric muscle runs from the lingual surface of the chin, near the midline to the hyoid bone. I cannot delineate this muscle from the surrounding tissue, but palpate superiorly the area this muscle transverses (Figure 3-17). If tenderness is observed, rule out an oral disorder causing this tenderness. If tenderness is not due to an oral disorder, referred pain may be generated by applying sustained pressure to the tender area.
Posterior digastric muscle	The posterior digastric muscle runs from the hyoid sling medial to the sternocleidomastoid muscle and attaches medial to the mastoid process. Place a fingertip posterior to the angle of the mandible and medial to the sternocleidomastoid muscle and apply the palpation force posteriorly (Figure 3-18). If tenderness is observed, referred pain may be generated by applying sustained pressure.
Sternocleidomastoid muscle	Bilaterally palpate the sternocleidomastoid muscles by squeezing each between the thumb and index finger. If tender, holding for 5 seconds may generate referred pain. Clinically, the more superior portions of the muscle are more likely to generate referred pain to the head and face (Figure 3-19).
Additional muscle cervical palpation	Place the palm of the nondominant hand above the patient's forehead and the four fingertips of the dominant hand just below the occipital protuberance. Press in several millimeters and slowly slide the fingertips down the neck muscles, feeling for tender nodules (Figure 3-20). To each tender nodule, apply firm, steady pressure up to patient tolerance for 5 seconds, inquiring about discomfort referred to other areas (Figure 3-21). Similar to the sternocleidomastoid muscle, clinically the superior region tends to refer to the head and face, whereas the inferior region tends to refer into the upper back and shoulders.
Lateral pterygoid area	Slide the fifth digit along the lateral side of the maxillary alveolar ridge to the most posterior region of the vestibule (the location for the posterior superior alveolar injection). Palpate by pressing superior, medial, and posterior direction (Figure 3-22). If tenderness is observed, referred pain may be generated by applying heavier sustained pressure.
Medial pterygoid muscle	Place the index finger at the traditional insertion site for an inferior alveolar injection and press laterally. If the patient gags, the finger is too posterior (Figure 3-23). If tenderness is observed, referred pain may be generated by applying heavier sustained pressure.
Cornoid process	Slide the index finger superiorly along the anteromedial border of the ramus; as the finger approaches the superior extent, palpate the temporalis muscle's tendon overlaying the coronoid process (Figure 3-24). If tenderness is observed, referred pain may be generated by applying heavier sustained pressure.
Stylomandibular ligament	Palpate with a blunt instrument or fingertip medial to the posterior border of the mandible and 10 to 15 mm above the angle of the mandible in an anteromedial direction (Figure 3-25). If tenderness is observed, referred pain may be generated by applying heavier sustained pressure.

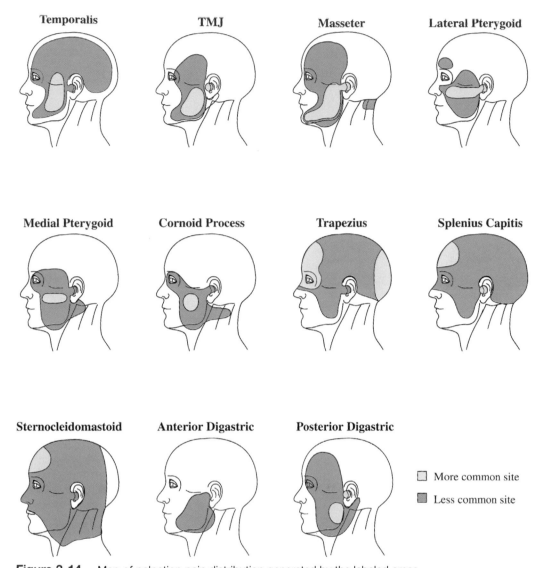

Figure 3-14.   Map of palpation pain distribution generated by the labeled areas.

titioner may find the maps of palpation pain distribution in Figure 3-14 helpful in determining the most probable structures that would reproduce the patient's pain.

The temporalis muscle can visually be divided into its three segments. The *middle region of the temporalis muscle* is palpated bilaterally in its central portion, approximately 2 inches above the TMJs (Figure 3-15). The *posterior region of the temporalis muscle* is similarly palpated bilaterally in its central portion, above and behind the ears

(Figure 3-16). If the practitioner suspects the patient's pain may be from these structures, the practitioner should find and load the tender nodules with momentary or sustained pressure to increase the pain intensities and probability of generating referred pain.

The digastric muscle has an anterior and posterior belly with an intermediate tendon that slides through a fibrous sling attached to the hyoid bone. These are primarily opening muscles, and clinically I cannot delineate

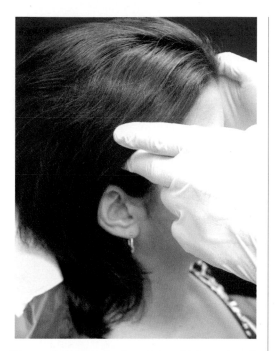

Figure 3-15. Palpation of the middle region of the temporalis muscle.

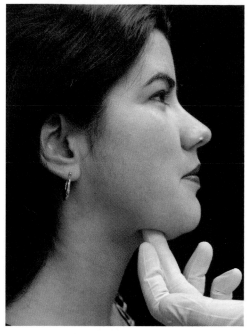

Figure 3-17. Palpation of the anterior digastric muscle.

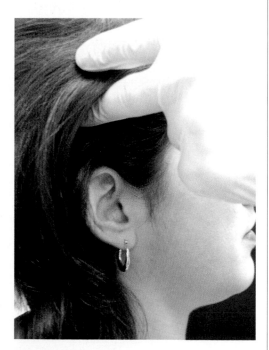

Figure 3-16. Palpation of the posterior region of the temporalis muscle.

these muscles from the surrounding tissue. The *anterior digastric muscle* attaches lingual to the chin and runs near the midline to the hyoid sling. Based on the anatomical knowledge, palpate the location that the anterior digastric muscle transverses and observe for tenderness (Figure 3-17). If there is tenderness in this region, the practitioner should consider and rule out an oral disorder as the cause of this tenderness.

The *posterior digastric muscle* runs from the hyoid sling, medial of the sternocleidomastoid muscle, and attaches medial to the mastoid process. Palpate this muscle by placing a fingertip posterior to the angle of the mandible and medial to the anterior edge of the sternocleidomastoid muscle and press posteriorly (Figure 3-18). If tenderness is observed, referred pain may be generated by applying heavier sustained pressure. Clinical experience has shown that the posterior digastric muscle may be very tender when a patient has recently developed a restricted opening (e.g., acute TMJ disc displacement

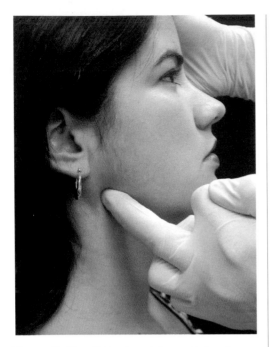

Figure 3-18. Palpation of the posterior digastric muscle.

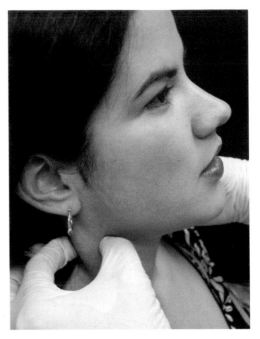

Figure 3-19. Palpation of the sternocleidomastoid muscle.

without reduction). In this situation, the posterior digastric muscle is most likely painful from the patient's repeated forcible attempts to open wider.

Referred pain to the temple, masseter, ear, and TMJ areas can be generated by the *sternocleidomastoid muscle*, although the splenius capitis and trapezius muscles more commonly refer pain to these sites.[14] Clinical experience has shown that the more superior region of the sternocleidomastoid muscle is more likely to generate referred pain to the head and face. Bilaterally palpate the sternocleidomastoid muscles by simultaneously squeezing each between the thumb and index finger along the length of the muscle (Figure 3-19). If it is suspected that a patient's pain may be from these structures, any tender region should be held and squeezed for 5 seconds in an attempt to generate referred pain.

The occipital protuberance area should have been assessed during the initial palpations, but the *additional cervical muscle palpation* can appraise the remainder of the neck muscles. The cervical musculature has several layers of muscles overlapping each other that are nearly impossible to differentiate. It is common for the most superficial muscle to indicate the region (e.g., trapezius muscle), although the designated problem may actually be located in one of the deeper muscles.

Tender nodules within the remainder of the neck can be identified and palpated. Begin by placing the palm of the nondominant hand above the patient's forehead and the four fingertips of the dominant hand just below the occipital protuberance. Press in several millimeters and slowly slide your fingertips down the neck muscles, feeling for tender nodules (Figure 3-20). For each tender nodule, apply firm, steady pressure up to patient tolerance for 5 seconds, inquiring about discomfort referred to another area (Figure 3-21). Continue this process throughout the cervical region, as each of the tender nodules may refer pain to a different location. Clinically the superior region tends to refer pain to the head and face, whereas

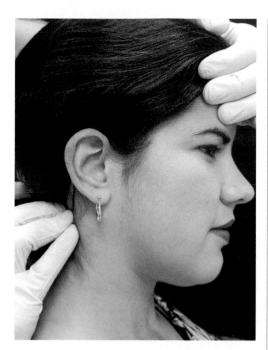

Figure 3-20. Palpation of additional cervical muscles.

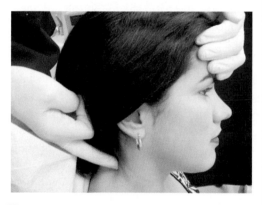

Figure 3-21. Firm, steady pressure applied to a tender nodule identified in the cervical musculature.

the inferior region tends to refer pain into the upper back and shoulders.

When lecturing in the U.S. Air Force, it was common to be asked to evaluate their TMD patients who were not responding to their therapies. One of these patients who had unilateral TMD symptoms localized to the masseter muscle region had received several years of TMD therapy, but the symp-

toms had not improved. During my initial recommended palpations and more intense palpation of the masseter muscle, the patient's pain could not be reproduced. While performing these additional cervical palpations, several tender nodules within the neck muscles were found that referred pain to distant locations, but only one of these nodules reproduced the patient's complaint. This experience confirmed the necessity to find and test each tender nodule. My evaluation suggested that the patient's masseter muscle region pain would respond best from the therapy directed to the neck.

⦿ **QUICK CONSULT**

Directing Therapy at the Source

If the patient's TMD pain is primarily from the neck, therapy primarily needs to be directed to the neck.

Even though cervical muscle palpation reproduces a patient's pain, the source of the neck muscle tenderness may actually be a disorder within the spinal column. Spinal column disorders tend to cause the muscles in the region to become painful, and similarly painful muscles tend to cause a malalignment of the spinal column. Dental practitioners can attempt to palpate the spinal column, but it is preferred to refer the patient to an individual who specializes in treating the cervical region and let the specialist determine the diagnoses, contributing factors, and treatment.

The *lateral* (external) *pterygoid muscle* cannot be directly felt or palpated, but pressure applied to the *lateral pterygoid area* appears to put pressure on structures that transmit the load to the lateral pterygoid muscle. Clinical experience has shown that, when the symptoms (e.g., the patient cannot close the posterior teeth together because of a lateral pterygoid myospasm) suggest the lateral pterygoid muscle should be relatively tender, the palpation of this area has shown corresponding tenderness. Functional tests for the

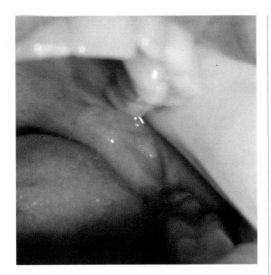

Figure 3-22. Palpation of the lateral pterygoid area.

lateral pterygoid muscle have not been found to be as reliable as palpating this area.

To palpate the lateral pterygoid area, slide the fifth digit along the lateral side of the maxillary alveolar ridge to the most posterior region of the vestibule (the location for the posterior superior alveolar injection). Palpate by pressing in a superior, medial, and posterior direction (Figure 3-22). If tenderness is observed, referred pain may be generated by applying heavier sustained pressure. Palpation of the lateral pterygoid area is generally tender for most TMD patients and also the most likely masticatory palpation to be tender for non-TMD patients.

A practitioner whose fingernails are not well trimmed will more likely to get a painful response. When asked, sometimes the patient will respond, "The pain was due to your fingernail digging into my gum." As an alternative, some practitioners use the head of a mouth mirror to palpate this area.

Room to palpate this area is limited, so the right or left fifth digit, which will flex to curve along the alveolar ridge, is used. Occasionally the patient is asked to move the mandible to the ipsilateral side to provide more room. If the practitioner finds space is still tight, the head of a mouth mirror can be used to palpate this area.

When teaching this palpation to residents, the fifth digit is placed on a skull in the area of the palpation. The skull is turned to view it from the bottom, visualize the lateral pterygoid muscle traversing from the lateral pterygoid plate to the fovea on the condyle neck's anteromedial surface, and discuss the relative closeness of this palpation to the muscle.

The *medial* (internal) *pterygoid muscle* is similar to the masseter muscle, but traverses medial to the ramus and therefore has very limited access. A small area of the medial pterygoid muscle can be palpated intraorally (at the insertion site for a traditional inferior alveolar nerve block), and the extreme inferior portion can be palpated extraorally. Clinical experience has shown that the extraoral palpation is not as reliable as the intraoral palpation.

Intraorally, to palpate the medial pterygoid muscle, place the index finger at the traditional insertion site for an inferior alveolar injection and press laterally (Figure 3-23). If the patient gags, the finger is too posterior. Extraorally the medial pterygoid muscle is palpated by sliding the index finger medial to the inferior border of the ramus, pressing superior until resistance is met, and then pulling lateral to load the medial pterygoid muscle. If tenderness is observed in the medial pterygoid muscle, and the patient's pain is suspected to be from this structure, heavier sustained pressure will generate more intense and possibly referred pain.

The temporalis muscle inserts into the mandible on the medial and anterior surfaces of the *cornoid process*. This is the portion of the cornoid process that is evaluated by this palpation. Palpate this structure by sliding the index finger superiorly along the anteromedial border of the ramus; as the finger approaches the superior extent, palpate the temporalis muscle's tendon overlying the cornoid process (Figure 3-24). If tenderness is observed, and the pain is suspected to be from this structure, heavier sustained pressure will generate more intense and possibly

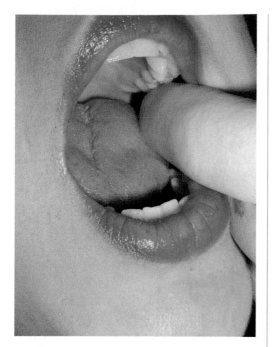

Figure 3-23. Palpation of the medial pterygoid muscle.

referred pain.

Tenderness of this structure suggests tendonitis, and clinically it correspondingly improves, with the other masticatory structures, from conservative TMD therapy. If the pain is limited to this area and is recalcitrant to TMD therapy, the practitioner may desire to prescribe an oral anti-inflammatory medication or inject an anti-inflammatory medication into the tendon.

Occasionally patients report the pain source is located medial to the ramus and 10 to 15 mm anterior and superior to the angle of mandible. Tendonitis of the *stylomandibular ligament* has been reported as a source of pain in this location, in addition to causing referred pain to other areas. The diagnosis of this disorder has been designated *Ernest syndrome*.[15]

Palpate this structure with a blunt instrument or fingertip medial to the posterior border of the mandible and 10 to 15 mm above the angle of the mandible anteromedially (Figure 3-25). It has been reported that hyperactive masticatory muscles cause this disorder.[10] Clinical experience has shown it

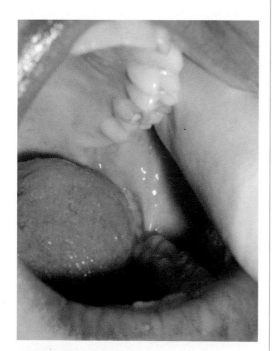

Figure 3-24. Palpation of the cornoid process.

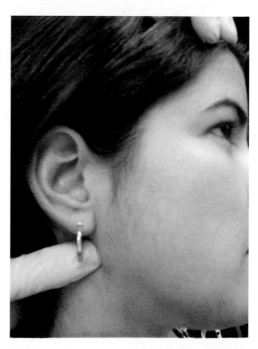

Figure 3-25. Palpation of the stylomandibular ligament.

correspondingly improves, with the other masticatory structures, from conservative TMD therapy. If the pain is limited to this area and is recalcitrant to therapy, the practitioner may desire to prescribe an oral administration and/or injection of anti-inflammatory medication.[10]

Referred pain frequently causes confusion for both the practitioner and the patient. There is the potential that the non-reproduced portion of the pain may be referred from a distant location. Referred pain is commonly seen with a heart attack; the site of the pain may be in the left arm or shoulder, while the pain's source is the heart. Treatment for the pain must be directed toward the source, not the site where it is felt.

To demonstrate the clinical relevance of determining a referred pain's source, assume that a patient with ear pain, whose physician has ruled out ear pathology, was referred to the dentist because the physician suspected the ear pain was due to TMD. During the TMD evaluation, the practitioner will need to determine the source of the ear pain. It is recommended the practitioner palpate the locations mapped in Figure 3-13 under "Ear." If the splenius capitis muscle was found to be the only area that could generate referred pain to the ear, this would suggest that therapy for the neck would have the highest probability of resolving the patient's ear pain. If palpating the masticatory muscles and/or the TMJ generated referred pain to the ear, but the ear pain could not be reproduced by palpating the cervical muscles, then TMD therapy would have the highest probability of resolving the ear pain.

If both the cervical and masticatory regions could generate referred pain to the ear, this would suggest that ear pain may be perceived when the patient stimulates either of these regions (e.g., cervical stimulation through poor posture or masticatory stimulation through oral habits). Therapy recommendations are a clinical judgment based on factors such as (a) understanding that TMD and cervical pain can negatively influence each other and treatment for one may benefit the other; (b) knowledge of the patient's symptom patterns (e.g., whether the masticatory or cervical region becomes painful first and then the pain moves to the other location); (c) knowledge of whether the masticatory or cervical region more readily reproduces the pain and is more tender to palpation; (d) efficacious experiences of the practitioner and patient for TMD and cervical treatments; and (e) understanding that many TMD patients report improvement of cervical symptoms following occlusal appliance therapy. Discussing this information with the patient, the practitioner may elect to institute TMD therapy first, cervical therapy first, or both together. Observational studies report that combining therapies enhances the potential for success.[16,17]

Cervical treatment and referrals are within a dentist's scope of clinical practice for TMD.[18] Many therapies have been shown to be beneficial in treating the cervical dysfunction, and clinical experience generally dictates the approach the practitioner uses, e.g., prescription of the practitioner's preferred medication, instruction on cervical exercises, referral to a physician, or referral to a physical therapist. Referrals for treatments that do not give patients the ability to control their cervical dysfunction on their own and require them to return continually to their provider for therapy are generally avoided.

When evaluating patients for TMD or TMD-like pain, sometimes palpation will not reproduce it. The practitioner needs to balance the discomfort created by the palpating and the probability of identifying the pain source through these palpations. If unable to reproduce the pain through these palpations, at some point the practitioner will need to proceed to the structures or tests described in "Intraoral Examination" and "Additional Evaluations," the next two sections in this chapter.

Intraoral Examination

The nervous system shares the neurological circuitry for deep pain (produced by musculoskeletal, neural, vascular, and visceral structures) among many structures. This enables pain from oral disorders to be perceived in the masticatory muscles and/or TMJs.[14,15,20] The responses to the "Initial Patient Questionnaire" should alert a practitioner that an oral disorder may be causing or contributing to a patient's TMD-like symptoms, but the questionnaire is not infallible. It is imperative that dentists observe for dental disorders contributing to pain, because nondentists treating patients for TMD generally assume that, if the patient has been evaluated by a dentist for TMD, a dental disorder has been ruled out.

It is recommended the practitioner begin the intraoral exam by performing a general oral screening. The oral cavity should be appraised for swelling, deflection of the soft palate, etc. Occasionally the practitioner may desire to palpate the back of the throat (e.g., evaluating for Eagle's syndrome) and may find the end of the mouth-mirror handle useful for this. If intraoral palpations were necessary, it is assumed these were previously performed.

A practitioner who is not aware of a patient's dental caries and periodontal disease status may desire to take dental radiographs in addition to clinically evaluating the teeth for cavities and periodontal disease. By far, the most common oral disorder that I see misdiagnosed as TMD is referred odontogenic pain. Bear in mind that a patient may have odontogenic pain even though the teeth are caries and restoration free and the periodontal health is within normal limits. Patients might have odontogenic pain from a tooth with a history of trauma or incomplete fracture.[21] Patients with an incomplete tooth fracture generally report a sharp lancinating pain upon biting or releasing tough or crunchy foods.[22]

⊙ **QUICK CONSULT**

Observing for an Odontalgia Contribution

By far, the most common oral disorder that I see misdiagnosed as TMD is referred odontogenic pain.

A dental disorder may not only contribute to a patient's pain, but may also alter the patient's treatment plan, for any restorations that are placed after the occlusal appliance is fabricated may require the practitioner to alter the appliance. If a patient is diagnosed with TMD and needs restorations, the practitioner may choose (a) to delay appliance therapy until the restorations are completed, (b) to fabricate the appliance on an arch that is (or becomes) caries free and adjust the appliance's occlusal surface as the opposing restorations are placed, or (c) to fabricate and adjust a temporary appliance (e.g., soft appliance) until the restorations are completed.

If odontogenic pain is suspected to be contributing to the pain, the dentist will need to search for the offending tooth. A few clinical observations may aid in locating the offending tooth. Anterior teeth (canine to canine) have been observed referring odontogenic pain bilaterally, whereas the bicuspids and molars have been observed referring pain only to the ipsilateral side.[23]

Bilateral pain does not exclude the possibility that the patient may have odontogenic pain from a posterior tooth. It is common to observe a patient with odontogenic pain whose complaint is bilateral ache, pressure, and/or dull pain in addition to unilateral throbbing pain. The offending tooth is subsequently identified as a posterior tooth on the throbbing side, and the bilateral ache, pressure, and/or dull pain is due to coexisting TMD.[23]

If a patient reports the pain increases when drinking hot or cold liquids, ask which tooth the liquid touches to cause the increase. The answer should indicate a quadrant to evaluate initially for a dental source. It is common for patients with symptomatic muscles to report that their pain increases when the muscles get chilled, so it is not surprising that some TMD patients report that their pain increases when the cold liquid touches the medial pterygoid muscle rather than a tooth. In this situation, an odontogenic contributor is usually not present.

☻ FOCAL POINT

If a patient reports that pain increases when drinking hot or cold liquids, this should lead the practitioner to suspect a tooth may be contributing to the pain.

The offending tooth should be identified through percussion and thermal tests (hot or cold, depending on which stimulus reproduces the pain). In a study of referred odontogenic pain, all patients diagnosed with odontogenic pain contributing to their complaint had tenderness to percussion of the offending tooth.[23] It is common for TMD patients to have multiple teeth tender to percussion, which is speculated to be a result of the high prevalence of clenching or bruxing among these patients.[10] Some patients with a positive thermal test relate it caused only lingering pain within the tooth (hyperresponsive reaction), and others relate it referred pain to the location of their chief complaint, whereas still others relate the test reproduced the sequential pain pattern they described during the interview.

If the thermal test is positive, a ligamentary injection to the suspected tooth will help determine the impact the hyperresponsive tooth may be having on the pain. When performing the thermal and anesthetic tests, it has been helpful for the patient to grade the pain intensity on a 0 to 10 scale, where 0 is no pain and 10 is the worst pain imaginable.

If the ligamentary injection dramatically reduces or eliminates the pain, odontogenic pain is apparently contributing significantly to the complaint. The ligamentary injection, rather than the traditional dental anesthetic injection, is recommended for the anesthetic test. A maxillary infiltration or inferior alveolar nerve block may cause symptom reduction due to the anesthetic's direct effect on the lateral pterygoid or medial pterygoid muscle.

☻ FOCAL POINT

If the ligamentary injection dramatically reduces or eliminates a patient's pain, odontogenic pain is apparently contributing significantly to the complaint.

It is important for practitioners to realize that a ligamentary injection does not anesthetize only the tooth injected. It provides intraosseous distribution of the anesthetic, which may cause pulpal anesthesia of as many as two teeth on each side of the injected tooth.[24] Therefore, prior to administering the injection, it is imperative to identify the offending tooth by percussion and thermal testing. Careful diagnostic testing must also be used to rule out adjacent teeth as possible contributors.

Recommended criteria for classifying a tooth as an odontogenic contributor to a patient's TMD pain are (if both are positive) (a) the thermal test caused lingering tooth pain or generated the TMD pain, and (b) the ligamentary injection dramatically reduced or eliminated the TMD pain.[23]

Once the offending tooth is identified, the practitioner must determine whether the odontogenic pain is due to a reversible or a nonreversible disorder. Examples of nonreversible conditions include deep caries or restorations for which endodontic therapy is indicated, an incomplete tooth fracture with pulpal involvement, and a combined periodontal-endodontic condition. Offending teeth with nonreversible conditions should receive the traditional dental treatments for the disorder, generally involving endodontic therapy or extraction.

Clinical experience has shown that a reversible pulpitis in an offending tooth is often caused by a patient continually aggravating this tooth with an opposing tooth. This could be from a habit of rubbing or bumping the opposing teeth together, a high restoration causing the tooth to be the first or only closure contact, etc.

⊚ **QUICK CONSULT**

Observing Teeth with Reversible Pulpitis

Clinical experience has shown when a TMD patient's pain is primarily from a reversible pulpitis, the pulpitis is often caused by the patient continually aggravating the tooth with an opposing tooth.

For patients whose offending tooth pain is believed to be caused by a habit, there are generally three choices of therapy: (a) Ask the patient to observe and break the rubbing or bumping habit. Some patients are unwilling or unable to do so, or it could be a nocturnal habit outside of the patient's ability to change. (b) Adjust the occlusion; e.g., remove the excursive contact on a posterior tooth. (c) Fabricate an occlusal appliance, which will interpose the opposing teeth so the habit cannot be performed.

Once the odontogenic pain is resolved, a significant reduction or elimination of the TMD symptoms should be observed.[21,23] If a patient is interested in pursuing treatment of the residual TMD symptoms, they have probably substantially changed, requiring the practitioner to reevaluate the remaining TMD symptoms and contributing factors.

It is common for both dental and TMD patients to have a combination of dental and TMD-type pains.[10,25] Patients generally focus their complaint on the aspect they believe is their pain source, but the two may be interrelated.

Patients with primarily dental pain should first be evaluated to identify whether the source is dental pathology, e.g., caries, periodontal disease, or incomplete tooth fracture. If these pathological conditions are ruled out as the source of the pain, other causes for dental pain should be considered, e.g., periodontal ligament inflammation secondary to parafunctional activity,[19,26-28] reversible pulpitis secondary to parafunctional activity,[19,28-30] or pain referred from the masticatory muscles or TMJs.[14,28,31]

The source(s) can often be identified by aggravating the suspected structure(s). If aggravating the structure reproduces or intensifies the pain, this would suggest the tested structure contributes to the complaint. If necessary and if the patient currently has the pain, local anesthetic to the structure(s) can further help verify the source(s).[10]

Periodontal ligament inflammation can be aggravated by applying an apical or lateral load to the tooth, e.g., by percussing the tooth with the end of a mouth-mirror handle.[19] The tooth pulp can be aggravated by applying hot or cold to the tooth (whichever the patient relates aggravates the pain). If the practitioner identifies the source as the periodontal ligament or the pulp, and concludes the primary cause for the pain is the patient's chronic parafunctional activity, the dentist will need to identify treatment options to mitigate these activities and their effect.

One of the goals in TMD therapy is to decrease the parafunctional activity and its effects on the masticatory system.[32] Therefore, many of the therapies used in treating TMD may also be beneficial for patients with dental pain caused by chronic parafunctional habits.

⊗ **FOCAL POINT**

One of the goals in TMD therapy is to decrease the parafunctional activity and its effects on the masticatory system. Therefore, many of the therapies used in treating TMD may also be beneficial for patients with dental pain caused by chronic parafunctional habits.

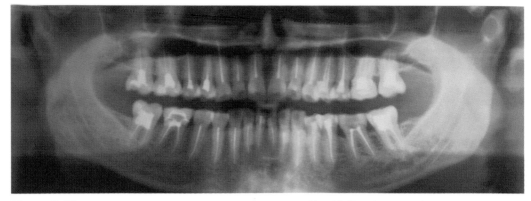

Figure 3-26. Radiograph of a TMD patient who perceived her TMD pain to be of pulpal origin and convinced dentists to treat her pain with endodontic therapy.

Similar to how the shared neurological circuitry can cause tooth pain to be perceived as TMD pain, TMD pain can also be perceived as dental pain.[10,14,33] If a patient complains of tooth pain and no dental pathology is identified, be cautious about proceeding with a root canal or extraction to appease the patient.[34] A TMD patient's panoramic radiograph in Figure 3-26 depicts what may happen if this is repeatedly performed.

⊚ **QUICK CONSULT**

Treating a Tooth without Dental Pathology

If a patient complains of tooth pain and no dental pathology is identified, be cautious about proceeding with a root canal or extraction to appease the patient; the pain may be due to referred masticatory muscle or TMJ pain.

By maintaining heavy palpation pressure on the masticatory muscles (preferably the myofascial trigger points) identified in Figure 3-13 and on the TMJs, one can usually identify whether TMD is contributing to tooth pain. This palpation aggravates these structures to the degree that, if they are causing or contributing to the dental pain, this will usually cause the pain to be reproduced or intensified.[14]

ADDITIONAL EVALUATIONS

During the patient interview, the practitioner may have developed suspicions for disorders that have not yet been evaluated and may not be within the practitioner's ability to evaluate. Sometimes the practitioner may prefer to refer patients directly to their physician for this, whereas at other times the practitioner may wish to obtain additional information to support or rule out the suspected disorder.

If one wishes to evaluate for sinus congestion, bear in mind that sinus congestion cannot be ruled out by palpating the maxillary and frontal sinuses. Even though a patient may have sinus congestion contributing to his or her pain, the maxillary and frontal sinuses are not always tender to palpation, and the congestion could be in a sinus that is not subject to palpation, e.g., the ethmoid sinus. Therefore, the practitioner may desire to test the patient's response with decongestants or refer the patient to his or her physician for evaluation and management of sinus congestion. As mentioned earlier, an increase in pain with bending forward may predict sinus congestion involvement, and some patients with masticatory muscle pain have been observed who received little relief with decongestants but had these symptoms eliminated completely after administration of antibiotics for treatment of sinus infection.

Some practitioners attempt to substantiate the suspicion of fibromyalgia by determining whether at least 11 of a possible 18 fibromyalgia tender points (different from trigger points) are tender to palpation. Palpation of fibromyalgia tender points is beyond the scope of this book, and it is recommended that a patient who has not been appropriately diagnosed or treated for widespread muscle pain (suggestive of fibromyalgia) be referred to his or her medical provider or to someone who specializes in this area. Patients diagnosed with fibromyalgia by rheumatologists have been observed whose fibromyalgia advanced to other disorders, such as multiple sclerosis.

If a patient's mouth opening is significantly restricted, the practitioner may be able to determine the restriction's origin by stretching the mouth wider, usually by placing the index finger over the incisal edges of the mandibular incisors and the thumb over the incisal edges of the maxillary incisors and pressing the teeth apart by moving the fingers in a scissor-type motion (Figure 1-1). The patient will usually feel tightness or pain at the location of the restriction. Clinical experience has shown that not all patients accurately point to the stretched discomfort location, and it is necessary to palpate the TMJ and musculature to reproduce the discomfort to identify its origin.

▼ **TECHNICAL TIP**
Determining Origin of Patient's Restricted Opening
If a patient's mouth opening is significantly restricted, the practitioner may be able to determine the restriction's origin by stretching the mouth wider.

Occasionally the information gathered during the patient interview suggests the patient has TMD, but palpating the masticatory and cervical muscles and TMJs (as described previously) cannot reproduce the pain. A less specific test can be used to stimulate the masticatory system in order to demonstrate that the pain is probably of masticatory origin. This involves asking the patient to put his or her teeth into MI and squeeze them together hard. The patient is asked to continue squeezing until the first sign that the pain is starting or until 1 minute elapses. This technique stimulates the masticatory system (including the dentition), so the practitioner needs to be sure the dentition is not the pain's source.

On rare occasions, the interview suggests the patient has TMD, and all other traditional causes for the pain are ruled out to the degree possible, but none of the aforementioned techniques can reproduce the pain. This generally occurs with a patient who only occasionally has the complaint. The patient is informed that a TMD origin for the pain could not be verified, but the signs, symptoms, aggravating activities, and alleviating activities are traditionally observed with TMD. The patient is offered a trial occlusal appliance to determine whether it might have a beneficial effect. If the practitioner observes that a trial appliance does not have a beneficial effect, it is recommended the patient be referred to someone with greater expertise in this area or to the patient's physician for evaluation for atypical causes of the pain.

The literature is filled with case reports of patients with TMD symptoms who actually had a brain tumor, eye disease, throat cancer, etc. Also, appliance therapy might reduce the TMD symptoms satisfactorily so that a comorbid disease becomes recognizable. Throughout TMD therapy, it is imperative to continually monitor the symptoms because the primary disorder may resolve and a secondary problem (e.g., cervical dysfunction) may become the primary disorder.

⊚ **QUICK CONSULT**

Monitoring Symptoms throughout Therapy

Throughout TMD therapy, it is imperative that the practitioner continually monitor the patient's symptoms because the primary disorder may resolve and a secondary problem (e.g., cervical dysfunction) may become the primary disorder.

REFERENCES

1. Ribeiro RF, Tallents RH, Katzberg RW, Murphy WC, Moss ME, Magalhaes AC, Tavano O. The prevalence of disc displacement in symptomatic and asymptomatic volunteers aged 6 to 25 years. J Orofac Pain 1997;11(1):37–47.

2. Egermark I, Carlsson GE, Magnusson T. A 20-year longitudinal study of subjective symptoms of temporomandibular disorders from childhood to adulthood. Acta Odontol Scand 2001;59(1):40–8.

3. Magnusson T, Egermark I, Carlsson GE. A longitudinal epidemiologic study of signs and symptoms of temporomandibular disorders from 15 to 35 years of age. J Orofac Pain 2000;14(4): 310–9.

4. Yatani H, Sonoyama W, Kuboki T, Matsuka Y, Orsini MG, Yamashita A. The validity of clinical examination for diagnosis of anterior disc displacement with reduction. Oral Surg Oral Med Oral Pathol Oral Radiol Endod 1998;85:647–53.

5. Schiffman E, Anderson G, Fricton J, Burton K, Schellhas K. Diagnostic criteria for intraarticular T.M. disorders. Community Dent Oral Epidemiol 1989;17(5):252–7.

6. Eriksson L, Westesson PL, Rohlin M. Temporomandibular joint sounds in patients with disc displacement. Int J Oral Surg 1985;14(5):428–36.

7. Stegenga B. Osteoarthritis of the temporomandibular joint organ and its relationship to disc displacement. J Orofac Pain 2001;15(3):193–205.

8. Bush FM, Abbott FM, Butler JH, Harrington WG. Oral orthotics: design, indications, efficacy and care. In: Hardin JF, ed. Clark's Clinical Dentistry, volume 2, chapter 39. Philadelphia: JB Lippincott, 1998:14.

9. Okeson JP, Hayes DK. Long-term results of treatment for temporomandibular disorders: an evaluation by patients. J Am Dent Assoc 1986;112(4): 473–8.

10. Okeson JP. Management of Temporomandibular Disorders and Occlusion, 5th edition. St Louis: CV Mosby, 2003:57–63, 153, 258–60, 276–7, 277–8, 292, 323, 461, 464–7, 471, 491–8.

11. Dworkin SF, LeResche L. Research diagnostic criteria for temporomandibular disorders: review, criteria, examinations and specifications, critique. J Craniomandib Disord 1992;6(4):301–55.

12. Austin DG, Pertes RA. Examination of the TMD patient. In: Pertes RA, Gross SG, eds. Clinical Management of Temporomandibular Disorders and Orofacial Pain. Chicago: Quintessence, 1995:148–9.

13. Sciotti VM, Mittak VL, DiMarco L, Ford LM, Plezbert J, Santipadri E, Wigglesworth J, Ball K. Clinical precision of myofascial trigger point location in the trapezius muscle. Pain 2001;93(3): 259–66.

14. Wright EF. Patterns of referred craniofacial pain in TMD patients. J Am Dent Assoc 2000;131(9): 1307–15.

15. Shankland II WE. Common causes of nondental facial pain. Gen Dent 1997;45(3):246–53.

16. Fricton JR, Dall'Arancio D. Myofascial pain of the head and neck: controlled outcome study of an interdisciplinary pain program. J Musculoske Pain 1994;2(2):81–99.

17. Gil IA, Barbosa CMR, Pedro VM, Silverio KCA, Goldfarb EP, Fusco V, Navarro CM. Multidisciplinary approach to chronic pain from myofascial pain dysfunction syndrome: a four-year experience at a Brazilian center. Cranio 1998;16(1):17–25.

18. Rosenbaum RS, Gross SG, Pertes RA, Ashman LM, Kreisberg MK. The scope of TMD/orofacial pain (head and neck pain management) in contemporary dental practice. Dental Practice Act Committee of the American Academy of Orofacial Pain. J Orofac Pain 1997;11(1):78–83.

19. Okeson JP. Bell's Orofacial Pains, 5th edition. Carol Stream, IL: Quintessence, 1995:129–31, 246.

20. Gremillion HA. Multidisciplinary diagnosis and management of orofacial pain. Gen Dent 2002;50(2):178–86.

21. Wright EF, Gullickson DC. Dental pulpalgia contributing to bilateral preauricular pain and tinnitus. J Orofac Pain 1996;10(2):166–8.

22. Wright EF. Diagnosis, treatment, and prevention of incomplete tooth fractures. Gen Dent 1992;40(5):390–9.

23. Wright EF, Gullickson DC. Identifying acute pulpalgia as a factor in TMD pain. J Am Dent Assoc 1996;127:773–80.

24. Walton RE. Distribution of solutions with the periodontal ligament injection: clinical, anatomical, and histological evidence. J Endod 1986;12: 492–500.

25. Falace DA, Reid K, Rayens MK. The influence of deep (odontogenic) pain intensity, quality, and duration on the incidence and characteristics of referred orofacial pain. J Orofac Pain 1996;10(3): 232–9.

26. Fricton JR. A unified concept of idiopathic orofacial pain: clinical features [Critical commentary 1]. J Orofac Pain 1999;13(3):185–9.

27. Shimizu N, Ozawa Y, Yamaguchi M, Goseki T, Ohzeki K, Abiko Y. Induction of COX-2 expression by mechanical tension force in human periodontal ligament cells. J Periodontol 1998;69(6): 670–7.

28. Yount K. Diagnosis and management of nondental toothache. Dent Today 2002;21(11)130–5.

29. Cooke HG. Reversible pulpitis with etiology of bruxism. J Endod 1982;8(6):280–1.

30. Wilson TG. Bruxism and cold sensitivity. Quintessence Int 2002;38(8):559.

31. Kreiner M, Okeson JP. Toothache of cardiac origin. J Orofac Pain 1999;13(3):201–7.

32. American Academy of Orofacial Pain, with Okeson JP (ed). Orofacial Pain: Guidelines for Assessment, Diagnosis and Management. Chicago: Quintessence, 1996:141.

33. Simons DG, Travell JG, Simons LS. Travell & Simons' Myofascial Pain and Dysfunction: The Trigger Point Manual, volume 1, 2nd edition. Baltimore: Williams & Wilkins, 1999:330–1, 350–1.

34. Farella M, Michelotti A, Gargano A, Cimino R, Ramaglia L. Myofascial pain syndrome misdiagnosed as odontogenic pain: a case report. Cranio 2002;20(4):307–11.

Chapter 4

Imaging

There is a wide choice of imaging procedures that can be used for patients with TMD, and they vary considerably in cost, availability, and information that can be obtained. This chapter provides an overview of these procedures, followed by imaging recommendations.

The osseous portion of the TMJ may be assessed with plain radiographs, panoramic radiograph, tomography, and computed tomography (CT). It is relatively common for TMD patients to have some observable radiographic osseous change[1] that occurs in response to TMJ inflammation, which is clinically identified by TMJ palpation tenderness or pain.[2] The clinical symptoms are generally caused by TMJ overload from activities such as parafunctional habits.[3] As the TMJ pain and inflammation resolve, demineralization correspondingly stops. The radiographic changes lag behind the clinical symptoms by as much as 6 months.[2,4] Therefore, treatment needs to be directed toward the patient's symptoms and not toward the radiographic findings.

⊙ QUICK CONSULT

Stopping Radiographic Osseous Changes

It is relatively common for TMD patients to have radiographic osseous changes, which are generally in response to TMJ inflammation from TMJ overload, i.e., parafunctional habits. As a patient's TMJ inflammation resolves, the demineralization correspondingly stops.

✪ FOCAL POINT

Radiographic changes generally lag behind the clinical symptoms by as much as 6 months.

The soft-tissue portion of the TMJ may be assessed with magnetic resonance imaging (MRI) and arthrography. Soft-tissue imaging is generally directed at identifying TMJ articular disorders, predominantly disc displacements.

PLAIN RADIOGRAPHS

Several plain radiographic projections can image the osseous portion of the TMJ. However, these images have such significant distortion and superimposition from other structures that they can be used only to screen for gross degenerative changes and to evaluate condylar translation. The significant distortion also makes it impossible to determine the condyle's position in the glenoid fossa.

In dental offices, the most commonly performed plain radiographic TMJ projection is the transcranial projection, which can be taken with the standard dental x-ray unit using a positioning device that is often available from the manufacturer. Typically the TMJ's degenerative changes begin on the condyle's lateral pole, and the image projected by this procedure enables the lateral pole to be evaluated for osseous changes.

PANORAMIC RADIOGRAPH

The panoramic radiograph provides a screening image of the TMJs, maxilla, mandible, maxillary sinuses, teeth, and periodontium. It can identify fractures (including a subcondylar fracture) and screen for gross degenerative changes of the TMJ and gross pathological changes of the maxilla and mandible. An old non-reduced condylar or subcondylar fracture is not suggestive that the fracture was missed by the provider, that the patient received poor treatment, or that it is the primary factor contributing to the patient's TMD. Open reduction may not have been indicated, and non-reduced condylar or subcondylar fractures rarely cause a problem.[5]

As the TMJ is being imaged, the x-ray beam travels from the posterior-inferior direction, causing the condyle's lateral pole to be superimposed within the head of the condyle and the medial pole to be projected as the condyle outline. Similarly the articular eminence is obstructed by superimposition on the panoramic radiograph. Superimposition of the glenoid fossa over the condyle can be minimized by asking the patient to open maximally during imaging, but this prevents most of the mandible from being imaged.

Some panoramic machines allow two to four projections of the TMJ to be imaged on one film, which may enable condylar mobility to be visualized. The x-ray beam for these images generally travels along the pathway of the panoramic image, projecting the medial pole as the condyle outline.[4]

⊙ **QUICK CONSULT**
Viewing Panoramic Radiographs
The condyle outline on the panoramic radiograph is the condyle's medial pole; this is generally the last portion of the condyle to exhibit osseous change.

It is common to view a well-circumscribed radiolucent area on the anterior aspect of the condyle in a panoramic radiograph (Figure 4-1). These condylar pseudocysts are formed primarily by the cupping of the condyle's lateral pterygoid muscle fovea, and one survey

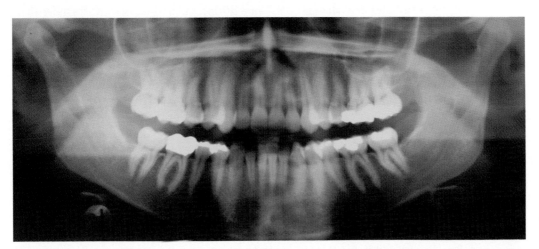

Figure 4-1. Condylar pseudocysts, formed primarily by the cupping of the condyle's lateral pterygoid muscle fovea, are common on panoramic radiographs.

found them in 18 percent of panoramic radiographs from children.[6]

TOMOGRAPHY (CORRECTED TOMOGRAPHY)

These radiographs are true lateral projections of the condyle without superimposition that enable practitioners to view osseous changes of the articular surface and the lateral and medial poles (through the sagittal view), in addition to condylar mobility and position. Condylar position has been shown not to be able to predict disc position reliably.[7,8]

Tomograms more accurately depict osseous changes than do the previously discussed radiographs, arthrograms, or MRI. Cost and inconvenience (tomography is rarely available in a dental office) are the primary disadvantages of these radiographs.

ARTHROGRAPHY

To obtain an arthrogram, radiopaque contrast medium must be injected into the TMJ. By observing the space outlines and for leakage of the contrast medium, the disc position, existence of a perforation, and sometimes disc condition can be identified. The procedure may be followed by a therapeutic TMJ lavage, which often provides symptom improvement and may change some of the identified information. Since the wide availability of MRI, TMJ arthrography is rarely performed, because of its discomfort, relatively high radiation levels, and invasiveness.

COMPUTED TOMOGRAPHY

CT scans may be useful for viewing TMJ ankylosis, neoplastic conditions, and anomalies. Although CT scans are valuable for identifying hard-tissue and soft-tissue abnormalities and pathology in the head and neck, their reliability is poor in identifying TMJ disc position. MRI best depicts the disc position, and tomography provides adequate viewing of the TMJ osseous structures, so CT scans are used only in special situations for TMD patients.

MAGNETIC RESONANCE IMAGING

MRI uses a magnetic field and radiofrequency impulses instead of radiation to produce its image. For TMD patients, it is primarily used to identify the disc position, usually viewed in both closed and maximal open positions. The accuracy of identifying the disc position may reach 95 percent.[9]

⊙ **QUICK CONSULT**
Viewing MRIs
The accuracy of identifying the disc position in an MRI may reach 95 percent.

Practitioners should bear in mind that the identification of a displaced disc does not suggest this is the source of the TMD symptoms, for patients who have received surgical correction rarely obtain long-term symptom resolution. In fact, MRIs taken on asymptomatic volunteers have shown that 25 to 38 percent have a displaced disc.[10,11]

Surgeons generally request an MRI prior to TMJ surgery. Clinical training experience has shown that, out of mere curiosity, some practitioners like to request the imaging they anticipate the surgeon will want. If a practitioner has decided to refer a TMD patient to a surgeon, it is recommended the practitioner not try to anticipate and prescribe the imaging, as the surgeon may desire a variation from the routine TMJ MRI and/or other imaging that could be obtained at the same imaging center.

IMAGING RECOMMENDATIONS

The patient interview and examination are the gold standard for determining the TMD diagnoses, contributing factors, and treatment plan.[12] Tumors in the TMJ are rare, and imaging to detect intraosseous lesions in asymptomatic individuals is neither cost effective nor biologically advisable.[13,14]

☻ FOCAL POINT

The patient interview and examination are the gold standard for determining the TMD diagnoses, contributing factors, and treatment plan.

It has been recommended that practitioners should image only if there is a reasonable expectation that the additional information will influence a patient's treatment approach.[9,15] Such selective imaging is advisable, and overimaging will hamper a practitioner's ability to provide cost-effective care. Other than imaging for suspected odontogenic pathology, imaging has rarely changed my treatment approach.

☻ FOCAL POINT

It has been recommended that practitioners should image only if there is a reasonable expectation that the additional information will influence a patient's treatment approach.

◉ QUICK CONSULT

Prescribing Imaging

Other than imaging for suspected odontogenic pathology, imaging has rarely changed my treatment approach.

The imaging indications that have been found useful are as follows:

1. If the practitioner is not aware of the patent's dental caries and periodontal disease status, the practitioner may desire to take dental radiographs.

2. A practitioner who suspects, based on the patient interview and clinical examination, that a patient may have pathology should not hesitate to take a screening radiograph, such as a transcranial or panoramic radiograph. Use common sense; e.g., a patient with facial pain and swelling after the

extraction of a mandibular tooth may have a fractured mandible.

◉ QUICK CONSULT

Prescribing for a Screening Radiograph

A practitioner who suspects, based on the patient interview and clinical examination, that a patient may have pathology should not hesitate to take a screening radiograph, such as a transcranial or panoramic radiograph.

3. If the patient's TMD symptoms began or greatly worsened with trauma, take a panoramic radiograph to rule out a fracture causing or contributing to the patient's pain. If the patient was not appropriately evaluated for a fracture following the trauma, and the practitioner suspects the patient may have a fracture in a bone that would not be revealed by the panoramic radiograph, then appropriate radiographs would be indicated.

◉ QUICK CONSULT

Observing for Trauma History

If the patient's TMD symptoms began or greatly worsened with trauma, take a panoramic radiograph to rule out a fracture causing or contributing to the patient's pain.

4. If the patient relates a progressively increasing open bite of the anterior teeth, the patient may have such severe TMJ osteoarthritis that it is causing the condyle to lose its vertical height. If the patient has such severe osteoarthritis, it should be visible in a screening radiograph, such as a transcranial or panoramic radiograph. A tomogram would provide a better view of the degenerative changes, but would not change the patient's treatment approach. The practitioner may desire a tomogram in order to better follow changes in the condyle's status throughout treatment. This disorder and its treatment are complicated and beyond the scope of this book. Practitioners observing

this complaint may desire to refer the patient to someone with greater expertise in this area.

5. If the patient has a progressively increasing posterior open bite, midline deviation, or observable preauricular swelling, the patient may have a neoplastic growth within the TMJ. Neoplasia arising in the TMJ are extremely rare,[14] but if this were to occur within the restricted space of the TMJ, it may cause the condyle to move inferior or anterior-inferior, thereby causing a progressively increasing posterior open bite and/or midline deviation. A neoplasm on or near the TMJ's lateral surface may clinically manifest as a progressively increasing observable preauricular swelling.

A posterior open bite or a change in the midline alignment are frequently observed among TMD patients. The occlusal change is typically caused by a disorder such as a lateral pterygoid myospasm or TMJ inflammation. These patients have pain (which may occur only when the patient attempts to occlude into maximum intercuspation), and the occlusal change fluctuates with the disorder's severity.

TMD patients also frequently relate a history of swelling over the region of their pain (e.g., preauricular swelling). The swelling caused by TMD is a minor indistinct elevation (usually only noticeable by the patient) that fluctuates with the disorder's severity.

If the practitioner suspects the patient may have a neoplastic growth within the TMJ or if this change is long-standing, the practitioner may desire to make a screening radiograph, such as a transcranial or panoramic radiograph. It is recommended, whether or not an abnormality is observed on the radiograph, that a patient with a history of a progressively increasing posterior open bite, midline deviation, or observable preauricular swelling be evaluated by someone with expertise in this area. The neoplasia may be slow growing, so a long-standing

persistent change should also be evaluated by someone with expertise in this area. Additional imaging is generally indicated.

6. TMJ implants composed of Teflon-Proplast and Silastic have a history of fragmenting, causing a foreign-body response that results in progressive degeneration of the condyle and glenoid fossa. A specific imaging and management protocol has been recommended for these implants and total joint prostheses, which is beyond the scope of this book.[16] If the practitioner is unsure of the implant type or management, it is recommended the practitioner refer the patient to, or work in conjunction with, someone who has greater expertise in this area.

7. If the patient does not respond to TMD therapy as anticipated, take a panoramic radiograph to screen for other possible pathology.

⊙ **QUICK CONSULT**

Observing Poor Therapy Response

▌If the patient does not respond to TMD therapy as anticipated, take a panoramic radiograph to screen for other possible pathology.

---

8. If the patient is being referred for a TMJ surgery evaluation, the surgeon will probably request imaging. Let the surgeon prescribe the desired imaging.

9. Occasionally a third-party payer requests that an MRI or other imaging be prescribed to document the status of the TMJ or for medicolegal reasons.

If the practitioner desires to use imaging to screen all TMD patients, then plain (e.g., transcranial) or panoramic radiographs would be the imaging of choice.

✆ **FOCAL POINT**

If the practitioner desires to use imaging to screen all TMD patients, then plain (e.g., transcranial) or panoramic radiographs would be the imaging of choice.

REFERENCES

1. Wiberg B, Wanman A. Signs of osteoarthrosis of the temporomandibular joints in young patients: a clinical and radiographic study. Oral Surg Oral Med Oral Pathol Oral Radiol Endod 1998;86:158–64.
2. Stegenga B. Osteoarthritis of the temporomandibular joint organ and its relationship to disc displacement. J Orofac Pain 2001;15(3):193–205.
3. American Society of Temporomandibular Joint Surgeons. White paper: guidelines for diagnosis and management of disorders involving the temporomandibular joint and related musculoskeletal structures. Cranio 2003;21(1):68–76.
4. Okeson JP. Management of Temporomandibular Disorders and Occlusion, 5th edition. St Louis: CV Mosby, 2003:292, 464–7.
5. Marker P, Nielsen A, Bastian HL. Fractures of the mandibular condyle. Part 2: Results of treatment of 348 patients. Br J Oral Maxillofac Surg 2000;38(5):422–6.
6. Collins TE, Laskin DM, Farrington FH, Shetty NS, Mourino A. Pseudocysts of the mandibular condyle in children. J Am Dent Assoc 1997;128(6):747–50.
7. Schiffman E, Anderson G, Fricton J, Burton K, Schellhas K. Diagnostic criteria for intraarticular T.M. disorders. Community Dent Oral Epidemiol 1989;17(5):252–7.
8. Kamelchuk L, Nebbe B, Baker C Major P. Adolescent TMJ tomography and magnetic resonance imaging: a comparative analysis. J Orofac Pain 1997;11(4):321–7.
9. Brooks SL, Brand JW, Gibbs SJ, Hollender L, Lurie AG, Omnell K-A, Westesson P-L, White SC. Imaging of the temporomandibular joint: a position paper of the American Academy of Oral and Maxillofacial Radiology. Oral Surg Oral Med Oral Pathol Oral Radiol Endod 1997;83:609–18.
10. American Academy of Orofacial Pain, with Okeson JP (ed). Orofacial Pain: Guidelines for Assessment, Diagnosis and Management. Chicago: Quintessence, 1996:33.
11. Emshoff R, Brandlmaier I, Gerhard S, Strobl H, Bertram S, Rudisch A. Magnetic resonance imaging predictors of temporomandibular joint pain. J Am Dent Assoc 2003;134(6):705–14.
12. Westesson P-L. Physical diagnosis continues to be the gold standard. Cranio 1999;17(1):3–4.
13. Howard JA. Imaging techniques for the diagnosis and prognosis of TMD. J Calif Dent Assoc 1990;18(3):61–71.
14. Fantasia JE. Neoplasia. In: Kaplan AS, Assael LA (eds). Temporomandibular Disorders: Diagnosis and Treatment. Philadelphia: WB Saunders, 1991:251–61.
15. Christiansen EL, Thompson JR. Radiographic evaluation of the TMJ. In: Pertes RA, Gross SG (eds). Clinical Management of Temporomandibular Disorders and Orofacial Pain. Chicago: Quintessence, 1995:161.
16. American Association of Oral and Maxillofacial Surgeons. Recommendations for management of patients with temporomandibular joint implants. Temporomandibular Joint Implant Surgery Workshop. J Oral Maxillofac Surg 1993;51(10):1164–72.

Chapter 5

TMD Diagnostic Categories

FAQ

Q: Why do people who have a displaced disc often do well even though their condyle continues to articulate on the retrodiscal tissue?

A: In the healthy TMJ, the repeated loading of the retrodiscal tissue causes adaptive changes within this tissue, making it comparable to the disc, and is sometimes called a pseudodisc.

Many TMD patients concurrently have muscle and TMJ pain in additional to TMJ noise.[1] Each of these findings represents a different TMD diagnosis; therefore, multiple TMD diagnoses are very common for TMD patients. To make the list of diagnoses meaningful, they are ranked as primary, secondary, tertiary, etc.

⊙ **QUICK CONSULT**

Ranking TMD Diagnoses

Since multiple TMD diagnoses are very common for TMD patients, they are ranked as primary, secondary, tertiary, etc.

The **primary TMD diagnosis** is the disorder most responsible for a patient's chief complaint. For example, if a patient's chief complaint is pain, the diagnosis for the structure that reproduces the pain is the primary diagnosis. When multiple structures reproduce a complaint, the structure that most readily reproduces it probably has the greatest impact on the it, and its diagnosis would be the primary diagnosis. The diagnoses for the other areas that reproduce the pain, followed by diagnoses involving tender structures that do not reproduce the pain, are the **secondary diagnosis**, **tertiary diagnosis**, etc.

When a patient has more than one complaint, these are also ranked; e.g., pain is the primary complaint, catching within the TMJ is secondary, and TMJ noise is tertiary. This complaint list is used to prioritize the diagnoses further. Ordering the diagnoses in this manner may sound complicated, but once practitioners have had a little practice formulating this list, it becomes simple and is very helpful in formulating the treatment recommendations.

Similar to many areas of medicine, TMD is plagued by inconsistent diagnostic categories and terminology. The American Academy of Orofacial Pain (AAOP) has published TMD diagnostic categories and criteria. This classification, which is the most widely accepted TMD terminology, is the terminology used in this book. The AAOP acknowledges that its classification and criteria are hampered by the limited knowledge about TMD disorders, the inability to develop diagnostic classifications for all TMD disorders, and the fact that no one set of criteria will satisfy all circumstances for the diagnosis.[2]

The diagnostic categories described in this chapter are separated into *TMJ articular disorders* and *masticatory muscle disorders*. The recommended diagnostic criteria represent *clinical diagnoses* based on information that can be obtained from a patient's history and clinical examination. They are not meant to be rigid criteria, but only provide guidance, and clinical judgment should be relied on for the final decision.[2]

TMJ ARTICULAR DISORDERS

This section covers which disorders can affect the TMJ and includes five articular disorders in addition to TMJ fractures, congenital or developmental disorders, and neoplasms.

Disc Displacement Disorders

These are the most common TMJ articular disorders. Autopsy, clinical, and imaging studies reveal that approximately 30 percent of asymptomatic volunteers have a displaced disc.[3] Since disc displacements are so prevalent among the normal population (as well as the TMD population), it may be considered a physiological accommodation without clinical significance for many individuals.

◉ **QUICK CONSULT**

Evaluating Disc Displacement Significance

Since disc displacements are so prevalent among the normal population (as well as the TMD population), it may be considered a physiological accommodation without clinical significance for many individuals.

To help explain disc displacement disorders, a "TMJ Disc Displacements" diagram is provided as Appendix 2. The diagram is broken into four sections, in which the top left section provides an overview and the top right section portrays the "normal" disc-condyle alignment.

For a disc to displace, the retrodiscal tissue (elastic ligament, in addition to its attachment complex) must stretch, allowing the disc to move anteriorly, as the disc-condyle alignment depicts in the top drawing in the bottom left section. Reports of the disc being posteriorly displaced are relatively rare.[4]

Once the disc is displaced, the portion of the retrodiscal tissue located where the disc used to be is subjected to repeated loading by the condyle. In a healthy TMJ, the repeated loading on this portion of the retrodiscal tissue causes adaptive changes, thereby providing most of the physical characteristics of the disc.[5] This is analogous to what happens to our hands when we increase our physical activity, which causes adaptive changes of the skin to develop calluses. This modified retrodiscal tissue functions well as the disc, withstands TMJ loading somewhat comparable to the disc, and has been referred to as a *pseudodisc*.[6,7]

There is no known anatomical mechanism for an anteriorly displaced disc to retract back to its normal disc-condyle relationship. People commonly relate that their TMJ clicking comes and goes; e.g., it occurs when the individual eats or is stressed and does not occur when relaxed. It is postulated that the TMJ anatomy (e.g., disc displacement with reduction) does not change, but clinically it appears the TMJ noise may vary with the degree of sustained joint loading.

Disc displacement with reduction is the most common diagnosis for patients with TMJ clicking or popping.[4,8,9] The top drawing in the bottom left section of the "TMJ Disc Displacements" diagram depicts a displaced disc. As the individual opens his or her mouth, the condyle translates forward and moves into the intermediate zone of the disc (called the *reduced position*, shown in the bottom drawing of the bottom left section), which may cause an opening click or pop. As the mouth continues to open, the condyle continues to translate forward with the disc and remains in the disc's intermediate zone.

✪ **FOCAL POINT**

Disc displacement with reduction is the most common diagnosis for patients with TMJ clicking or popping.

As the individual closes, the condyle *retrudes* and moves back under the posterior band onto the retrodiscal tissue, which may cause a closing click or pop. As the mouth continues to close, the condyle remains on the retrodiscal tissue. If both opening and closing noises are present, the opening click or pop occurs at a wider opening than the closing click or pop.

Sometimes the patient and practitioner cannot determine which TMJ is generating the click or pop, since the vibration can travel through the mandible and be perceived in the contralateral TMJ. The TMJ that is generating the noise can usually be determined by having the patient start in maximum intercuspation and move laterally to the one side several times and then laterally to the other side several times. The click or pop is generated during the translation phase, and whichever TMJ is translating when the noise is generated is the source of the noise.

▼ **TECHNICAL TIP**

Determining Origin of a Patient's TMJ Noise

If the practitioner cannot determine which TMJ is generating the click or pop, the TMJ can usually be identified by asking the patient to start in maximum intercuspation and move laterally to the one side several times and then laterally to the other side several times. The click or pop is generated during the translation phase, and whichever TMJ is translating when the noise is generated is the source of the noise.

Most individuals with a click or pop have a TMJ disc displacement with reduction, but a smaller percentage have a normal disc-condyle position or a disc displacement without reduction.[4,8] Conversely some patients without any noise have a disc displacement with reduction.[4,8] There are no clinical criteria to differentiate these individuals, but it has been shown that, if an individual has an opening and closing click or pop with the opening noise occurring at a wider opening than the closing noise, he or she has a high probability of having a disc displacement with reduction.[8,9]

◉ **QUICK CONSULT**

Understanding Variability of Disc Displacement with Reduction

Some patients without any TMJ noise have a disc displacement with reduction.

The clinical criteria a practitioner chooses to use for a diagnosis of disc displacement with reduction may vary from a single click or pop to an opening and closing click or pop in which the opening noise occurs at a wider opening. Personally I use the following clinical criteria: (a) the palpable presence of a click or pop; (b) if the noise is not palpable during the exam, then a relatively recent history of a click or pop that tends to fluctuate in its presence; or (c) if an opening and closing click or pop is present, then the opening noise occurs at a wider opening.

A more accurate assessment can be obtained by a TMJ magnetic resonance imaging (MRI) at maximal intercuspation and opening positions, but the findings rarely change the practitioner's treatment approach, and MRI is rarely indicated to confirm this diagnosis. Spending extensive time or using specialized equipment to verify the noise is also not warranted.

Disc displacement with reduction generally does not progress to disc displacement without reduction unless the patient has pain.[5] If the noise is the only complaint and is not an embarrassment or problem for the patient, then it is recommended the practitioner provide no therapy beyond education. The "TMJ Disc Displacements" diagram is used to explain the cause and inform the patient that TMJ noise is common, similar to noise in other joints of the body.

⊙ **QUICK CONSULT**

Understanding Progression of a Disc Displacement with Reduction

Disc displacement with reduction generally does not progress to disc displacement without reduction unless the patient has pain.

The effect of TMD therapy on TMJ noise is variable, because there are no established predictors to suggest which patients will receive noise improvement. As a general conservative guide, it is estimated that approximately one-third of patients provided occlusal appliance therapy will report significant noise improvement or elimination, one-third will report minor noise improvement, and one-third will report no noise improvement.

Acute disc displacement without reduction (also known as *closed lock*) may be diagnosed when a patient has sudden onset of a persistent marked limited opening (less

than 35 mm).[2] Patients with this disorder are often aware that the TMJ is blocked at the opening where the TMJ normally clicked or popped. Many report a history of their TMJ catching at that location or intermittently having had this problem (lasting seconds to days), which suddenly released and allowed them to regain their normal opening.

This disorder is demonstrated in the bottom right section of the "TMJ Disc Displacements" diagram. As the mouth opens, the condyle first rotates then attempts to translate forward, but it cannot slide under the disc's posterior band and cannot reduce onto the disc. The translation is limited by the disc, and typically the patient is initially able to open only between 20 and 30 mm.[10]

In theory, as the patient attempts to open wider, the ipsilateral TMJ translation is restricted by the disc while the contralateral TMJ can translate beyond that point, and the practitioner would observe the mandible deflecting to the affected side. Also during the range-of-motion evaluation, the practitioner would observe a marked limitation to the contralateral side. Clinically these findings are not always observed, because patients tend to guard against moving their mandible into painful positions, and the contralateral side may also have pain limiting a patient's movements.

A marked limited opening can also be caused by a muscle disorder, but a limited opening from a muscle disorder would typically exhibit a gradual onset (hours to days). One may be able to determine the origin of the restriction for a patient with a marked limited opening by stretching the mouth beyond a comfortable opening, as described in "Additional Evaluations" in Chapter 3.

Patients with a lateral pterygoid myospasm often present with similarities to the acute disc displacement without reduction disorder. These patients often have a marked limited opening in which the ipsilateral condyle has a limited ability to translate. One of the major differentiation factors is that patients with an acute disc displacement without reduction can generally put their teeth into maximum intercuspation without pain, whereas patients with a lateral pterygoid myospasm usually relate that they cannot close or that they have significant pain when closing into maximum intercuspation. Additional information on diagnosing and treating the lateral pterygoid myospasm is provided in Chapter 9, "Lateral Pterygoid Myospasm."

◉ **QUICK CONSULT**
Observing Lateral Pterygoid Myospasm Presentation
Patients with a lateral pterygoid myospasm often present with similarities to the acute disc displacement without reduction disorder.

If the sudden limited opening is due to external trauma, the limited opening may be due to a muscle injury, TMJ inflammation, or other causes in addition to an acute disc displacement without reduction. A more accurate assessment can be obtained by TMJ MRI at maximum intercuspation and maximum opening, but this clinical diagnosis can be determined by history and clinical examination. Recommended treatments for acute disc displacement without reduction are provided in Chapter 10, "Acute TMJ Disc Displacement without Reduction."

Chronic disc displacement without reduction may be diagnosed when a patient has a history of sudden-onset limited opening that gradually increased to greater than 35 mm. This history suggests the patient has an acute disc displacement without reduction, and over time the retrodiscal tissue stretched, enabling the disc to move further forward so that the patient could regain an adequate translation and opening.

◉ **QUICK CONSULT**
Diagnosing Chronic Disc Displacement without Reduction
Chronic disc displacement without reduction may be diagnosed when a patient has a history of sudden-onset limited opening that gradually increased to greater than 35 mm.

The mechanism for this transition is activated every time the individual attempts to open beyond the restriction. This causes the condyle to bump the posterior side of the disc, which puts a stretching force on the retrodiscal tissue. Repeatedly bumping the disc in this manner will often sufficiently stretch the retrodiscal tissue over time, allowing the disc to move forward so that the normal translation and opening are eventually regained. Many individuals can move through this transition without treatment (some with minimal discomfort), but others cannot.[11,12] This transition is often reported to take a few weeks to months and may have occurred many years ago.[7] This may not have been a significant event for the patient or may have occurred with trauma, so a patient with this disorder may not remember such a history.

Course crepitus is the most common noise associated with this disorder, but some patients have no noise, or a single click or a reciprocal click.[8] Personally the clinical criteria of the patient reporting this history or having course crepitus is used to clinically diagnose this disorder. Traditional TMD therapies have been shown to benefit patients with this disorder.

Dislocation (Also Known as Subluxation)

A dislocation is diagnosed when a patient presents with or relates a history of momentary or prolonged inability to close the mandible from a maximal open position. In this disorder, the condyle is caught in front of the articular eminence. It may be due to the articular eminence obstructing the posterior movement of the disc-condyle unit, the disc obstructing the posterior movement of the condyle, or a combination of the two.[13] Conservative treatments for TMJ dislocation are discussed in Chapter 11, "TMJ Dislocation."

Inflammatory Disorders

These are diagnosed when the TMJ is tender to palpation at one or more of the three palpation locations described in "Palpation" in Chapter 3. This disorder, referred to as **TMJ inflammation**, may be localized to the TMJ or be due to a systemic condition also affecting other joints of the body.

Synovitis and **capsulitis** can cause TMJ tenderness or pain, and they cannot be clinically differentiated. The collective term *TMJ inflammation* is used to signify either or both and is diagnosed whenever there is TMJ tenderness. Traditional TMD therapies have been shown to benefit patients with TMJ inflammation.

Polyarthritides is a systemic condition that may cause TMJ inflammation as well as tenderness and/or pain in other joints of the body, e.g., rheumatoid arthritis. The systemic condition may go through acute flare-up and remission phases. As these changes occur, observing the degree to which the TMJ inflammation follows the course of inflammation in other joints may suggest whether the TMJ involvement is related more to the systemic condition or to traditional TMD contributing factors. The systemic condition should be treated by a physician while the local component caused by TMD contributing factors should be treated with traditional TMD therapies. TMJ involvement is often treated by combining medical and dental therapies, and the TMD treatment may help to minimize the medications the physician needs to prescribe.

▼ **TECHNICAL TIP**
Working with Physicians

The systemic portion of a polyarthritides should be treated by a physician while the local component caused by TMD contributing factors should be treated with traditional TMD therapies.

Osteoarthritis

This condition, in which TMJ inflammation causes degeneration of the articular tissue and bone,[3] is diagnosed when the TMJ is tender to palpation and hard-tissue imaging reveals bony changes, i.e., subchondral sclerosis, osteophyte formation, or erosion. The bony changes are active when the TMJ is painful or tender and the radiographic changes lag behind the active disorder by as much as 6 months.[2,3,14] Therefore, the practitioner should treat the patient's symptoms to bring this disorder under control and not rely on the radiographic findings.

If radiographs are not taken, this disorder would be diagnosed as TMJ inflammation. Not having the radiographic support to diagnose osteoarthritis is not a problem because the treatment goal for both disorders is to treat the TMJ inflammation pain. As the inflammation resolves, the osseous degeneration concurrently resolves and adaptive remodeling occurs.[2]

◎ **QUICK CONSULT**
Failing to Image for Osteoarthritic Changes

Osteoarthritic changes are active when the TMJ is painful or tender. If radiographs were not taken, the same treatment objective would be sought—decrease the TMJ inflammation. As the inflammation resolves, the osseous degeneration concurrently resolves and adaptive remodeling occurs.

Occasionally the osteoarthritis is so severe that the osseous degeneration will cause the condyle to lose its vertical height. As the condylar height collapses, the most posterior ipsilateral tooth becomes the first tooth to contact, acts as a fulcrum, and progressively creates an open bite for the remaining dentition. The open bite generally begins on the contralateral anterior teeth and progressively spreads bilaterally until only the most posterior ipsilateral tooth makes contact. In this situation, the patient initially observes a progressively increasing open bite of the anterior teeth that progresses to the posterior teeth. This disorder and its treatment are complicated and beyond the scope of this book. A practitioner observing this complaint may desire to refer the patient to someone with greater expertise in this area.

TMJ osteoarthritis is subdivided into primary and secondary osteoarthritis, which are differentiated by their etiologic factors. Primary and secondary osteoarthritis are both generally referred to as *TMJ osteoarthritis.*

1. **Primary osteoarthritis** is diagnosed when there is no identifiable etiologic factor, and therefore the TMJ inflammation is presumed to be due to TMJ overloading from parafunctional habits, etc.[15] Traditional TMD therapies have been shown to reduce TMJ inflammation, thereby inactivating the degenerative process.[16]

2. **Secondary osteoarthritis** is diagnosed when there is an identifiable etiologic factor for the disorder, i.e., direct trauma, TMJ infection, or active systemic arthritis. If the etiologic factor can be resolved (e.g., TMJ infection), that should be accomplished first. If TMJ inflammation remains or the etiologic factor cannot be adequately altered, then traditional TMD therapies should be implemented. This has been shown to reduce TMJ inflammation and will thereby inactivate the degenerative process.

Ankylosis

This is the firm restriction of the TMJ due to fibrous bands or osseous union within the TMJ and is generally not associated with pain. It can be the result of direct trauma, systemic disease, surgery, etc. As a patient with TMJ ankylosis attempts to open beyond the restriction, the ankylosed TMJ will have limited translation, the contralateral TMJ will continue to translate, and the practitioner should observe the mandible deflecting to the affected side. During the range-of-motion evaluation, the practitioner should also observe a marked limitation to the contralateral side. Digital palpation of the affected TMJ during maximal movements will also reflect no or very limited translation of the condyle.[2,6]

⊙ **QUICK CONSULT**

Understanding TMJ Ankylosis

Ankylosis is the firm restriction of the TMJ due to fibrous bands or osseous union within the TMJ and is generally not associated with pain.

1. **Fibrous ankylosis** is associated with a limited opening and ability to translate. Treatment depends on the degree of dysfunction and discomfort. If the patient has adequate function and minimal discomfort, no treatment is indicated. If the patient desires to have the disc-condyle assembly released, TMJ surgery (e.g., arthroscopic or open joint surgery) will be needed.[6]

2. **Bony ankylosis** is caused by the union of the osseous structures within the TMJ, causing an extremely limited ability for the patient to open or the condyle to translate or possibly even rotate. This condition is rare, and treatment involves open joint surgery to release and recontour the osseous structures.[2,6]

Fracture

TMJ fracture may first be noticed on a routine panoramic radiograph taken for a non-TMD purpose. The patient may not have any symptoms associated with the fracture or be aware of the fracture. Subcondylar fractures are the most common, and the condyle may even be dislocated out of the glenoid fossa. Most patients with condylar fractures do well with only conservative therapy, with a higher risk associated with bilateral fractures and the condyle being dislocated out of the fossa.[17,18]

Congenital or Developmental Disorders

These disorders rarely cause TMD symptoms. The chief complaint may be esthetics or function, and the disorder may be inadvertently observed on a panoramic image taken for a non-TMD purpose.

1. **Aplasia** is the faulty or incomplete development of mandible or cranial bone.
2. **Hypoplasia** is the underdevelopment of mandible or cranial bone.
3. **Hyperplasia** is the overdevelopment of mandible or cranial bone.
4. **Neoplasia** is abnormal tissue growth. Reports of malignant and benign lesions developing within the TMJ, causing TMD symptoms, are rare.

MASTICATORY MUSCLE DISORDERS

TMD patients commonly complain about masticatory muscle pain.[19] This section lists four muscle disorders, a fifth muscle classification (local myalgia) for muscle pain that does not fall within the other categories, and an additional classification for muscle neoplasms.

Myofascial Pain

Myofascial pain is most commonly described by patients as an ache, pressure, and/or dull pain, but can be throbbing when more severe. These muscles are tender to palpation, and ideally the practitioner would identify trigger points to arrive at this diagnosis, but they may be difficult to discern, even for practitioners experienced in palpating muscles.[20]

⊗ FOCAL POINT

Myofascial pain is the most common cause for muscle palpation tenderness and is most commonly described by patients as an ache, pressure, and/or dull pain, but can be throbbing when more severe.

A practitioner may be able to identify one or more trigger points or nodules of spot tenderness by palpating the full extent of a muscle with myofascial pain. These are localized, firm, tender nodules that feel like firm knots within the muscle and are more tender than the surrounding muscle. Palpation of these tender nodules may generate pain within that structure, pain beyond the structure, referred pain to a distant location, and/or autonomic responses.[2] Firm, sustained palpation on the tender nodules maximizes the generated effect.

Muscle pain is often aggravated by the patient's stimulating these tender nodules through muscle function, stress, etc. Sometimes practitioners prefer to inactivate these nodules in an attempt to confirm the diagnosis, identify the degree of pain that is being generated by the nodule, or provide temporary pain relief. Temporary inactivation can be attempted through a trigger-point anesthetic injection, vapocoolant spray, transcutaneous electrical stimulation (TENS), etc.[2]

Myofascial pain is frequently the cause of regional pain in any part of the body and is generally described as muscle pain in the masticatory region, neck, shoulders, low back, etc. It involves the muscle and/or fascia, and many dentists incorrectly call it *myofacial* pain rather than *myofascial* pain.

From a clinically practical viewpoint, if the muscle is tender to palpation and none of the other masticatory muscle disorders better describe the patient's condition, it is recommended the muscle tenderness be diagnosed as myofascial pain. Among the TMD patients I have seen who have muscle tenderness, it is estimated that more than 95 percent of the time I diagnose the muscle tenderness as myofascial pain. Traditional TMD therapies have been shown to reduce masticatory myofascial pain.

Diagnosing Myofascial Pain
From a clinically practical viewpoint, if the muscle is tender to palpation and none of the other masticatory muscle disorders better describe the patient's condition, it is recommended the muscle tenderness be diagnosed as myofascial pain.

Myositis

This disorder is characterized by inflammation of the muscle due to a spreading infection, external muscle trauma, or muscle strain. Patients often relate the symptom onset directly to this event. The symptoms are constant acute pain within the muscle, which may additionally be swollen and red, with an overlying increased temperature. The muscle is tender to palpation and may cause a limited range of motion. If the inflammation involves the tendon or tendon-muscle attachment, the diagnosis may be tendonitis or tendomyositis.[2,21]

If an infection is the etiology of the myositis, then treatment must involve identifying and resolving the infection, and antibiotic therapy may be advisable. Additionally the myositis should be treated with nonsteroid anti-inflammatory drugs (NSAIDs), limiting the use of the masticatory muscles (e.g., soft diet or avoiding oral habits), and possibly using ice over the affected area for the first 48 hours after traumatic injury.[21] Practitioners may find the "TMD Self-management Therapies" handout provided in Appendix 3 helpful in explaining these therapies.

Myospasm

This is the involuntary contracture of a muscle, causing pain and interfering with its ability to move. This disorder has awakened many of us in the middle of the night with a cramp in the calf muscle. A myospasm can occur in any of the masticatory muscles, but it alarms patients (and unaware practitioners) the most when it occurs in the inferior lateral pterygoid muscle.

A myospasm of the inferior lateral pterygoid muscle causes constant involuntary contraction at a partially shortened position. Similar to an individual awaking with a calf myospasm that causes difficulty and increased pain when attempting to move the foot up or down, the individual with a lateral pterygoid myospasm has difficulty and increased pain when attempting to translate the condyle forward or retrude the jaw so the teeth fit into maximum intercuspation. The patient usually complains of the inability to put the ipsilateral posterior teeth together without excruciating pain (the teeth are usually separated by a fraction of a millimeter to a few millimeters), and the first tooth contact is in the area of the contralateral canine (if the patient has normal tooth alignment). Since the patient has difficulty translating forward, he or she also usually has a marked limited opening. A diagnostic test and treatments for the lateral pterygoid myospasm are provided in Chapter 9, "Lateral Pterygoid Myospasm."

Lateral pterygoid and closure muscle (e.g., medial pterygoid) myospasms are the only myospasms that I can recall treating. Myospasm treatments of the closure muscles may progress in a tiered approach while observing whether the recommended initial therapies adequately resolve the problem. The practitioner may desire to begin with the "TMD Self-management Therapies" handout provided in the appendix, muscle-stretching exercises, and medications.

The masticatory closure muscle should be actively stretched gradually to tolerance while ensuring the muscle is not aggravated by this procedure. It is recommended that

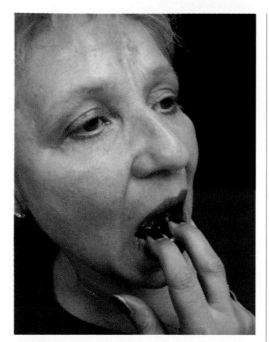

Figure 5-1. Stretching exercise recommended for a masticatory closure muscle myospasm, myofibrotic contracture, or an acute TMJ disc displacement without reduction. This exercise is recommended rather than the "Jaw Muscle-stretching Exercise" in Appendix 5, because these conditions require more forceful stretching, which may cause the digastric muscles to become painful.

the muscle be stretched and held by the index and middle fingers for 30 to 60 seconds, ten or more times times a day (Figure 5-1). Patients usually benefit from an analgesic (e.g., 800 mg ibuprofen, t.i.d.) and a muscle relaxant (e.g., 5 mg diazepam, 1 to 2 tablets h.s.). If these initial therapies do not resolve the myospasm or if it continues to recur, then traditional TMD therapies (e.g., occlusal appliance therapy, or identifying and changing contributing factors) should be implemented and have been shown to be beneficial.

▼ TECHNICAL TIP
Treating Myospasm
Myospasm is usually improved by gradual active stretching of the muscle; this can be performed with the masticatory closure muscle with the index and middle fingers between the maxillary and mandibular anterior teeth.

Myofibrotic Contracture

This is a painless disorder in which the muscle is incapable of stretching to its normal length. When this condition involves a closure muscle (e.g., masseter), then it limits a patient's ability to open wide, and forcibly attempting to stretch the muscle beyond its firm limitation elicits pain.[2,21]

Myofibrotic contracture is the result of fibrous adhesions within the muscle and may be caused by trauma, inflammation, or the muscle not being stretched beyond this limited range for an extended period, enabling the fibrous adhesions to develop.[14,21]

Generally the fibrous adhesions cause a permanent limitation to the muscle's range of motion, and traditional conservative TMD therapies would not help patients to regain the muscle's range of motion. Clinically, limited improvement has been achieved by patients using tongue depressors to stretch the muscle forcibly beyond its firm limitation. Surgical detachment and reattachment of the muscle may be indicated if the impairment is severe.[14,21]

A similar disorder, *myostatic contracture*, presents similarly, but the muscle does not have fibrous adhesions restricting its range of motion. Closure muscles with this disorder may be slowly stretched to regain the opening.[14,21] For a closure muscle with this condition, it is recommended that the mandible be stretched and held by the index and middle fingers for 30 to 60 seconds, six times a day (Figure 5-1). Additional supportive therapy may be needed, i.e., the "TMD Self-management Therapies" handout provided in the appendix, an analgesic (e.g., 800 mg ibuprofen, t.i.d.), and/or a muscle relaxant (e.g., 5 mg diazepam, 1 to 2 tablets h.s.).

Local Myalgia

This is a diagnostic category for additional muscle pain disorders that do not have sufficient distinguishing clinical characteristics to be given separate categories, e.g., protective splinting muscle pain, delayed-onset muscle soreness, muscle fatigue, and muscle pain from ischemia.[2]

Neoplasia

This is abnormal tissue growth, which may be malignant or benign, and may be painful or pain free. Neoplasms of the masticatory muscles are extremely rare.

REFERENCES

1. Fricton JR, Schiffman E. Management of masticatory myalgia and arthralgia. In: Lund JP, Lavigne GJ, Dubner R, Sessle BJ (eds). Orofacial Pain: From Basic Science to Clinical Management. Chicago: Quintessence, 2001:235.

2. American Academy of Orofacial Pain, with Okeson JP (ed). Orofacial Pain: Guidelines for Assessment, Diagnosis and Management. Chicago: Quintessence, 1996:127–41.

3. Stegenga B. Osteoarthritis of the temporomandibular joint organ and its relationship to disc displacement. J Orofac Pain 2001;15(3):193–205.

4. Yatani H, Sonoyama W, Kuboki T, Matsuka Y, Orsini MG, Yamashita A. The validity of clinical examination for diagnosis of anterior disc displacement with reduction. Oral Surg Oral Med Oral Pathol Oral Radiol Endod 1998;85:647–53.

5. Greene CS, Laskin DM. Long-term status of TMJ clicking in patients with myofascial pain and dysfunction. J Am Dent Assoc 1988;117:461–5.

6. Pertes RA, Gross SG. Disorders of the temporomandibular joint. In: Pertes RA, Gross SG (eds). Clinical Management of Temporomandibular Disorders and Orofacial Pain. Chicago: Quintessence, 1995:78, 85–6.

7. Isberg A, Stenstrom B, Isacsson G. Frequency of bilateral temporomandibular joint disc displacement in patients with unilateral symptoms: a 5-year follow-up of the asymptomatic joint—a clinical and arthrotomographic study. Dentomaxillofac Radiol 1991;20(2):73–6.

8. Schiffman E, Anderson G, Fricton J, Burton K, Schellhas K. Diagnostic criteria for intraarticular T.M. disorders. Community Dent Oral Epidemiol 1989;17(5):252–7.

9. Eriksson L, Westesson PL, Rohlin M. Temporomandibular joint sounds in patients with disc displacement. Int J Oral Surg 1985;14(5):428–36.

10. Fricton JR, Schellhas KP, Braun BL, Hoffmann W, Bromaghim C. Joint disorders: derangements and degeneration. In: Fricton JR, Kroening RJ, Hathaway KM (eds). TMJ and Craniofacial Pain: Diagnosis and Management. St Louis: Ishiyaku EuroAmerica, 1988:85–130.

11. Kurita K, Westesson PL, Yuasa H, Toyama M, Machida J, Ogi N. Natural course of untreated symptomatic temporomandibular joint disc displacement without reduction. J Dent Res 1998;77(2):361–5.

12. Minakuchi H, Kuboki T, Matsuka Y, Maekawa K, Yatani H, Yamashita A. Randomized controlled evaluation of non-surgical treatments for temporomandibular joint anterior disk displacement without reduction. J Dent Res 200180(3):924–8.

13. Yoda T, Imai H, Shinjyo T, Sakamoto I, Abe M, Enomoto S. Effect of arthrocentesis on TMJ disturbance of mouth closure with loud clicking: a preliminary study. Cranio 2002;20(1):18–22.

14. Okeson JP. Management of Temporomandibular Disorders and Occlusion, 5th edition. St Louis: CV Mosby, 2003:461, 464–7, 491–8.

15. American Society of Temporomandibular Joint Surgeons. White paper: guidelines for diagnosis and management of disorders involving the temporomandibular joint and related musculoskeletal structures. Cranio 2003;21(1):68–76.

16. Wexler GB, McKinney MW. Temporomandibular treatment outcomes within five diagnostic categories. Cranio 1999;17(1):30–7.

17. Marker P, Nielsen A, Bastian HL. Fractures of the mandibular condyle. Part 1: Patterns of distribution of types and causes of fractures in 348 patients. Br J Oral Maxillofac Surg 2000;38(5):417–21.

18. Marker P, Nielsen A, Bastian HL. Fractures of the mandibular condyle. Part 2: Results of treatment of 348 patients. Br J Oral Maxillofac Surg 2000;38(5):422–6.

19. Gremillion HA. The prevalence and etiology of temporomandibular disorders and orofacial pain. Tex Dent J 2000;117(7):30–9.

20. Sciotti VM, Mittak VL, DiMarco L, Ford LM, Plezbert J, Santipadri E, Wigglesworth J, Ball K. Clinical precision of myofascial trigger point loca-tion in the trapezius muscle. Pain 2001;93(3):259–66.

21. Fricton JR, Gross SG. Muscle Disorders. In: Pertes RA, Gross SG (eds). Clinical Management of Temporomandibular Disorders and Orofacial Pain. Chicago: Quintessence, 1995:91–108.

Chapter 6

Contributing Factors

TMD contributing factors are the elements that directly or indirectly contribute to the TMD symptoms, impacting both muscle and TMJ pain. They can be subcategorized into predisposing, initiating, and perpetuating contributing factors.[1-3] The **predisposing contributing factors** are the elements that make an individual more susceptible to developing TMD, e.g., fingernail biting, clenching, and biting on objects. The individual who is very predisposed to developing TMD may be the one who develops TMD from a slight occlusal change, e.g., from the placement of a pit and fissure sealant.

☯ FOCAL POINT

Predisposing contributing factors are the elements that make an individual more susceptible to developing TMD, e.g., fingernail biting, clenching, and biting on objects. An individual who is very predisposed to developing TMD may be the one who develops TMD from a slight occlusal change, e.g., from the placement of a pit and fissure sealant.

The **initiating contributing factor** is the event that caused the TMD symptoms to occur, e.g., trauma to the jaw or the placement of a crown. A total of 230 sequential TMD patients were asked what they perceived as the cause of their TMD symptoms, and it was found that most (61 percent) did

not associate the onset of their symptoms with any particular occurrence. Seven percent related it to dental treatment (orthodontic and other dental procedures) (see Table 6-1).

Some individuals who have developed TMD from dental treatment may have received treatments for which the average individual would not have had any problem, but these individuals may have been very predisposed to developing TMD. With the relatively high percentage of patients associating their TMD symptoms with dental treatment, it would be prudent for dentists to inquire about TMD symptoms and perform a cursory TMD evaluation prior to performing dental treatment, e.g., during the periodic dental examination. A cursory TMD evaluation can be done by measuring the patient's opening and checking for tenderness in the temporalis and masseter muscles,

Table 6-1. Events that patients related to TMD onset ($n = 230$)

61% No reason
17% Stress or stressful situation
4% Orthodontic treatment
4% Trauma
3% Other dental procedures
3% Motor vehicle accident
7% Other events

TMJs, and lateral pterygoid areas, as described in "Palpation" in Chapter 3 (Tables 3-1 and 3-2).

◉ **QUICK CONSULT**
Varying Patient Response
Some individuals who have developed TMD from dental treatment may have received treatments for which the average individual would not have had any problem, but these individuals may have been very predisposed to developing TMD.

The **perpetuating contributing factors** are the elements that directly or indirectly aggravate the masticatory system and prevent the TMD symptoms from resolving.[1,2,4] It is important to attempt to identify these factors and determine the degree they are contributing to a patient's symptoms. It is recommended to the patient that those which are the easiest to change and that should provide the greatest impact on the symptoms be initially changed.

◐ **FOCAL POINT**
Perpetuating contributing factors are the elements that directly or indirectly aggravate the masticatory system and prevent TMD symptoms from resolving.

Attempt to change the perpetuating contributing factors that are the easiest to change and that should provide the greatest impact on the patient's symptoms.

The daily variation in symptoms will often give an indication of when these factors are occurring. For example, a situation in which a patient awakes with the TMD symptoms that rapidly resolve would suggest the primary perpetuating contributing factors are occurring at night. It is recommended that the factors that should first be considered changing are sleeping position (if the patient sleeps on his or her stomach) and nocturnal parafunctional habits.

◉ **QUICK CONSULT**
Observing for Variation in Daily Symptoms
The daily variation in symptoms will often give an indication of when the perpetuating contributing factors are occurring.

Conversely, if the patient awakes symptom free with the symptoms occurring later in the day, this would suggest the primary perpetuating contributing factors are transpiring during the day and are under the patient's conscious control. At the initial evaluation, patients are rarely aware of their daytime parafunctional habits or the frequency with which they perform them. For example, some patients relate they lightly rest their teeth together throughout the day but are unaware that they squeeze the teeth together when they are busy, frustrated, or concentrating on other activities, e.g., using a computer or driving.

Clinically some residual effect of the TMD contributing factors appears to carry over to the other portions of the day. The contributing factors are widely diverse and unique to each patient. For ease of comprehending the broad continuum of contributing factors, they can be thought about in biological, behavioral, emotional, cognitive, social, and environmental categories.[2]

◉ **QUICK CONSULT**
Observing Treatment Effect on Daily Pattern
Clinically some residual effect of TMD contributing factors appear to carry over to the other portions of the day.

Biological contributing factors are the elements that mechanically or biologically contribute to TMD. They can include neck pain, poor posture, malocclusion, insomnia, and systemic diseases (e.g., fibromyalgia or rheumatoid arthritis). Behavioral contributing factors are habits a patient frequently performs that negatively impact TMD, e.g., clenching, fingernail biting, lip biting, stomach sleeping, or telephone cradling. Biological and behavioral contributing factors tend to influence the TMD symptoms directly, whereas emotional, cognitive, and social factors tend to convey their influence indirectly.[2]

⊙ **QUICK CONSULT**

Observing Contributing Factor Influence

Biological and behavioral contributing factors tend to influence the TMD symptoms directly, whereas emotional, cognitive, and social factors tend to convey their influence indirectly.

Emotional contributing factors are prolonged negative emotions such as depression, worry, anxiety, and anger. Cognitive factors are harmful thought processes or low cognitive skills, e.g., negative self-statements, or poor reasoning skills making it difficult for the patient to work with the self-management or other instructions. Social contributing factors are related to interactions with others, e.g., coworker difficulties, lack of social support, or secondary gain.

Environmental contributing factors can have a direct effect (e.g., a food additive directly causing a migraine headache) or an indirect effect (e.g., seasonal affective disorder causing depression and thereby contributing to TMD symptoms). These factors are usually quite difficult to identify and therefore are infrequently explored among TMD patients.[2]

Generally TMD therapies are not directed toward physically or biochemically changing the TMD diagnosis (e.g., myofascial pain), but are directed at changing the contributing factors. With the reduction in the intensity and frequency of the perpetuating contributing factors, the body heals itself. This is similar to a patient who has mild generalized periodontal disease. A practitioner would not surgically intervene to change this condition, but would try to determine the factors that have caused this disease to develop, e.g., not properly brushing or flossing, smoking, or poor nutrition. Once these factors have been identified, the practitioner would educate and motivate the patient to make sufficient behavioral changes to enable the body to reverse the disease. The practitioner would follow the patient's case to ensure adequate behavioral changes have been made to resolve the disease.[2]

✪ **FOCAL POINT**

With the reduction in the intensity and frequency of the perpetuating contributing factors, the body heals itself.

Identifying the TMD contributing factors, in addition to educating and motivating the patient to change the TMD contributing factors, is one of the most challenging aspects of treating TMD patients. When one is having difficulty identifying the contributing factors, a technique that has been helpful is asking the patient to hourly track the pain and other events that are occurring in the patient's life. This has often helped patients to identify events associated with the pain. For example, a TMD patient who also had moderately severe hip pain was being evaluated as to whether the disorder was benign or malignant. Using the diary, the patient found a direct association between her hip and TMD symptoms. Upon discussing this, the patient thought that, when her hip pain increased in severity, she tightened her masticatory muscles in response to the pain and started worrying about her hip disorder. She chose to use her hip pain as a cue to alert herself consciously to keep her jaw muscles relaxed. With this and other conservative therapies, she obtained satisfactory relief of her TMD pain.

◉ **QUICK CONSULT**

Challenging Segments of Therapy

Identifying the TMD contributing factors, in addition to educating and motivating the patient to change them, is one of the most challenging aspects of treating TMD patients.

▼ **TECHNICAL TIP**

Identifying Contributing Factors through a Diary

When one is having difficulty identifying the contributing factors, a technique that can be helpful is asking the patient to hourly track the pain and other events that are occurring in the patient's life.

A 64-year-old lady who had recently developed daytime TMD symptoms several days a week also found the diary helpful. At the initial appointment, when asked about new stresses, irritations, frustrations, or concerns in her life, she stated that she has a superb life, she doesn't work, all of her children have left home, and she and her husband have a wonderful relationship. After using the diary, she found her pain was related to thoughts regarding her 90-year-old father who lives alone (about an hour's drive from her home) and is becoming forgetful. She related that, in the previous week, he left his house for several hours with the flame burning on his stove. She also periodically receives telephone calls from her siblings re-

minding her that she lived the closest to him, it was her responsibility to watch over him and, if anything went wrong, she would receive the blame. It was speculated that, when she had concerned thoughts about her father, she tended to tighten her masticatory muscles sufficiently to manifest her TMD symptoms. She worked with a psychologist who taught her coping strategies and how to deal better with her siblings, in addition to my instructions on breaking her masticatory muscle-tightening habits, and her symptoms resolved after a few weeks.

REFERENCES

1. Fricton JR. Establishing the problem list: an inclusive conceptual model for chronic illness. In: Fricton JR, Kroening RJ, Hathaway KM (eds). TMJ and Craniofacial Pain: Diagnosis and Management. St Louis: Ishiyaku EuroAmerica, 1988:21–6.
2. Fricton JR, Chung SC. Contributing factors: A key to chronic pain. In: Fricton JR, Kroening RJ, Hathaway KM (eds). TMJ and Craniofacial Pain: Diagnosis and Management. St Louis: Ishiyaku EuroAmerica, 1988:27–37.
3. McNeill C, Mohl ND, Rugh JD, Tanaka TT. Temporomandibular disorders: diagnosis, management, education, and research. J Am Dent Assoc 1990;120(3):253–63.
4. American Academy of Orofacial Pain, with Okeson JP (ed). Orofacial Pain: Guidelines for Assessment, Diagnosis and Management. Chicago: Quintessence, 1996:142–3.

Part II

Common Acute TMD Conditions and Treatments

Most new TMD patients report having *chronic* rather than acute TMD symptoms; they have had the pain at least several months, and the pain intensity generally fluctuates over time. When considering medications for a patient with chronic symptoms, generally assume they will be used long term. Therefore, avoid prescribing muscle relaxants and primarily use tricyclic antidepressants and sometimes use nonsteroid anti-inflammatory drugs (NSAIDs) on an as-needed basis.

It is believed that patients with chronic TMD symptoms should change their parafunctional habits in addition to other perpetuating contributing factors, i.e., not coping well with life's stresses, anxiety, and depression. Clinical experience has demonstrated there is a tendency for patients with chronic symptoms who are prescribed muscle relaxants to rely on these medications for pain relief rather than attempting to change their contributing factors.

An *acute TMD condition* can be the recent onset of TMD symptoms or an acute flare-up of a chronic condition. For these patients, I am much more likely to prescribe short-term use of a muscle relaxant and/or anti-inflammatory medications. A few patients, who occasionally (every 1 or 2 years) develop mild TMD symptoms related to temporary stressful events, prefer to use only TMD self-management therapy and medication. It is recommended that these cases be followed to ensure the symptoms adequately resolve and the patients do not need additional TMD therapy.

✪ FOCAL POINT

An acute TMD condition can be the recent onset of TMD symptoms or an acute flare-up of a chronic condition.

Chapter 7

TMD Secondary to Trauma

FAQ

Q: What would you do if a patient who developed TMD from trauma was provided your initial recommended therapy and returned requesting stronger medications?

A: If the patient returns requesting stronger medications after having been provided the initial recommended therapy, there is probably some other pathology involved, e.g., pulpalgia from an incomplete tooth fracture.

Trauma is a force to the masticatory system whose intensity or duration exceeds the normal functioning forces of this system. It can occur in three forms: (a) **direct trauma** (macrotrauma), e.g., blow to jaw; (b) **indirect trauma** (nonimpact jolt to the jaw), e.g., occurring in conjunction with cervical whiplash; and (c) **microtrauma**, e.g., chronic parafunctional habits.[1]

⊙ **QUICK CONSULT**
Understanding Trauma
Trauma to the masticatory system can occur in three forms: (a) direct trauma (macrotrauma), (b) indirect trauma (nonimpact jolt to the jaw), and (c) microtrauma.

Direct and indirect trauma have identifiable events a patient normally reports as the initiating cause of the TMD symptoms. Microtrauma generally reflects unconscious

habits, which may predispose an individual to develop TMD from direct or indirect trauma and make it more difficult to resolve the manifested symptoms. This chapter focuses on direct and indirect trauma, and uses the term *trauma* to encompass both forms.

⊙ **QUICK CONSULT**
Understanding Trauma
This chapter focuses on direct and indirect trauma, and uses the term *trauma* to encompass both forms.

Trauma can cause muscle pain, TMJ pain and inflammation, and intracapsular changes. It can stretch ligaments supporting the TMJ's smooth mechanical movements, causing or predisposing an individual to develop one of the disc displacements or a dislocation. It can create irregularities in the smooth condyle, fossa, or disc surfaces, thereby causing roughness or catching during TMJ movements. Additionally, trauma can precipitate bleeding within the TMJ, leading to adhesion formation.[2-5]

☻ FOCAL POINT

Trauma can cause muscle pain, TMJ pain and inflammation, and intracapsular changes.

The "Initial Patient Questionnaire" asks when the problem began and whether the patient has suffered whiplash or trauma to the head or neck. These responses will alert the practitioner as to whether the patient has acute TMD symptoms secondary to trauma. These patients may have complaints of muscle pain, TMJ pain, other pains, new TMJ noises, and/or disruption of smooth TMJ movements. These symptoms may not manifest until weeks to months after the traumatic event.[3]

◉ QUICK CONSULT
Observing for Trauma History

The "Initial Patient Questionnaire" responses will alert the practitioner as to whether the patient has acute TMD symptoms secondary to trauma.

Many factors can cause or contribute to these complaints and need to be considered when trauma is the initiating contributing factor or has greatly exacerbated chronic symptoms. The more common possibilities include bone fracture, referred odontogenic pain secondary to tooth trauma, comorbid cervical disorder, and psychosocial issues related to the trauma or treatment for the trauma. The literature reports many other less common disorders that have been related to traumatic events. If the patient has signs and/or symptoms suggestive of disorders beyond the practitioner's ability, the practitioner should refer the patient to someone with greater expertise in this area.

Even though a patient has only an acute problem, the TMD examination should be performed as recommended in Chapter 3, "Clinical Examination." Cervical pain is even more prevalent among patients whose TMD is secondary to trauma from a motor vehicle accident.[2,6] It is recommended a panoramic radiograph be taken to rule out a fracture causing or contributing to the pain. If the patient was not appropriately evaluated for a fracture following the trauma and the practitioner suspects the patient may have a fracture in a bone that would not be revealed by the panoramic radiograph, then appropriate radiographs are indicated.

◉ QUICK CONSULT
Evaluating Patients with History of a Motor Vehicle Accident

Among patients whose TMD is secondary to trauma from a motor vehicle accident, cervical pain is more likely to be present.

▽ TECHNICAL TIP
Contributing Factor of Trauma

When trauma is the initiating contributing factor or has greatly exacerbated chronic symptoms, it is recommended a panoramic radiograph be taken to rule out a fracture causing or contributing to the patient's pain.

Depression, anger, and hostility are significantly more common with these patients.[7] Sometimes patients angrily complain about the injustice of their situation, whereas others may disclaim these feelings but also internally stew with these thoughts. Some practitioners routinely refer all patients with significant trauma to a psychologist to evaluate for such perpetuating contributing factors.

◉ QUICK CONSULT
Observing for Psychosocial Contributors

Depression, anger, and hostility are significantly more common with patients whose TMD symptoms were initiated by trauma.

Significant trauma may cause patients to have neuropsychological and cognitive functioning deficits that may comprise memory and concentration impairment, rapid mental fatigue, weakness, sleep disturbances, anxiety, etc.[6,8,9] Patients with such deficits should be evaluated and treated with a multidisciplinary approach by medical personnel trained in this area. In conjunction with these therapies, traditional TMD therapy can be provided for the masticatory system.

The trauma's severity and the patient's TMD perpetuating contributing factors are major determinants for how readily the TMD symptoms will resolve. The patient may require anything from no or minimal treatment to very extensive multidisciplinary therapies; even with extensive therapy, some patients with trauma-induced TMD do not improve.[10]

✪ FOCAL POINT

The trauma's severity and the patient's TMD perpetuating contributing factors are major determinants for how readily the TMD symptoms will resolve.

Initial therapy for many of these patients may encompass discussing TMD self-management instructions and prescribing a muscle relaxant, anti-inflammatory, and/or analgesic medications. The "TMD Self-management Therapies" handout (Appendix 3) recommends that patients limit use of the masticatory system by eating a soft diet, eliminating oral habits, etc. It also recommends the use of heat and cold, but the practitioner may desire to alter these instructions verbally to using cold over the affected area for the first 48 hours after injury and then applying heat as needed.

▼ TECHNICAL TIP
Determining Initial Therapy

Initial therapy for many of these patients may encompass discussing TMD self-management instructions and prescribing a muscle relaxant, anti-inflammatory, and/or analgesic medications.

As a general pharmaceutical guide, I tend to prescribe the following for patients with constant pain at these intensities. This will vary with the patient's fluctuating pain intensity pattern, the patient's palpation tenderness, and the emotional impact these are causing. If the patient has a low level of pain (3/10 or below), I would tend to prescribe the patient 800 mg ibuprofen, t.i.d. If the pain is greater and primarily of muscle origin, I would tend to prescribe 5 mg diazepam, 1 to 2 tablets h.s. If the patient has significant daytime muscle pain, I would consider discussing the possibility of the patient taking 1/2 tablet in the morning and afternoon; the potential side effects and ramifications must be discussed. If the pain is above 3/10 and primarily of TMJ origin, I consider prescribing 500 mg naproxen, b.i.d. If the pain is above 6 to 7/10 and primarily of TMJ origin, I consider prescribing the Medrol Dosepak-naproxen regimen discussed in "Anti-inflammatory Medications" in Chapter 17. In healthy adults, the anti-inflammatory and the muscle relaxant can be taken together; if additional analgesic relief is needed, acetaminophen can be added.

After providing this therapy, if the patient returns requesting stronger medications, some other pathology is probably involved, e.g., pulpalgia from an incomplete tooth fracture. Based on the patient's history and practitioner's experience, the practitioner may elect to provide additional temporary TMD therapies (e.g., temporary soft appliance) or initiate long-term therapy (e.g., making impressions for an acrylic appliance). Comparative studies reveal considerable variability as to whether patients with posttraumatic TMD respond differently to TMD therapies than do patients whose TMD developed independently of trauma.[9-13]

REFERENCES

1. American Academy of Orofacial Pain, with Okeson JP (ed). Orofacial Pain: Guidelines for Assessment, Diagnosis and Management. Chicago: Quintessence, 1996:120.
2. Kolbinson DA, Epstein JB, Senthilselvan A, Burgess JA. A comparison of TMD patients with or without prior motor vehicle accident involvement: initial signs, symptoms, and diagnostic characteristics. J Orofac Pain 1997;11(3):206–14.
3. Burgess JA, Kolbinson DA, Lee PT, Epstein JB. Motor vehicle accidents and TMDs. J Am Dent Assoc 1996;127(12):1767–72.
4. Okeson JP. Management of Temporomandibular Disorders and Occlusion, 5th edition. St Louis: CV Mosby, 2003:337–8, 419–20.
5. Okeson JP. Bell's Orofacial Pains, 5th edition. Carol Stream, IL: Quintessence, 1995:285, 310–1.
6. Goldberg MB. Posttraumatic temporomandibular disorders. J Orofac Pain 1999;13(4):291–4.
7. Krogstad BS, Jokstad A, Dahl BL, Soboleva U. Somatic complaints, psychologic distress, and treatment outcome in two groups of TMD patients, one previously subjected to whiplash injury. J Orofac Pain 1998;12(2):136–44.
8. Grossi M, Goldberg MB, Locker D, Tenenbaum HC. Reduced neuropsychologic measures as predictors of treatment outcome in patients with temporomandibular disorders. J Orofac Pain 2001;15(4):329–39.
9. Romanelli GG, Mock D, Tenenbaum HC. Characteristics and response to treatment of post-traumatic temporomandibular disorder: a retrospective study. Clin J Pain 1992;8(1):6–17.
10. Kolbinson DA, Epstein JB, Senthilselvan A, Burgess JA. A comparison of TMD patients with or without prior motor vehicle accident involvement. J Orofac Pain 1997;11(4):337–45.
11. De Boever JA, Keersmaekers K. Trauma in patients with temporomandibular disorders: frequency and treatment outcome. J Oral Rehabil 1996;23(2):91–6.
12. Epstein JB. Temporomandibular disorders, facial pain and headache following motor vehicle accidents. J Can Dent Assoc 1992;58(6):488–9, 493–5.
13. Steed PA, Wexler GB. Temporomandibular disorders: traumatic etiology vs. nontraumatic etiology—a clinical and methodological inquiry into symptomatology and treatment outcomes. Cranio 2001;19(3):188–94.

Chapter 8

TMD Secondary to Dental Treatment

FAQs

Q: If a dental patient develops TMD after a dental procedure, was the dental treatment the cause of the symptoms?

A: A patient's propensity for developing TMD may play a major role for one individual manifesting TMD after dental treatment, whereas a dentist using excessive and/or prolonged forces on the mandible may play a major role for another individual manifesting TMD after dental treatment.

Q: If a patient returns to my office with a medial pterygoid myospasm and the patient is provided the therapy you recommend, how long will it take the disorder to resolve?

A: Depending on its severity, this disorder generally takes 5 to 10 days to resolve.

Q: Do most patients prefer to take the medication prior to the appointment or after the appointment?

A: Some patients may desire premedication, others prefer postoperative medication, and some may need both.

When 230 sequential TMD patients were asked what they perceived as the cause for their symptoms, most (61 percent) did not associate the onset of their symptoms with any particular event, whereas 4 percent related it to orthodontic treatment and 3 percent related it to other dental procedures (see Table 6-1).

Observing the Onset of TMD Symptoms

Most patients with TMD do not associate the onset of their symptoms with any particular event.

For many TMD patients, their pain appears to develop slowly and worsen in a fluctuating pattern until a severity is reached for which they desire to obtain relief. For other individuals, TMD symptoms may fluctuate over time, but never develop the severity for which therapy is desired. The propensity for any one individual to develop TMD from dental treatment may vary with the degree of low-level or subclinical symptoms.

The propensity for any one individual to develop TMD from dental treatment may vary with the degree of low-level or subclinical symptoms.

A dentist can also provide dental therapy appropriately for an individual who is in the midst of developing TMD, but may not even be aware of it because of such minor symptoms. Because of the patient's propensity for developing TMD, the dental treatment may cause this individual to manifest TMD from the dental treatment. Conversely it is possible for a dentist to place such excessive and/or prolonged forces on the jaw that someone who is not predisposed to developing TMD would develop the disorder.

Understandably it would be prudent for dentists to inquire about TMD symptoms and perform a cursory TMD evaluation prior to performing dental treatment, e.g., during the periodic dental examination. A cursory TMD evaluation can be done by measuring the patient's opening and checking for tenderness in the anterior region of the temporalis and masseter muscles, TMJs, and lateral pterygoid areas (Table 8-1).

Table 8-1. Cursory TMD evaluation palpations for dental patients

Anterior region of the temporalis muscle	Bilaterally palpate approximately 1½ inches behind the eye canthus and ½ inch above the zygomatic arch (Figure 3-6).
TMJ	Three areas of the TMJ need to be palpated bilaterally, and any one of these can be tender without tenderness of the others (a common mistake is not having the patient open sufficiently to palpate the TMJ adequately): (a) Ask the patient to open approximately 20 mm and palpate the condyle's lateral pole. (b) Ask the patient to open as wide as possible and palpate the depth of the depression behind the condyle with the fingertip. (c) With the finger in the depression, pull forward to load the posterior aspect of the condyle (Figure 3-7).
Masseter muscle	Bilaterally palpate the center of the masseter muscle (Figure 3-8). If the practitioner is unsure of the muscle's extent, ask the patient to clench, and its extent can easily be felt.
Lateral pterygoid area	Slide the fifth digit along the lateral side of the maxillary alveolar ridge to the most posterior region of the vestibule (the location for the posterior superior alveolar injection). Palpate by pressing superior, medial, and distal (Figure 3-22). If tenderness is observed, referred pain may be generated by applying heavier sustained pressure.

Protecting Yourself

It is recommended dentists inquire about TMD symptoms prior to dental treatment, measure the patient's opening, and check for tenderness in the anterior region of the temporalis and masseter muscles, TMJs, and lateral pterygoid areas.

Many elements of dental treatment in addition to excessive and/or prolonged opening can initiate TMD symptoms or aggravate a chronic TMD condition. For example, a medial pterygoid myospasm may occur from piercing the medial pterygoid muscle during an inferior alveolar injection, a myositis may occur from extracting an infected tooth, and generalized muscle and/or TMJ pain may occur from placing a restoration with an inharmonious occlusion.

If a patient returns to the practitioner's office and complains of TMD pain after a dental procedure, the pain may also be postoperative dental pain referring to the masticatory muscles and/or TMJ. An example of referred pain that dentists frequently observe is among patients with a mandibular third-molar osteitis, for which TMJ and/or ear pain is a common complaint. Referred pain to the masticatory muscles or TMJ may be observed from any tooth or deep structure that is causing postoperative dental pain.

TMD symptoms secondary to dental treatment can be limited to one muscle, the TMJ, or be present in a generalized fashion. The following two sections of this chapter discuss pain that may occur in the medial pterygoid muscle and disorders that can cause a patient to be unable to close into maximum intercuspation after dental treatment. Two sections then discuss TMD sequelae generated from placing occlusally inharmonious restorations (usually presents as generalized pain) and suggestions that can be used to prevent TMD symptoms secondary to dental treatment. The last section discusses TMD symptoms secondary to ob-structive sleep apnea appliances and treatment suggestions.

MEDIAL PTERYGOID MUSCLE PAIN

The most common disorder observed for the medial pterygoid muscle is a *medial pterygoid myospasm* induced by trauma from the needle piercing the medial pterygoid muscle during an inferior alveolar injection.[1,2] The myospasm may involve the entire muscle or be limited to the traumatized portion of the muscle.[3] The majority of patients treated for this disorder previously received multiple inferior alveolar injections, but some only had a single injection.

A patient who develops this disorder typically returns to the practitioner's office 1 or 2 days after a dental procedure that required an inferior alveolar injection. The patient complains of significant pain in the medial pterygoid muscle region and limited opening. Palpation of the masticatory muscles and TMJs typically reveals no or minimal tenderness, until the medial pterygoid muscle is palpated. The patient's limited opening often makes it difficult to palpate the medial pterygoid muscle, but, once this is palpated, the patient's eyes usually "light up" and there is no doubt that this is the source of the pain.

For these patients, I generally prescribe 800 mg ibuprofen, t.i.d., and 5 mg diazepam, 1 to 2 tablets h.s. If the pain is severe, it is recommended the patient also take acetaminophen and consider discussing the possibility of the patient taking $1/2$ tablet of 5 mg diazepam in the morning and afternoon. If diazepam is prescribed for daytime use, the potential side effects and ramifications must be discussed with the patient.

▼ **TECHNICAL TIP**

Prescribing Medication for a Medial Pterygoid Myospasm

For patients with a medial pterygoid myospasm, I generally prescribe 800 mg ibuprofen, t.i.d., and 5 mg diazepam, 1 to 2 tablets h.s.

Additionally the "TMD Self-management Therapies" handout is reviewed, and the patient is requested to stretch the medial pterygoid muscle (up to tolerance) ten or more times a day with the index and middle fingers and hold the stretch for 30 to 60 seconds, as demonstrated in Figure 5-1. Anatomically it appears that heat applied to the lateral surface of the mandible would not penetrate to the medial pterygoid muscle, but these patients report they have a beneficial effect from its use.

Depending on its severity, this disorder generally takes 5 to 10 days to resolve. On one occasion, a patient who had only minimal improvement with his limited opening was asked to implement a more aggressive stretching technique. This entailed him using wooden tongue depressors to stretch the medial pterygoid muscle more actively (up to tolerance), ten or more times a day, and hold the stretch for 1 minute. He inserted as many wooden tongue depressors that would fit between his maxillary and mandibular incisors, and held them together with a rubber band. He next inserted an additional tongue depressor at the far end and slowly slid it between the others, providing additional stretch to his medial pterygoid muscle, as demonstrated in Figure 8-1. He continued to insert tongue depressors up to tolerance and eventually regained his normal opening. Tongue depressors could similarly be held together by placing them inside a finger cot or the finger of a glove.

Clinically a *medial pterygoid myositis* presents in a similar manner as a myospasm. The myositis can be due to a bacterial infection of the muscle, which can occur from procedures such as extracting an infected tooth.[4] A practitioner might have to attempt to differentiate whether a patient has a medial pterygoid myospasm or myositis, if the

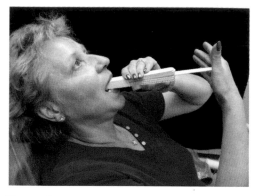

Figure 8-1. Forceful stretching procedure that may be desired for a resistant medial pterygoid myospasm, myofibrotic contracture, or fibrous ankylosis.

patient had an inferior alveolar injection to extract an infected tooth and returned complaining of significant medial pterygoid muscle pain limiting opening. If the patient has a fever or lymphadenopathy, this would suggest an infection is present, and antibiotics are indicated.

◉ **QUICK CONSULT**

Observing a Medial Pterygoid Myositis

Clinically patients with a medial pterygoid myositis present similarly to those with a medial pterygoid myospasm.

The importance of following the cases of TMD patients and their symptoms cannot be overemphasized. An oral surgeon once referred me a patient who had TMD symptoms (generalized unilateral pain and palpation tenderness) after a tooth extraction. Based on the patient interview and clinical examination, the patient's symptoms were diagnosed as TMD. Two or three weeks later, she returned complaining that her airway was starting to become restricted. At my request, the patient returned that day to the oral surgeon, and a computed tomogram he took revealed this was caused by a space infection. Once her infection was treated, her TMD symptoms resolved.

INABILITY TO CLOSE INTO MAXIMUM INTERCUSPATION

Occasionally at the end of a dental procedure, some patients have difficulty putting their teeth into maximum intercuspation (MI). This can be a momentary or prolonged problem and can make it nearly impossible for the practitioner to adjust the occlusion of a new restoration.

Holding the mouth open wide for an extended period tends to fatigue a susceptible inferior lateral pterygoid muscle and inflame a susceptible TMJ. If either is predisposed to developing this problem, the susceptible structure may be the source. Palpating the TMJs and lateral pterygoid areas (Table 8-1) should enable the practitioner to determine the source; this problem may be unilateral or bilateral. The top left section of the "TMJ Disc Displacements" diagram (Appendix 2) may help practitioners explain the cause and symptoms to patients.

◉ **QUICK CONSULT**

Observing Susceptible Muscles and TMJs

Having a dental patient hold his or her mouth open wide for an extended period tends to fatigue a susceptible inferior lateral pterygoid muscle and inflame a susceptible TMJ.

▼ **TECHNICAL TIP**

Explaining Cause and Symptoms to Patients

The top left section of the "TMJ Disc Displacements" diagram (Appendix 2) may help practitioners explain the cause and symptoms to patients.

If only the lateral pterygoid muscles are tender, they are probably fatigued (almost certainly due to the aggravation of preexisting myofascial pain) and unable to stretch to their normal relaxed length. Therefore, they hold the condyles in a slightly translated position, and the first occlusal contact is often on the anterior teeth. In this situation, the TMJs are not tender to palpation, and the practitioner may be able to stretch the lateral pterygoid muscles, enabling the patient to close into MI. Stretching of the lateral pterygoid muscles is demonstrated in Chapter 9, "Lateral Pterygoid Myospasm." If pain occurs in the TMJ while performing this stretch, there is probably some TMJ inflammation, and continued stretching will probably aggravate the inflammation.

▼ **TECHNICAL TIP**

Stretching the Lateral Pterygoid Muscle

If only the lateral pterygoid muscles are tender, stretching them often enables patients to close into MI.

If only the TMJs are tender to palpation, the diagnosis is TMJ inflammation, and an anti-inflammatory medication should help prevent or resolve this problem. If both the lateral pterygoid areas and TMJs are tender to palpation, then both problems are probably present. If the TMJs are considerably more tender than the lateral pterygoid areas, the lateral pterygoid muscles may be sore from holding the condyles forward to protect the inflamed TMJs (protective muscle splinting) and, once the TMJ inflammation is treated, the muscle splinting usually resolves.

▼ **TECHNICAL TIP**

Reducing TMJ Inflammation

If only the TMJs are tender to palpation, an anti-inflammatory medication should help prevent or resolve this problem.

Patients who report that this problem occurs every time they receive dental treatment would probably benefit from using applicable suggestions in the section on "Preventing Aggravation from Dental Treatment." If this does not provide adequate improvement, the practitioner may desire the patient to take medication prior to the appointment. Some patients may report they have TMD symptoms also at other times that are significant enough for them to desire TMD therapy.

As a general premedication guide, I tend to prescribe patients who have TMJ inflammation an anti-inflammatory (e.g., 500 mg naproxen) and those who have muscle fatigue (probably aggravation of preexisting myofascial pain) a muscle relaxant (e.g., 5 mg diazepam). The dosing varies with the severity of the symptoms; i.e., if symptoms are mild, ask the patient to take the medication 1 hour prior to the appointment, but, if symptoms are severe, ask the patient to start the night before the appointment, 1 hour prior to appointment, and an appropriate time after the appointment. If the patient is to take a muscle relaxant during the day, the potential side effects and ramifications must be discussed.

◉ **QUICK CONSULT**

Prescribing Anti-inflammatory and Muscle Relaxant Medications

I tend to prescribe patients who have TMJ inflammation an anti-inflammatory (e.g., 500 mg naproxen) and those who have muscle fatigue a muscle relaxant (e.g., 5 mg diazepam).

If a patient requests medication for the discomfort from the dental procedure, the practitioner may desire to consider the patient taking the medication for a few days postoperatively. In healthy adults, the anti-inflammatory and muscle relaxants may be taken together; if additional analgesic relief is needed, acetaminophen can be added.

The inability to close into MI is not exclusively associated with dental treatment, but may be a chronic fluctuating problem for some individuals, with the source being either the TMJ or the lateral pterygoid muscle. In fact, some dentists have informed me

that they themselves experience having this problem after providing certain difficult dental procedures, after stressful events, or after a stressful day.

◉ **QUICK CONSULT**

Observing Chronic Inability to Close into Maximum Intercuspation

The inability to close into MI is not exclusively associated with dental treatment, but may be a chronic fluctuating problem for some individuals, with the source being either the TMJ or the lateral pterygoid muscle.

A lateral pterygoid muscle that is overused and remains fatigued might develop a myospasm.[5] The myospasm can occur independently of dental treatment and may cause a prolonged inability for the patient to close into MI. The diagnosis and treatment for this are discussed in Chapter 9, "Lateral Pterygoid Myospasm."

Some patients may be able to close into MI immediately after the dental procedure, but develop this inability hours to days later. One patient was referred to me with this symptom pattern in addition to constant severe pain and tenderness in the lateral pterygoid area. The practitioner had unknowingly placed a large restoration over a maxillary bicuspid with an acute pulpalgia. The patient also had bicuspid pain to a lesser degree and a PDL injection along the bicuspid provided temporary relief of the lateral pterygoid pain. It is believed the pulp's deep pain input caused a myospasm of the lateral pterygoid muscle.[5] Once the practitioner endodontically cleaned the bicuspid's canal, the constant pain and inability to close into MI resolved.

OCCLUSAL INTERFERENCE SEQUELAE

Many studies have demonstrated that placing a restoration with an occlusion that is not in harmony with the rest of the dentition may cause patients to develop TMD symptoms.[6-8] These may develop relatively rapidly, occur on the ipsilateral and/or contralateral side of the restoration, and consist of masticatory muscle pain, TMJ pain, and/or TMJ clicking. The inharmonious change may be as minor as a pit and fissure sealant.

◉ **QUICK CONSULT**

Placing an Inharmonious Restoration

Placing a restoration inharmonious with the rest of the occlusion may cause TMD symptoms, which develop relatively rapidly, occur on the ipsilateral and/or contralateral side of the restoration, and consist of masticatory muscle pain, TMJ pain, and/or TMJ clicking.

When a patient returns to the practitioner's office and complains of TMD symptoms that the practitioner believes are due to the recent placement of an occlusally inharmonious restoration, clinical experience has shown the restoration should be adjusted until the patient relates it feels comfortable. The interference may be located in MI or any other position.

If the complaint is with a posterior tooth, first check whether the MI contacts on the new restoration are too heavy. Once it is observed the MI contacts are evenly distributed on the dentition, then check whether the tooth strikes in the eccentric positions. It is recommended the tooth's other contacts be marked with a thin red articulating film in the following manner: manipulate the patient's mandible into centric relation and ask the patient to squeeze so his or her teeth slide into MI, help the patient to return to centric relation and ask the patient to rub side to side on that tooth, ask the patient to bite down (into MI) and rub side to side, and finally ask the patient to slide the mandible forward. Next use thin black articulating film and ask the patient to tap in MI. Clinical experience has shown that

highly polished crowns reflect the red oral mucosa, making it difficult to observe the red marks on the crown, so a different color may be needed in this situation.

Reduce the new restoration wherever the red marks are located. The tooth should be adjusted so it feels comfortable to the patient. Occasionally a restoration is adjusted as described, but the patient relates that it still feels uncomfortable. Clinically it has been observed that nonrestored portions of the tooth may need to be adjusted in the same manner prior to the patient relating that it feels comfortable. It is speculated this may occur because these teeth become tender to percussion,[9] and prior nonideal contacts may no longer be perceived as comfortable.

An anterior tooth may also need to be adjusted in centric and excursive movements. Observe whether the new restoration has heavier contacts than the other anterior teeth and adjust so it feels comfortable to the patient. If it appears the adjustments may compromise the patient's esthetics, the practitioner may need to discuss the possibility of providing minor adjustments of the opposing teeth.

Once the tooth feels comfortable to the patient, the TMD symptoms generally resolve rapidly. There is not a direct relationship between a newly placed interference and the development of TMD symptoms. In studies, some patients did not develop TMD symptoms from the placement of an interference, some in the control group (who unknowingly only had the placement of an interference simulated) developed TMD symptoms, and a few patients took up to 6 weeks to obtain symptom resolution after the interference was removed.[6,10]

◉ **QUICK CONSULT**

Adjusting an Inharmonious Restoration

Once the tooth feels comfortable to the patient, the TMD symptoms generally resolve rapidly.

It is suspected that some of the control patients who developed TMD and the patients whose symptoms took an inordinate amount of time to resolve had a high predisposition for developing TMD symptoms. The likelihood of a patient's TMD symptoms not resolving once the tooth feels comfortable is low, but it is possible.[9]

A patient who does not respond well to refining the occlusion, and for whom referred pain from the tooth has been ruled out, may have had his or her masticatory system aggravated during the dental procedure (e.g., from prolonged opening). Initial therapy for such patients may encompass discussing TMD self-management instructions and prescribing muscle relaxants and/or anti-inflammatory medications. If medications are desired, as a general guide I tend to prescribe patients who have TMJ inflammation an anti-inflammatory (e.g., 500 mg naproxen, 1 tablet b.i.d.) and those who have muscle pain a muscle relaxant (e.g., 5 mg diazepam, 1 to 2 tablets h.s.). The patient's case should be followed to ensure the symptoms resolve, and, if they do not, traditional TMD therapies should be instituted.

⊙ **QUICK CONSULT**

Failing to Relieve Symptoms

A patient who does not respond well to refining the occlusion, and for whom referred pain from the tooth has been ruled out, may have had his or her masticatory system aggravated during the dental procedure (e.g., from prolonged opening).

PREVENTING AGGRAVATION FROM DENTAL TREATMENT

Prolonged or extensive opening of the mouth in addition to forces applied to the mandible may aggravate the masticatory muscles and TMJs. Some individuals relate they have TMD symptoms only after aggravating events such as dental treatment, whereas other TMD patients continue to suffer flare-ups from dental treatment despite considerable benefit from TMD therapy. Many techniques are available to decrease the aggravation that patients may experience from dental treatment.

Some patients relate their masticatory muscles and TMJs become sore or stiff during dental treatment and would appreciate the opportunity to take a break periodically to move their jaw. The practitioner may wish to inform patients they are "allowed" to take stretching breaks and devise a form of communication so patients can notify the practitioner when they would like a break.

A number of patients find they have less TMD discomfort after using a bite block, whereas others relate its use aggravates their symptoms. If a bite block is used, the practitioner should place it so the patient is open no further than will be needed for most of the intended procedure. The practitioner can periodically ask the patient to open wider and, as the patient requests, periodically remove it for stretching breaks. Once the bite block is placed, the patient should be informed that this is all the wider the practitioner needs him or her to open (at this time), that the patient should rest the teeth only lightly on the block (not bite it), and that the patient should indicate whenever a break is desired. Patients who previously found that the use of the bite block aggravated their symptoms may want to try it again using these recommendations.

Make a patient's appointments for when the patient has minimal symptoms. If the patient has a daily symptom pattern, make the appointment for the portion of the day when the symptoms will be minimal. If the patient can predict future stressful or relaxing times, these usually affect the TMD symptoms, so appointments can be scheduled when the symptoms will be minimal. Some patients prefer short appointments, whereas others may prefer longer appointments that enable them to suffer through the postoperative discomfort fewer times.

Making Appointments
Make a patient's appointments for when the patient has minimal symptoms.

Some patients may desire premedication, others prefer postoperative medication, and some may need both. Many patients who develop mild to moderate TMD pain from dental procedures receive adequate relief from 800 mg ibuprofen, t.i.d. Depending on the severity of their symptoms, they may desire to start 1 or 2 days before the procedure and take it afterward for as long as needed. If ibuprofen does not provide adequate relief, I tend to prescribe patients who have TMJ inflammation 500 mg naproxen, 1 tablet b.i.d. If the pain is primarily of muscle origin, I tend to prescribe 5 mg diazepam and dose as needed; if the patient is to take it during the day, the potential side effects and ramifications must be discussed.

The fear of symptom aggravation may cause TMD patients to be reluctant to seek routine dental care and perform routine oral hygiene.[11] Empathy for their disorder and encouragement to obtain routine dental care and perform routine oral hygiene are usually quite beneficial for these patients.

If a patient has TMD symptoms, but needs to have restorations placed prior to occlusal appliance fabrication, the patient may desire to have a temporary appliance (e.g., soft appliance) fabricated until the restorations are completed. An alternative is to complete the restorations on the arch that needs the least treatment, fabricate an appliance for this arch, and adjust the appliance's occlusal surface as the opposing restorations are placed.

With all patients, be cautious not to overly strain the masticatory system. Whenever force is applied to the mandible, a balancing force should be applied with the nondominant hand to support the mandible. Some patients are more prone to developing TMD, and forces that do not bother most patients may cause TMD symptoms among patients more predisposed to the disorder. The occlusion of all new restorations must be adjusted so they are in harmony with the rest of the dentition or the patient may develop TMD symptoms.

OBSTRUCTIVE SLEEP APNEA APPLIANCES

Obstructive sleep apnea (OSA) appliances have been shown to help patients manage snoring and OSA. TMD symptoms (muscle pain, TMJ pain, and/or TMJ noise) are reported by up to 40 percent of patients using these appliances and are the most common reason they discontinue using their appliances.[12-15]

⊙ FOCAL POINT
TMD symptoms are reported by up to 40 percent of patients using obstructive sleep apnea appliances and are the most common reason patients discontinue using their appliances.

Many techniques are used to reduce the TMD symptoms associated with these appliances. Some practitioners use analgesics (e.g., ibuprofen) and ask patients to increase the appliance wear slowly up to tolerance, whereas others ask patients to reduce the appliance use and perform stretching exercises.[14,16]

Occlusal changes are another common complaint among patients wearing these appliances.[12,14] Some are thought to be permanent occlusal changes, whereas others are due to muscle and/or TMJ dysfunction and resolve on their own after the appliance is removed or after jaw-stretching exercises.[14,15]

Clinically it has been observed that patients who develop TMD symptoms from the use of these appliances receive benefit from a stabilization appliance (the standard flat-plane appliance). It is recommended patients alternate the use of these appliances at their discretion, using their judgment to balance the appliance wear with their TMD and snoring or sleep apnea symptoms.

Some clinicians believe the two-piece OSA appliance that allows the patient freedom to move the jaw laterally is less likely to cause TMD symptoms. Intuitively this seems plausible, but the only comparative study performed did not find a difference with the TMD symptom development.[16,17]

If TMD symptoms are derived from holding the mandible forward, limiting the mandibular advancement to the amount that satisfactorily relieves the snoring or obstructive sleep apnea may reduce the likelihood of these patients developing symptoms. Based on this hypothesis, it appears an adjustable mandibular advancement appliance where the patient would adjust the appliance to titrate between his or her TMD and snoring or sleep apnea symptoms would provide the most satisfactory results. The results of comparative studies evaluating TMD symptoms are not yet available.

Since OSA appliances aggravate the masticatory musculoskeletal system, it is conceivable that traditional TMD therapies may reduce the propensity for patients developing symptoms and benefit patients who develop symptoms from wearing these appliances. It is speculated that the TMD therapies shown to be more beneficial for morning pain (e.g., employing a relaxation exercise just prior to sleep) would have greater benefit for these patients.[18] Traditional TMD therapies are discussed in Part IV, "Multidisciplinary Treatment Approach."

Some practitioners find their patients can obtain satisfactory OSA relief with a single arch appliance that increases only the vertical and does not hold the mandible in a protruded position.[19] This may reduce the TMD problems associated with the OSA appliances, but comparative studies need to be performed.

Randomized clinical trials comparing the presented hypotheses will facilitate our ability to more effectively help patients manage their snoring and obstructive sleep apnea, while minimizing their TMD symptoms.

REFERENCES

1. Madan GA, Madan SG, Madan AD. Failure of inferior alveolar nerve block: exploring the alternatives. J Am Dent Assoc 2002;133(7):843–6.
2. Blanton PL, Jeske AH. Avoiding complications in local anesthesia induction: anatomical considerations. J Am Dent Assoc 2003;134(7):888–93.
3. Mense S, Simons DG, Russell IJ. Muscle Pain: Understanding Its Nature, Diagnosis, and Treatment. Philadelphia: Lippincott Williams & Wilkins, 2001:117, 120, 122.
4. Okeson JP. Bell's Orofacial Pains, 5th edition. Carol Stream, IL: Quintessence, 1995:285, 310–1.
5. Okeson JP. Management of Temporomandibular Disorders and Occlusion, 5th edition. St Louis: CV Mosby, 2003:337–8, 419–20.
6. Randow K, Carlsson K, Edlund J, Oberg T. The effect of an occlusal interference on the masticatory system: an experimental investigation. Odontol Revy 1976;27(4):245–56.
7. Riise C, Sheikholeslam A. The influence of experimental interfering occlusal contacts on the postural activity of the anterior temporal and masseter muscles in young adults. J Oral Rehabil 1982;9:419–25.
8. Le Bell Y, Jamsa T, Korri S, Niemi PM, Alanen P. Effect of artificial occlusal interferences depends on previous experience of temporomandibular disorders. Acta Odontol Scand 2002;60(4):219–22.
9. Clark GT, Tsukiyama Y, Baba K, Watanabe T. Sixty-eight years of experimental occlusal interference studies: what have we learned? J Prosthet Dent 1999;2:704–13.
10. Magnusson T, Enbom L. Signs and symptoms of mandibular dysfunction after introduction of experimental balancing-side interferences. Acta Odontol Scand 1984;42:129–35.
11. Humphrey SP, Lindroth JE, Carlson CR. Routine dental care in patients with temporomandibular disorders. J Orofac Pain 2002;16(2):129–34.
12. Clark GT, Sohn J-W, Hong CN. Treating obstructive sleep apnea and snoring: assessment of an anterior mandibular positioning device. J Am Dent Assoc 2000;131(6):765–71.
13. Friedlander AH, Walker LA, Friedlander IK, Felsenfeld AL. Diagnosing and comanaging pa-

tients with obstructive sleep apnea syndrome. J Am Dent Assoc 2000;131(8):1178–84.

14. Pantin CC, Hillman DR, Tennant M. Dental side effects of an oral device to treat snoring and obstructive sleep apnea. Sleep 1999;22(2):237–40.

15. Lindman R, Bondemark L. A review of oral devices in the treatment of habitual snoring and obstructive sleep apnoea. Swed Dent J 2001;25(1): 39–51.

16. George PT. Selecting sleep-disordered-breathing appliances, biomechanical considerations. J Am Dent Assoc 2000;132(3):339–47.

17. Bloch KE, Iseli A, Zhang JN, Xie X, Kaplan V, Stoeckli PW, Russi EW. A randomized, controlled crossover trial of two oral appliances for sleep apnea treatment. Am J Respir Crit Care Med 2000;162(1):246–51.

18. Lavigne GJ, Goulet J-P, Zuconni M, Morisson F, Lobbezoo F. Sleep disorders and the dental patient: an overview. Oral Surg Oral Med Oral Pathol Oral Radiol Endod 1999;88:257–72.

19. Bailey DR. Oral device therapy for TMD and sleep disordered breathing conditions: combination therapy. In: 27th Scientific Meeting on Orofacial Pain and Temporomandibular Disorders, April 18-21, 2002, San Antonio. Mt Royal, NJ: American Academy of Orofacial Pain, 2002.

Chapter 9

Lateral Pterygoid Myospasm

This is the most common disorder seen among the emergency TMD patients I am referred. Patients and their dentists are often frantic because it develops relatively rapidly, and the patient can no longer close his or her teeth into maximum intercuspation (MI) and can no longer open wide. The patient also has constant pain and palpation tenderness of the lateral pterygoid area.

⊙ QUICK CONSULTS

Observing Emergency TMD Patients

The lateral pterygoid myospasm is the most common disorder seen among the emergency TMD patients I am referred.

Observing for Lateral Pterygoid Myospasm

Lateral pterygoid myospasm develops relatively rapidly, the patient can no longer close his or her teeth into maximum intercuspation, can no longer open wide, has constant pain, and has palpation tenderness of the lateral pterygoid area.

A *myospasm* is the involuntary contracture of a muscle, causing pain and interfering with the muscle's ability to move. This disorder has awakened many of us during the middle of the night with a painful cramp in one's calf muscle.[1]

When the inferior lateral pterygoid muscle has a myospasm, it is in a partially shortened state and holds the condyle in a translated position. This is generally far enough forward that the teeth no longer mesh into MI. Additionally the slope of the articular eminence dictates that, with the condyle translated, there is a space that forms between the ipsilateral posterior teeth (see Figure 9-1).

Similar to awaking with a calf myospasm in which the individual has difficulty and increased pain when attempting to move the foot up or down, the person with a lateral pterygoid myospasm has difficulty and increased pain attempting to translate the condyle forward or retrude the jaw so the teeth fit into MI. The patient usually complains of the inability to put the ipsilateral posterior teeth together without excruciating pain, and the first tooth contact is in the area of the contralateral canine (if the patient has a normal tooth alignment). Since the patient also has difficulty translating, he or she usually has a marked limited opening.

The severity of the myospasm may vary, so the extent of these symptoms will differ from patient to patient; e.g., a patient with minimal symptoms may complain about pain only when closing into MI. The overview drawing (top left) of the "TMJ Disc Displacements" diagram (Appendix 2)

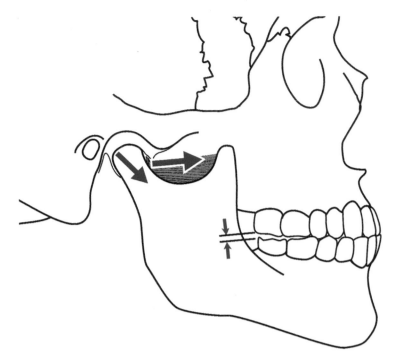

Figure 9-1. Lateral pterygoid myospasm often causes a gap between the ipsilateral posterior teeth.

is used to visually explain the lateral pterygoid myospasm symptoms to the patient.

Explaining Lateral Pterygoid Myospasm Symptoms

The overview drawing (top left) of the TMJ Disc Displacements diagram (Appendix 2) is used to visually explain the lateral pterygoid myospasm symptoms to the patient.

The condyle could also be held in a partially translated location by TMJ inflammation or a combination of both disorders. A simple test tentatively to differentiate these is first to ask the patient to bite on the posterior ipsilateral teeth. If the patient has a lateral pterygoid myospasm, as he or she bites, the gap between the teeth closes, the teeth are forced toward MI, the inferior lateral pterygoid muscle stretches, and the patient's pain is aggravated. If the patient has TMJ inflammation, the TMJ is loaded and also aggravating the pain. This initial bite enables the patient to register the amount of pain elicited by the exerted force.

Next, place two or three wooden tongue depressors (three are needed with more severe symptoms) over the occlusal surfaces of the posterior teeth, as shown in Figure 9-2, and ask the patient to bite on the tongue depressors. The tongue depressors prevent the interdigitation of the teeth and are usually sufficiently thick to support the gap between

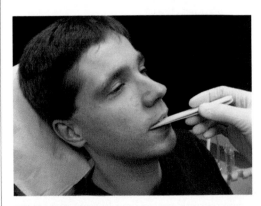

Figure 9-2. Wooden tongue depressors used to test for lateral pterygoid myospasm.

the teeth so the lateral pterygoid muscle is not stretched.[2] Clinical experience has shown that, if the patient has no pain when biting on the depressors, the lateral pterygoid myospasm is more probably the primary cause for the symptoms, and the tentative diagnosis is lateral pterygoid myospasm.

Clinically it appears biting on the tongue depressors allows sufficient loading of the TMJ so that, if TMJ inflammation is contributing to the patient's pain, biting aggravates the TMJ pain. Clinical experience has shown that, if the patient reports similar pain when biting on the tongue depressors as without them, TMJ inflammation is more probably the primary cause of the patient's symptoms, and the tentative diagnosis is TMJ inflammation. Sometimes patients report biting on the depressors hurts less than without them, in which case it is generally observed that both lateral pterygoid myospasm and TMJ inflammation are contributing to the patient's symptoms.

Finally the tentative diagnosis is confirmed by palpating the TMJ and lateral pterygoid area as described in "Palpation" in Chapter 3. Tenderness should correspond to the tentative diagnosis derived from the tongue depressor test. Based on the two tests, diagnose lateral pterygoid myospasm, TMJ inflammation, or a combination (the more severe being the primary diagnosis and the other being the secondary diagnosis).

▼ TECHNICAL TIP
Differentiating Lateral Pterygoid Myospasm and TMJ Inflammation
Diagnose lateral pterygoid myospasm, TMJ inflammation, or a combination, based on a patient's symptoms, the tongue depressor test, and palpation tenderness.

Practitioners need to keep in mind that other, rarely observed disorders may cause similar symptoms and are beyond the scope of this book. I once observed an individual who had an external ear infection that caused a similar inability to close into MI. The patient clearly knew the ear was the source of his pain and recognized the inability to close into MI; additionally the opening was not restricted. If a patient does not adequately respond to initial therapy or there is cause for other concerns, the practitioner may want to take a screening image of the TMJ with a plain radiograph (e.g., transcranial radiographs) or panoramic radiograph.

It is recommended that lateral pterygoid myospasm treatment be provided in a tiered approach and the initial therapies be observed to determine whether they adequately resolve the problem. Initially provide the patient with the "TMD Self-management Therapies" handout (Appendix 3) and with an exercise to stretch the lateral pterygoid muscle. If the muscle pain is severe enough to justify medications, patients usually benefit from an analgesic (e.g., 800 mg ibuprofen, t.i.d.) and a muscle relaxant (e.g., 5 mg diazepam, 1 to 2 tablets h.s.).

◉ QUICK CONSULTS
Providing Tiered-approach Treatment
It is recommended that lateral pterygoid myospasm treatment be provided in a tiered approach and the initial therapies be observed to determine whether they adequately resolve the problem.

TMD-stretching exercises (as in Appendix 5) are generally for closure muscles and will tend to aggravate a painful lateral pterygoid muscle. To stretch the inferior lateral pterygoid muscle, place the thumb on the most posterior ipsilateral teeth and wrap the fingers around the mandible, as depicted in Figure 9-3. One may prefer to use the dominant or nondominant hand. Some practitioners like to place gauze between the patient's teeth and their thumb to prevent discomfort from pressing on the cusp tips.

Push down with the thumb and pull up

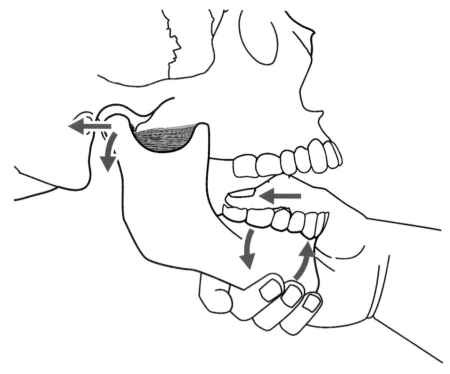

Figure 9-3. Stretching the lateral pterygoid muscle.

on the chin. This rotates the mandible, distracts the condyle, and provides more room to mobilize the condyle. While distracting the condyle, slowly push the mandible posteriorly up to approximately 4 pounds of force and hold for about 30 seconds. Release the force, but maintain the hand position on the mandible.

After about 10 seconds, repeat the 30-second stretch of the lateral pterygoid muscle. Perform six of these stretches, remove the hand, and ask the patient to close lightly. The patient generally relates that the teeth fit together better and the pain has decreased. Ask the patient to practice this stretch on himself or herself, and advise the patient on performing the maneuver as needed.

Patients who have TMJ inflammation may have their pain aggravated when the mandible is pushed posteriorly. If the patient has TMJ inflammation in conjunction with the lateral pterygoid myospasm, slowly stretch the lateral pterygoid muscle and ask

the patient whether you are applying too much force.

The patient should perform this gradual active stretch of the inferior lateral pterygoid muscle up to tolerance, ensuring that neither the muscle nor the TMJ is aggravated from this procedure. It is recommended the patient perform a series of six stretches, six times a day, and hold each stretch for 30 seconds.

If the patient cannot perform the stretches in this manner or prefers not to place his or her fingers in the mouth, an alternative technique has been recommended in which the patient uses a tongue depressor to disengage the teeth and help retrude the mandible. The patient performs this exercise by placing a tongue depressor between the maxillary and mandibular incisors with the extraoral end of the tongue depressor tipped down at an angle of approximately 45° to the vertical. The patient slowly protrudes the mandible along the tongue depressor, then relaxes the jaw and retrudes the mandible up the incline,[3] and holds the retruded position as recommended previously.

At the follow-up appointment, the great majority of my patients with lateral pterygoid myospasm report that the exercises have resolved or are controlling their symptoms and they have no desire to escalate therapy. If these initial therapies do not resolve the myospasm or if the myospasm continues to recur, then traditional TMD therapies (e.g., occlusal appliance therapy, or identifying and changing contributing factors) should be implemented and have been shown to be beneficial.

◉ **QUICK CONSULTS**
Reducing Symptoms of Lateral Pterygoid Myospasm

The great majority of my patients with lateral pterygoid myospasm report that the stretching exercises have resolved or are controlling their symptoms and they have no desire to escalate therapy.

If the diagnosis includes TMJ inflammation, it is generally recommended that the patient be provided an anti-inflammatory medication. If there is only mild TMJ inflammation in comparison to the lateral pterygoid myospasm, I consider prescribing 500 mg naproxen, b.i.d. If the primary diagnosis is TMJ inflammation, if the condition is of recent onset or an acute aggravation of a chronic condition, and if the pain is mild to moderate, I provide the patient with "TMD Self-management Therapies" handout and tend to prescribe 500 mg naproxen, b.i.d. If the pain is a 6/10 or above, I consider prescribing the Medrol Dosepak-naproxen regimen discussed in "Anti-inflammatory Medications" in Chapter 17, in addition to the "TMD Self-management Therapies" handout (Appendix 3). The patient's case should be followed to ensure the symptoms resolve; otherwise, traditional TMD therapies should be initiated and have been shown to be beneficial in resolving TMJ inflammation.

Since the inability to close into MI is due to a temporary condition, it is important the practitioner does not adjust the occlusion at this transitory position.

REFERENCES

1. American Academy of Orofacial Pain, with Okeson JP (ed). Orofacial Pain: Guidelines for Assessment, Diagnosis and Management. Chicago: Quintessence, 1996:140.
2. Okeson JP. Bell's Orofacial Pains, 5th edition. Carol Stream, IL: Quintessence, 1995:283.
3. Gray RJ, Davies SJ. Emergency treatment of acute temporomandibular disorders: part 1. Dent Update 1997;24(4):170–3.

Chapter 10

Acute TMJ Disc Displacement without Reduction

FAQ

Q: If a patient has an acute TMJ disc displacement without reduction, should the practitioner attempt to "unlock" the TMJ?

A: The longer the patient has had the acute TMJ disc displacement without reduction, the less likely the dentist will be able to "unlock" the TMJ. There is no distinct time limit after which this procedure should not be attempted.

Patients with this disorder present with some similarities to patients with a lateral pterygoid myospasm; i.e., both patients have limited opening, and their contralateral and protrusive movements are generally restricted. Fortunately there are many differences that enable practitioners to separate these diagnoses clinically; e.g., a patient with an acute TMJ disc displacement without reduction generally can close his or her teeth into maximum intercuspation without pain.

◉ **QUICK CONSULT**

Observing for Acute TMJ Disc Displacement without Reduction

Patients with this disorder present with some similarities to patients with a lateral pterygoid myospasm; i.e., both patients have limited opening, and their contralateral and protrusive movements are generally restricted.

Differentiating from Lateral Pterygoid Myospasm

Patients with an acute TMJ disc displacement without reduction present with many differences from patients with a lateral pterygoid myospasm, the primary one being that the former can generally close their teeth into maximum intercuspation without pain.

The symptoms known to be associated with an acute TMJ disc displacement without reduction have been shown to be a reliable clinical indicator for this condition.[1] The condition occurs suddenly and includes restriction of mouth opening and of contralateral and protrusive movements; deflection of the mandible toward the ipsilateral side as the patient attempts to open maximally; and elimination of clicking, popping, or transient locking.[1]

This sudden onset is an immediate change; e.g., the patient may have been eating a meal with a normal opening and suddenly on the next bite the TMJ blocks the opening at the location where the TMJ normally clicked, popped, or transiently locked. Patients are usually aware that the TMJ's translation is blocked in this manner and typically have an initial restricted opening of approximately 20 to 30 mm.[2]

◉ QUICK CONSULT
Asking Patients about Symptoms
Patients are usually aware that the TMJ's translation is blocked in this manner and typically have an initial restricted opening of approximately 20 to 30 mm.

Clinically it has been observed that some patients with this disorder cannot or are reluctant to demonstrate the deviation upon maximal opening or the expected restricted movements. This may be due to pain on the contralateral side or guarding of the painful TMJ.

This disorder is demonstrated in the bottom right section of the "TMJ Disc Displacements" diagram (Appendix 2). As the individual opens and the condyle attempts to translate, the condyle is blocked by the disc's posterior band and cannot reduce onto the disc. As the patient repeatedly bumps into this restriction or attempts to open beyond it, the retrodiscal tissue is forcibly stretched, releasing inflammatory and pain mediators into the synovial fluid. This causes TMJ inflammation and is the basis for the TMJ pain.[3]

▼ TECHNICAL TIP
Explaining Acute TMJ Disc Displacement without Reduction
This disorder is demonstrated in the bottom right section of the "TMJ Disc Displacements" diagram (Appendix 2), which should be helpful in explaining the disorder to patients.

◖ FOCAL POINT
As the patient repeatedly bumps into this restriction or attempts to open beyond it, the retrodiscal tissue is forcibly stretched, releasing inflammatory and pain mediators into the synovial fluid.

The patient generally points to the TMJ as the source of the pain, and the TMJ is generally the most palpation-tender masticatory structure. The masticatory muscles often tighten in response to the TMJ pain (protective muscle splinting), so they are also frequently tender and painful. If there is a question about the source of the restriction, the patient's mouth can be stretched to aggravate the restricting structure (as discussed in "Additional Evaluations" in Chapter 3).

Some patients with this disorder also complain about painful anterior and/or posterior digastric muscles, which are small jaw-opening muscles that are not developed to provide repeated forceful contractions. These muscles are generally painful from the patient repeatedly opening his or her mouth, pushing against the disc, in an attempt to free or stretch this restriction. Occasionally these muscles are as painful as the TMJ.

Direct trauma occasionally causes an acute TMJ disc displacement without reduction.[4] If the patient relates the sudden limited opening is due to external trauma, then muscle injury, TMJ inflammation, and fracture should also be considered as possible causes of the restriction. In this situation, a panoramic radiograph should be taken to rule out a fracture.

This disorder's onset is most commonly related to repeated loading of the TMJ through activities such as parafunctional habits.[5,6] Thinning of the retrodiscal tissue is speculated to cause the disorder,[3,7] and parafunctional habits as well as loading of the TMJ can decrease the joint space.[8,9]

An easy manner in which to explain this disorder to patients is through the use of the

"TMJ Disc Displacements" diagram (Appendix 2). Start by orientating the patient to the diagrams and explain the mechanism of the disc displacement with reduction (which the vast majority of patients had prior to the onset) in the bottom left diagram. Explain that the condyle repeatedly loaded the retrodiscal tissue (through parafunctional habits, eating tough foods, etc.), thereby thinning the tissue so the condyle is now higher in the mandibular fossa. For the condyle to reduce onto the disc, it must now fall further to travel below the posterior band. This is more difficult, and in the patient's situation the condyle cannot move below the posterior band. The posterior band now blocks the condyle from translating forward, as shown in the bottom right diagram.

Depending on how I plan to treat the disorder, I may inform the patient that the tension held in the muscles (the closure muscles: masseter, temporalis, and medial pterygoid) contributes to the continuation of the disorder by bracing the condyle higher in the mandibular fossa. I also might inform the patient that the tension held in the muscles continues to load the retrodiscal tissue, aggravating the TMJ. This tension is usually related to stress, parafunctional habits, or eating.

Some patients complain that this disorder occurs only intermittently and is not present at the time of the dental appointment. It is recommended that this be diagnosed as *intermittent acute TMJ disc displacement without reduction*, the mechanical problem just discussed be reviewed, and inquiry made about the type of events that seem to precede or initiate the disorder. Patients commonly report an increase in clicking and/or intermittent locking severity associated with daytime parafunctional habits, nocturnal parafunctional habits, or eating.[3]

If the patient awakes with the intermittent disorder, nocturnal parafunctional habits are probably the primary contributor,

and it is recommended that the practitioner (a) review the "TMD Self-management Therapies" (Appendix 3), with special emphasis on sleep posture; and (b) provide the patient with an occlusal appliance that is worn at night. If the disorder is not adequately resolved by these therapies, other traditional TMD therapies should benefit this disorder (see "Integration of Conservative Therapies" in Chapter 19).

◉ **QUICK CONSULT**

Observing Waking Intermittent Symptoms

If the patient awakes with the intermittent disorder, nocturnal parafunctional habits are probably the primary contributor.

If the intermittent disorder occurs during the day, the primary contributors are probably daytime muscle tension and/or parafunctional habits. In addition to the TMD self-management instructions, it is recommended that the patient become aware of the daytime muscle tension and parafunctional habits, and learn to break them (breaking these parafunctional habits is discussed in "Breaking Daytime Habits" in Chapter 14). If this does not adequately resolve the disorder, I would ask a psychologist to help the patient break the daytime parafunctional habits (as discussed in "Breaking Daytime Habits" in Chapter 16). If the patient needed additional assistance, it is recommended that therapy be escalated by fabricating an appliance for the patient to wear at night to decrease the impact any nocturnal parafunctional habits may have on the problem. Until the patient learns to control the daytime muscle tension and parafunctional habits, the appliance may also be worn for a limited time during the day, especially in situations the patient relates to preceding or initiating the disorder (except for eating). If these techniques do not adequately resolve the disorder, other traditional TMD therapies should benefit this disorder (see

"Integration of Conservative Therapies" in Chapter 19).

Observing Daytime Intermittent Symptoms

If the intermittent disorder occurs during the day, the primary contributors probably are daytime muscle tension and/or parafunctional habits.

For patients with the intermittent disorder, three techniques can be discussed that they may find beneficial in "unlocking" their TMJ. About half of my patients can "unlock" their TMJ by placing their finger about 1/2 inch anterior to their TMJ, pressing medially and slightly posterior, and moving the mandible side to side. It is speculated this pressure tends to push tissue between the condyle and fossa, helping to distract the condyle, enabling it to slide more easily under the posterior band of the disc.

Unlocking an intermittent Acute TMJ Disc Displacement without Reduction

For patients with the intermittent disorder, three techniques can be discussed that they may find beneficial in "unlocking" their TMJ.

A second procedure is for patients consciously to relax and massage the temporalis and masseter muscles. As these muscles relax, ask patients to move the mandible side to side. It is speculated that the closure muscles are often tight when the intermittent disorder occurs, bracing the condyle higher in the fossa. As these muscles relax, the condyle distracts slightly, enabling it to slide more easily under the posterior band of the disc as the patient moves the mandible to the contralateral side.

A third technique some find beneficial is to slide the mandible as far as possible to the contralateral side and then open maximally.[4] This attempts to forcibly reduce the condyle onto the disc and may cause discomfort as this vigorous reduction occurs.

It is recommended patients first try pressing in front of the TMJ, because this is a quick nonaggravating maneuver. If that does not unlock the TMJ, then try relaxing and massaging the temporalis and masseter muscles while moving the mandible side to side. It is recommended the third maneuver be used as a last resort because of the discomfort that can occur when the condyle abruptly reduces.

It is recommended patients with the intermittent disorder be treated with conservative therapies in an attempt to resolve their intermittent locking and TMD pain. Otherwise, it is feared that the disorder may progress from intermittent to continuous, and TMD pain severity appears to be one of the factors predicting which patients will be thus affected.[10]

In treating patients who have the continuous disorder, some practitioners attempt to unlock the TMJ if it has been a problem for less than several weeks. There is no distinct time limit after which this procedure should not be attempted, but the longer the patient has had this disorder, the less likely the dentist will be able to unlock the TMJ.[3,4] The practitioner can easily tell whether the unlocking procedure was clinically successful, because the patient immediately regains the normal opening, even though findings on magnetic resonance imaging often show complete reduction is not obtained.[11]

One technique is to first have the patient attempt to self-unlock. Ask the patient to consciously relax and massage the closure muscles, and then make several attempts at unlocking the TMJ by moving the mandible to the contralateral side as far as possible and opening maximally. If this is unsuccessful, the practitioner can manually distract the TMJ by placing the thumb on the most posterior ipsilateral teeth, wrapping the fingers

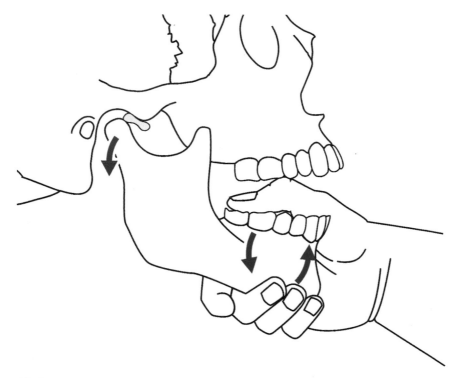

Figure 10-1. Manually distracting the TMJ.

around the mandible, and pressing down on the posterior teeth and up on the chin (Figure 10-1). This motion is similar to removing the cap from a soda pop bottle. Some practitioners like to place gauze between the teeth and their thumb to prevent discomfort from pressing on the cusp tips. While distracting the TMJ, ask the patient to repeat the prior movements several times.[4] If this is unsuccessful, while continuing to distract the TMJ, the practitioner can attempt to move the condyle forward and medial (the usual location of the disc) in an attempt to unlock the TMJ (Figure 10-2).

If these were unsuccessful and the patient and practitioner would like to continue attempting to unlock the TMJ, many additional procedures can be used in conjunction with the manipulation. They attempt to decrease the patient's pain (which reduces the patient guarding) and/or relax the patient (which reduces the tension in the closure muscles). These procedures include nitrous oxide–oxygen inhalation, lateral pterygoid muscle anesthetic injection, lateral pterygoid and masseter muscle anesthetic injection, TMJ anesthetic injection, and an oral anti-inflammatory and/or muscle relaxant prescription.[3,12-14] Once these medication(s) have taken effect, the practitioner can attempt to unlock the TMJ by the same manipulations described previously.

If the practitioner is successful at unlocking the TMJ, the patient often needs to wear an anterior positioning appliance to hold the condyle in the reduced position (Figure 10-3). Otherwise, the condyle will tend to lock again when it is retruded off the disc. A quick, easy technique for fabricating a temporary anterior positioning appliance is to use the putty that is used for crown and bridge impressions.[15] Ask the patient to place the anterior teeth end to end, which provides a stable reproducible position where the condyle is usually reduced on the disc. Mix the putty into the shape of a thick rope

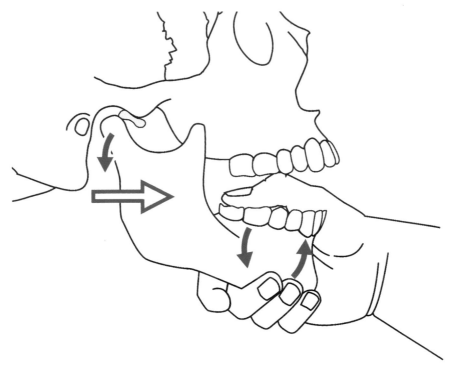

Figure 10-2. Moving the condyle forward and medial while manually distracting the TMJ.

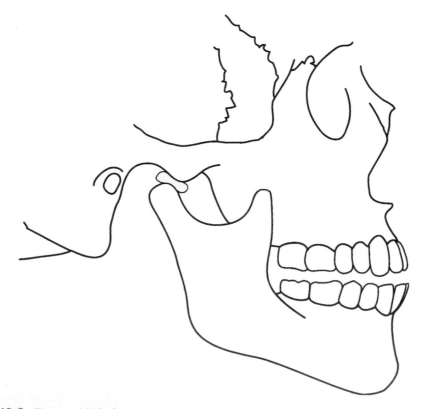

Figure 10-3. The condyle in the reduced position.

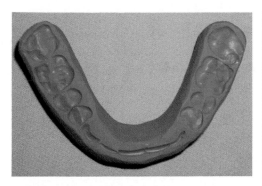

Figure 10-4. Mandibular view of the temporary anterior positioning appliance.

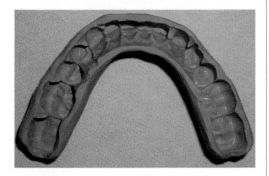

Figure 10-5. Maxillary view of the temporary anterior positioning appliance.

4 to 5 inches long, ask the patient to open, place the material along the occlusal-incisal surfaces of the teeth, and ask the patient to close back to the end-to-end position. Adjust the appliance so it is retentive for the mandibular teeth and has only approximately 1- to 2-mm-deep incisal indentations for the maxillary teeth (Figures 10-4 and 10-5).

▼ TECHNICAL TIP
Fabricating a Temporary Anterior Positioning Appliance
A quick, easy technique for fabricating a temporary anterior positioning appliance is to use the putty that is used for crown and bridge impressions.

The need to wear this appliance will vary with a patient's propensity for redeveloping this disorder. Initially many patients need to wear the appliance 24 hours a day, including while eating. If a patient does not have a stabilization appliance because of the time needed for its fabrication, the practitioner may desire to make impressions as soon as the patient can tolerate it. After a week or so, the patient may be able to transition from the anterior positioning appliance to wearing the stabilization appliance 24 hours a day, but this needs to be modulated by the patient's propensity for redeveloping the disorder. Similarly, over time, the patient can slowly reduce the wear of the stabilization appliance, modulated by this propensity. Depending on the pain severity associated with this disorder, the practitioner may desire to prescribe an anti-inflammatory and/or muscle relaxant (as discussed below and in Chapter 17, "Pharmacological Management").

Clinically I am not successful in unlocking the TMJs for many patients with this disorder. Even though the TMJ could not be unlocked or the practitioner does not feel comfortable attempting these manipulations or managing the patient once the TMJ unlocks, the vast majority of these patients do well with conservative TMD therapy.[12,16] In fact, many patients with this disorder improve without treatment;[17,18] the symptoms tend to gradually fade away over a few weeks or months.[1]

◉ QUICK CONSULT
Unlocking the TMJ
Clinically I am not successful in unlocking the TMJs for many patients with this disorder.

☻ FOCAL POINT
Even if patients' TMJs are not unlocked, the vast majority do well with conservative TMD therapy.

One study followed the cases of individuals who chose not to have treatment for this disorder (their symptoms tended to be mild) and found the approximate portions of the group at 6 months, 12 months, and 18 months whose symptoms had resolved were one-third, one-half, and two-thirds, respectively.[18] The investigators found that younger individuals more readily become asymptomatic without treatment.[19]

It is speculated that the reason people can progress through this disorder is that they often unintentionally apply a stretching force to their retrodiscal tissue. Every time an individual with this disorder opens to the restriction, the condyle pushes the disc forward. This may unintentionally occur when the person talks, laughs, puts food in the mouth, etc. Repeatedly bumping or pushing the disc in this manner will often sufficiently stretch the retrodiscal tissue over time. As the retrodiscal tissue is stretched, the disc moves forward, eventually the disc is pushed out of the condyle's translation path, and the individual regains the normal opening. As this progression occurs, the retrodiscal tissue typically gets stretched less often, and the amount of inflammatory and pain mediators released into the synovial fluid is correspondingly reduced, allowing the TMJ inflammation to improve proportionally. If the microtrauma to the retrodiscal tissue (from parafunctional habits, muscle tension, etc.) is satisfactorily small, the TMJ inflammation may totally resolve.

⚉ **FOCAL POINT**
Every time an individual with this disorder opens to the restriction, the condyle pushes the disc forward. Repeatedly bumping or pushing the disc in this manner will often sufficiently stretch the retrodiscal tissue over time.

Even though many individuals can progress through this disorder with minimal treatment, others have excruciating pain and desperately need help. Conservative treatment for this disorder primarily attempts to reduce the TMJ inflammation and TMJ loading. This promotes a synovial fluid environment that facilitates more rapid adaptive alterations of the retrodiscal tissue. Additionally patients often benefit from adjunctive stretching to help mobilize the disc out of the condyle's translation path.

Sufficient studies have not been completed to suggest a specific conservative therapy regimen, and conservative therapy's success is highly variable from patient to patient.[6] Most patients with this disorder are successfully treated with conservative TMD therapies, but some patients will not satisfactorily improve and will need to have their level of therapy escalated.

The amount of conservative therapy I initially provide these patients varies with the level of their pain, the length of time they have had the disorder, and whether their limited opening has improved. It is recommended all of these patients be provided with the explanation discussed earlier and a "TMD Self-management Therapies" handout (Appendix 3), emphasizing the importance of observing for and breaking any daytime contributing habits.

◉ **QUICK CONSULT**
Proving Conservative Therapy
The amount of conservative therapy I initially provide these patients varies with the level of their pain, the length of time they have had the disorder, and whether their limited opening has improved.

Most of my patients receive a stretching exercise unless they have such TMJ pain that it is believed performing the exercise will be too painful at the time, or a patient has rapidly regained most of the opening and the exercise is considered unnecessary. The exercise tends to aggravate the TMJ, but most patients are prescribed an anti-inflammatory medication, so they generally can tolerate the exercise. The patient is instructed to perform the exercise as shown in Figure 5-1, hold the stretch 30 to 60 seconds, and sporadically perform this approximately six times throughout the day. The patient needs to balance the amount of force, length of time the stretch is held, and number of times the stretch is performed throughout the day, so the resulting TMJ pain is tolerable.[4] Patients are asked, when possible, to preheat the TMJ with a heating pad prior the exercise.[20]

As a general pharmaceutical guide, I tend to prescribe the following for patients with constant pain. This will vary with a patient's fluctuating pain-intensity pattern, the TMJ palpation tenderness, and the emotional impact of the disorder. If the patient has a low level of TMJ pain (3/10 or below), I tend to prescribe 500 mg naproxen, b.i.d. If the TMJ pain is above 5/10, I consider prescribing the Medrol Dosepak-naproxen regimen discussed in "Anti-inflammatory Medications" in Chapter 17. If nocturnal parafunctional habits appear to be contributing to the TMJ inflammation (the patient awakes with greater TMJ pain), I also tend to prescribe 5 mg diazepam, 1 to 2 tablets h.s., to decrease the nocturnal parafunctional habits until a stabilization appliance can be inserted.

If there is muscle pain, I tend to prescribe 5 mg diazepam, 1 to 2 tablets h.s. If the patient has significant muscle pain causing a substantial amount of daytime pain, I consider discussing the possibility of the patient also taking 1/2 tablet in the morning and afternoon; the potential side effects and ramifications must be discussed. I maintain the patient on 5 mg diazepam, 1 to 2 tablets h.s., and/or nonsteroid anti-inflammatory drugs as long as it appears they are beneficial. This is the only TMD disorder for which I might continue prescribing diazepam for longer than 2 to 3 weeks.

The longer patients have had this disorder, the less likely they are to do well with conservative therapy.[6] Therefore, at the initial exam, if a patient reports having had the disorder for more than 2 months or so, especially if the patient has not observed improvement in limited opening, I tend to include a stabilization appliance as part of my initial therapy. A stabilization appliance, in addition to these other therapies, generally provides greater benefit for these patients.[6,16]

If a patient cannot open wide enough that an adequate mandibular impression can be made, the provider has several options: (a) make only a maxillary impression and fabricate an appliance that does not need an opposing cast, e.g., soft appliance; or (b) make the mandibular impression after removing a portion of the tray's lingual flange. If this results in an inadequate impression and a mandibular appliance is preferred, (c) fabricate a temporary mandibular appliance (e.g., soft appliance) and, if desired, replace it once the opening sufficiently improves.

During treatment, closely monitor the opening and pain level to ensure the patient is responding well to the initial therapy. If it appears the patient is not responding quite positively to this therapy over the next 1 or 2 weeks, and a stabilization appliance is not being used, escalate therapy by adding the appliance.

While under therapy, it is not uncommon for a patient to report that his or her TMJ has unlocked. This situation is different than when a practitioner manipulates a patient to unlock his or her TMJ, for in this situation the TMJ does not tend to relock immediately and therefore an anterior positioning appliance is not needed. Even though the TMJ unlocked, it is important that the patient continue therapy and become as asymptomatic as possible, for patients with greater pain appear to have a greater propensity for redeveloping this disorder.[10]

If a patient does not appear to be improving from the conservative therapy or is frustrated with the slow progress, the practitioner may desire to escalate treatment to an invasive procedure.[21] Studies show that conservative therapy, arthrocentesis, and arthroscopic surgery provide a similar degree of improvement for this disorder.[16,22] Flushing the pain and inflammatory mediators out of the TMJ through arthrocentesis or arthroscopic surgery appears to enable patients to rapidly stretch the retrodiscal tissue. If the perpetuating contributing factors (parafunctional habits, etc.) were never adequately controlled, though, TMD pain may return after the surgery and the contributing factors would need be addressed.[23,24]

◉ **QUICK CONSULT**
Escalating to an Invasive Procedure

If a patient does not appear to be improving from the conservative therapy or is frustrated with the slow progress, the practitioner may desire to escalate treatment to an invasive procedure.

Additionally referral for these procedures should not be unnecessarily delayed when it becomes evident that conservative therapy will not be successful; the longer the patient has this disorder, the less likely it is much benefit will be derived from arthrocentesis and the more likely it is arthroscopic surgery (more expensive and invasive) may be needed.[25] TMJ injections with anesthetic, steroid, and/or sodium hyaluronate (not yet approved by the FDA for use in the TMJ) have also been recommended and are also reasonable considerations for treating this disorder.[26,27]

An alternative hypothesis for this disorder has been presented in the literature, in which TMJ loading causes a breakdown of the synovial fluid, potentiating the tendency for the superior portion of the disc to adhere to the articular eminence in a fashion similar to a suction cup. It is theorized that the anterior displacement is caused by the disc adhering to the articular eminence while the condyle is translated and, as the condyle retrudes, the disc remains anchored anteriorly. Conservative therapy can decrease the TMJ loading and inflammation, allowing

the reconstitution of the "healthy" synovial fluid, thereby promoting the release of the adhered disc. Pressure injections and arthrocentesis can be beneficial for treatment of this condition and are recommended if conservative therapy is not successful.[21,28-30] As more information is obtained about this condition, it may become recognized as an independent TMD disorder.

Practitioners must bear in mind that a patient's inability to translate may be due to a neoplastic growth within the TMJ.[31] Neoplasia arising within the TMJ are extremely rare,[31] but the practitioner may desire to make a screening radiograph, such as a transcranial or panoramic radiograph, during the initial evaluation or if the initial therapy does not improve the patient's condition.

REFERENCES

1. Isberg A, Stenstrom B, Isacsson G. Frequency of bilateral temporomandibular joint disc displacement in patients with unilateral symptoms: a 5-year follow-up of the asymptomatic joint—a clinical and arthrotomographic study. Dentomaxillofac Radiol 1991;20(2):73–6.

2. Fricton JR, Schellhas KP, Braun BL, Hoffmann W, Bromaghim C. Joint disorders: derangements and degeneration. In: Fricton JR, Kroening RJ, Hathaway KM (eds). TMJ and Craniofacial Pain: Diagnosis and Management. St Louis: Ishiyaku EuroAmerica, 1988:85–130.

3. Pertes RA, Gross SG. Disorders of the temporomandibular joint. In: Pertes RA, Gross SG (eds). Clinical Management of Temporomandibular Disorders and Orofacial Pain. Chicago: Quintessence, 1995:75–8.

4. Okeson JP. Management of Temporomandibular Disorders and Occlusion, 5th edition. St Louis: CV Mosby, 2003:448–53.

5. Molina OF, dos Santos J Jr, Nelson SJ, Nowlin T. A clinical study of specific signs and symptoms of CMD in bruxers classified by the degree of severity. Cranio 1999;17(4):268–79.

6. Stiesch-Scholz M, Fink M, Tschernitschek H, Rossbach A. Medical and physical therapy of temporomandibular joint disk displacement without reduction. Cranio 2002;20(2):85–90.

7. Okeson JP. Bell's Orofacial Pains, 5th edition. Carol Stream, IL: Quintessence, 1995:310.

8. Kuboki T, Azuma Y, Orsini MG, Takenami Y, Yamashita A. The effect of sustained unbilateral molar clenching on the temporomandibular joint space. Oral Surg Oral Med Oral Pathol Oral Radiol Endod 1996;82(6):616–24.

9. Ito T, Gibbs CH, Marguelles-Bonnet R, Lupkiewicz SM, Young HM, Lundeen HC, Mahan PE. Loading on the temporomandibular joints with five occlusal conditions. J Prosthet Dent 1986;56(4):478–84.

10. Lundh H, Westesson P-L, Kopp S. A three-year follow-up of patients with reciprocal temporomandibular joint clicking. Oral Surg Oral Med Oral Pathol 1987;63(5):530–3.

11. Segami N, Murakami K, Iizuka T. Arthrographic evaluation of disk position following mandibular manipulation technique for internal derangement with closed lock of the temporomandibular joint. J Craniomandib Disord 1990;4(2):99–108.

12. Mongini F, Ibertis F, Manfredi A. Long-term results in patients with disc displacement without reduction treated conservatively. Cranio 1996;14(4):301–5.

13. Helkimo M, Hugoson A. Nitrous oxide–oxygen sedation in the diagnosis and treatment of temporomandibular joint locking: a clinical and methodological study. Cranio 1988;6(2):148–55.

14. Mongini F. A modified extraoral technique of mandibular manipulation in disk displacement without reduction. Cranio 1995;13(1):22–5.

15. Hicks NA. An efficient method for constructing a soft interocclusal splint. J Prosthet Dent 1989;61(1):48–50.

16. Schiffman E, Look J, Fricton J, Swift J, Wikes C, Templeton B, Anderson Q. TMJ disk displacement without reduction: a randomized clinical trial [abstract 3004]. J Dent Res (Special Issue) 1997;76:389.

17. Minakuchi H, Kuboki T, Matsuka Y, Maekawa K, Yatani H, Yamashita A. Randomized controlled evaluation of non-surgical treatments for temporomandibular joint anterior disk displacement without reduction. J Dent Res 200180(3): 924–8.

18. Sato S, Kawamura H, Nagasaka H, Motegi K. The natural course of anterior disc displacement without reduction in temporomandibular joint: follow-up at 6, 12, and 18 months. J Oral Maxillofac Surg 1997;55:234–8.

19. Sato S, Goto S, Kawamura H, Motegi K. The natural course of nonreducing disc displacement of the TMJ: relationship of clinical findings at initial visit to outcome after 12 months without treatment. J Orofac Pain 1997;11(4): 315–20.

20. Lentell G, Hetherington T, Eagan J, Morgan M. The use of thermal agents to influence the effectiveness of a low-load prolong stretch. J Orthop Sports Phys Ther 1992;16(5):200–7.

21. Reston JT, Turkelson CM. Meta-analysis of surgical treatments for temporomandibular articular disorders. J Oral Maxillofac Surg 2003;61(1): 3–10.

22. Murakami K, Hosaka H, Moriya Y, Segami N, Iizuka T. Short-term treatment outcome study for the management of temporomandibular joint closed lock: a comparison of arthrocentesis to nonsurgical therapy and arthroscopic lysis and lavage. Oral Surg Oral Med Oral Pathol Oral Radiol Endod 1995;80(3):253–7.

23. Schiffman E. Five-year followup of RCT comparing surgical and non-surgical TMJ acute locks. In: 26th Scientific Meeting on Orofacial Pain and Temporomandibular Disorders, March 23–25, 2001, Washington DC. Mt Royal, NJ: American Academy of Orofacial Pain, 2001.

24. Dimitroulis G. A review of 56 cases of chronic closed lock treated with temporomandibular joint arthroscopy. J Oral Maxillofac Surg 2002;60(5): 519–24.

25. Sakamoto I, Yoda T, Tsukahara H, Imai H, Enomoto S. Comparison of the effectiveness of arthrocentesis in acute and chronic closed lock: analysis of clinical and arthroscopic findings. Cranio 2000;18(4):264–71.

26. Sato S, Sakamoto M, Kawamura H, Motegi K. Disc position and morphology in patients with nonreducing disc displacement treated by injection of sodium hyaluronate. Int J Oral Maxillofac Surg 1999;28(4):253–7.

27. Suarez OF, Ourique SAM. An alternate technique for management of acute closed locks. Cranio 2000;18(3):168–73.

28. Nitzan DW, Etsion I. Adhesive force: the underlying cause of the disc anchorage to the fossa and/or eminence in the temporomandibular joint—a new concept. Int J Oral Maxillofac Surg 2002;31(1):94–9.

29. Nitzan DW, Samson B, Better H. Long-term outcome of arthrocentesis for sudden-onset, persist-

ent, severe close lock of the temporomandibular joint. J Oral Maxillofac Surg 1997;55:151–7.

30. Nitzan DW. Arthrocentesis for management of severe close lock of the temporomandibular joint. Oral Maxillofac Surg Clin North Am 1994;6:245–57.

31. Fantasia JE. Neoplasia. In: Kaplan AS, Assael LA (eds). Temporomandibular Disorders: Diagnosis and Treatment. Philadelphia: WB Saunders, 1991:251–61.

Chapter 11

TMJ Dislocation

A TMJ dislocation is diagnosed when a patient presents with or relates a history of momentary or prolonged inability to close the mandible from a maximal open position. This is due to the condyle being trapped in front of the articular eminence.[1] The entrapment may be from the articular eminence obstructing the posterior movement of the disc-condyle unit, the disc obstructing the posterior movement of the condyle, or a combination of the two.[2]

Diagnosing TMJ Dislocation

A TMJ dislocation is diagnosed when the patient presents with or relates a history of momentary or prolonged inability to close the mandible from a maximal open position.

It is very common for individuals to have this disorder and self-reduce.[3,4] Some define the self-reducing condition as *subluxation*,[3] but in this book (and as defined by the American Academy of Orofacial Pain) *dislocation* includes both when an individual is able or needs someone else to reduce the condyle.[1]

This disorder is extremely easy to diagnose. The patient relates a history of a sudden catching or locking near maximal opening (e.g., from a yawn, dental procedure, or yelling). If the duration is more than momentary, the closure muscles become painful, tend to develop spasms, and make it progressively more difficult to reduce the condyle over time. As individuals are unable to self-reduce, they often become distressed because the pain increases as they attempt to close their mouth.[4,5]

If a patient has a dislocation, the sooner the condyle is manipulated, the easier it is for the practitioner to reduce the dislocation. If the dislocation just recently occurred, it will probably be fairly easy to reduce through manipulation. However, few patients who have had the dislocation for a month or more can have it reduced through manipulation.[4]

Observing Ease of Manipulation

If a patient has a dislocation, the sooner the condyle is manipulated, the easier it is for the practitioner to reduce the dislocation.

Prior to attempting to reduce a patient's dislocation, explain to the patient how the temporalis and masseter muscles are tight and bracing the condyle in front of the articular eminence. Explain that he or she will need to concentrate and relax the muscles as the condyle is pushed down and around the eminence. While the patient is concentrating to relax his or her closure muscles, put gauze bilaterally over the mandibular molars, place your thumbs over the gauze (some practitioners place their thumbs on the buccal shelves), and wrap your fingers around the chin. Ask the patient to open wider, which physiologically causes the closure muscles to relax. As he or she attempts to open wider, bilaterally press down on the molars, press up on the chin, and slowly slide the mandible posteriorly.[5,6] Fortunately, so far, I have always been successful with this maneuver.

If this is unsuccessful, some practitioners recommend having an assistant activate the gag reflex by touching the patient's soft palate with a couple of cotton-tip applicators, while the practitioner reattempts the maneuver.[5,6] The gag reflex should more vigorously stimulate the opening muscles, providing a greater physiological inactivation of the closure muscles.

If this fails to reduce the condyle, medications may enable the manipulation to be successful. The medications are used in an attempt to relax the patient (which reduces the tension in the closure muscles) and/or decrease the pain (which reduces the patient's guarding). They may include nitrous oxide–oxygen inhalation, TMJ anesthetic injection, intravenous sedation, or general anesthesia.[4,5] Adjunctive procedures with manipulation have also been recommended, i.e., arthrocentesis, arthroscopic surgery, or open joint surgery.[3,7,8]

At this stage of therapy escalation, many practitioners refer the patient to someone with greater expertise in this area. An oral surgeon would be a reasonable choice.

Patients whose condyles were successfully reduced or who have a dislocation history may desire to prevent this from recurring. In this situation, it is recommended that preventative therapy be provided in an escalating fashion. First educate the patient about the mechanical problem; explain that, if the patient learns not to open too wide, the problem will not occur. The top left diagram of the "TMJ Disc Displacements" handout

(Appendix 2) may help to explain TMJ dislocation visually to patients. Warn them to be very cautious when they yawn, yell, and have dental treatment.

Some find this satisfactorily prevents the dislocation, whereas others have difficulty remembering to restrict their opening and thus desire to escalate therapy. The next therapy recommended is a stabilization appliance worn at night, which clinical experience has shown and others have observed generally reduces the frequency and intensity of a dislocation.[7,9] This may be due to the appliance's capability to decrease the TMJ loading, thereby improving the quality of the TMJ's lubricant (sodium hyaluronate).[7] Others theorize the dislocation is primarily due to a muscular disorder and the appliance decreases the dislocation's frequency and/or intensity through improvement of the muscle disorder.[9]

⊙ **QUICK CONSULT**

Reducing Dislocation's Frequency and Intensity

Wearing a stabilization appliance at night generally reduces the frequency and intensity of a dislocation.

If the appliance does not satisfactorily diminish the dislocation, it is recommended that the practitioner discuss three other options and let the patient decide which of these he or she is interested in pursuing: (a) If the patient desires help remembering to restrict the opening, it is recommended the patient be offered a referral to an orthodontist to have buttons placed on the molars. Plastic fishing line or elastics are placed around the buttons, so when the patient tries to open wide, he or she is reminded to restrict the opening. The patient wears this for 2 months.[6] (b) If the patient has trouble reducing when the dislocation occurs, it is recommended the patient be taught how to distract and reduce his or her condyle.[5] (c) If the dislocation is a significant problem, it is

recommended the patient be offered a referral to an oral surgeon to discuss a surgical
treatment for the dislocation.

▼ **TECHNICAL TIP**
Self-reducing a TMJ Dislocation
Sometimes I teach the patient how to distract
and reduce his or her condyle.

REFERENCES

1. American Academy of Orofacial Pain, with Okeson
   JP (ed). Orofacial Pain: Guidelines for Assessment,
   Diagnosis and Management. Chicago: Quintessence, 1996:134.
2. Yoda T, Imai H, Shinjyo T, Sakamoto I, Abe M,
   Enomoto S. Effect of arthrocentesis on TMJ disturbance of mouth closure with loud clicking: a
   preliminary study. Cranio 2002;20(1):18–22.
3. Shorey CW, Campbell JH. Dislocation of the
   temporomandibular joint. Oral Surg Oral Med
   Oral Pathol Oral Radiol Endod 2000;89(1):
   29–34.
4. Caminiti MF, Weinberg S. Chronic mandibular
   dislocation: the role of non-surgical and surgical
   treatment. J Can Dent Assoc 1998;64(7):484–91.
5. Pertes RA, Gross SG. Disorders of the temporomandibular joint. In: Pertes RA, Gross SG (eds).
   Clinical Management of Temporomandibular
   Disorders and Orofacial Pain. Chicago: Quintessence, 1995:80–1.
6. Okeson JP. Management of Temporomandibular
   Disorders and Occlusion, 5th edition. St Louis:
   CV Mosby, 2003:457–8.
7. Nitzan DW. Temporomandibular joint "open lock"
   versus condylar dislocation: signs and symptoms,
   imaging, treatment, and pathogenesis. J Oral
   Maxillofac Surg 2002;60(5):506–11.
8. Esposito C, Clear M, Veal SJ. Arthroscopic surgical
   treatment of temporomandibular joint hypermobil-
   ity with recurrent anterior dislocation: an alternative to open surgery. Cranio 1991;9(3):286–92.
9. Kai S, Kai H, Nakayama E, Tabata O, Tashiro H,
   Miyajima T, Sasaguri M. Clinical symptoms of
   open lock position of the condyle: relation to anterior dislocation of the temporomandibular joint.
   Oral Surg Oral Med Oral Pathol 1992;74(2):
   143–8.

Part III

Occlusal Appliance Therapy

Occlusal appliances have been used to improve TMD symptoms for over 100 years.[1] They generally provide a beneficial effect for masticatory muscle pain, TMJ pain, TMJ noise, and jaw mobility.[2] Their effectiveness was demonstrated in one study in which 81 percent of the patients provided a **stabilization appliance** (the traditional occlusal appliance) in conjunction with TMD self-management instructions reported at least a 50 percent improvement in their TMD pain at their 6-month follow-up.[3]

> ✪ **FOCAL POINT**
> Occlusal appliances generally provide a beneficial effect for masticatory muscle pain, TMJ pain, TMJ noise, and jaw mobility.

Some dentists limit their TMD therapy to occlusal appliances, most probably because they have not been taught how and/or when to provide other therapies. Occlusal appliances alone will not provide many TMD patients satisfactory treatment and will not provide any relief for some. These appliances should be thought of as only one of many potential conservative TMD therapies. Effective integration of conservative TMD therapies is discussed in "Integrating Conservative Therapies" in Chapter 19.

> ✪ **FOCAL POINT**
> Occlusal appliances alone will not provide many TMD patients with satisfactory treatment and will not provide any relief for some.

> ◉ **QUICK CONSULT**
> **Providing Conservative TMD Therapies**
> Occlusal appliances should be thought of as only one of many potential conservative TMD therapies.

Occlusal appliances can cause irreversible changes with jaw movement and occlusion. This problem is generally limited to patients who wear their appliance long term for more than 12 hours a day, especially if their appliance covers only part of the dental arch. Patients who do not maintain their appliance or oral hygiene sufficiently may develop caries, gingival inflammation, and/or mouth odors.[4]

Practitioners use a vast number of appliance variations. Therefore, when one begins studying occlusal appliances, the subject matter appears overwhelming. Basically appliances can only be fabricated to vary (a) whether the appliance allows the mandible to slide freely from maximum intercuspation (e.g., stabilization appliance) or holds the mandible in a predetermined condylar position (e.g., anterior positioning appliance), (b) the condyle's position when a patient occludes in maximum intercuspation on the appliance, and (c) the physical aspects of the appliance, i.e., whether it covers all of the teeth in the arch, whether it covers the maxillary or mandibular teeth, the type of material it is fabricated with, its thickness, and its form of retention.

The two most common appliances used to treat TMD patients are the stabilization and anterior positioning appliances. The **stabilization appliance** has a flat surface occluding with the opposing dentition, which provides a gnathologically stable occlusal environment. This appliance enables patients to move freely from maximum intercuspation and is most commonly used for patients with tooth attrition or TMD symptoms.

The **anterior positioning appliance** is primarily used for patients who have a disc displacement with reduction and holds the mandible in an anterior location where the condyle is reduced onto the disc. In this manner, the disc-condyle mechanical disturbances are temporarily eliminated, and any forces loading the condyle are transmitted through the disc's intermediate zone rather than the retrodiscal tissue.

The reason occlusal appliances are clinically effective is not fully understood. This section uses the occlusal appliance literature and clinical observations to provide a better understanding of these appliances, so practitioners may use them more effectively with their TMD patients.

◉ **QUICK CONSULT**

Understanding the Mechanism for Effectiveness

The reason occlusal appliances are clinically effective is not fully understood.

REFERENCES

1. Goodwillie DH. Arthritis of the temporomaxillary articulation. Arch Med 1881;5:259–63.
2. Bush FM, Abbott FM, Butler JH, Harrington WG. Oral orthotics: design, indications, efficacy and care. In: Hardin JF (ed). Clark's Clinical Dentistry, volume 2, chapter 39. Philadelphia: JB Lippincott, 1998:1–33.
3. Suvinen TI, Hanes KR, Reade PC. Outcome of therapy in the conservative management of temporomandibular pain dysfunction disorder. J Oral Rehabil 1997;24(10):718–24.
4. American Academy of Orofacial Pain, with Okeson JP (ed). Orofacial Pain: Guidelines for Assessment, Diagnosis and Management. Chicago: Quintessence, 1996:150–3.

Chapter 12

Stabilization Appliance

FAQs

Q: Do you recommend practitioners use a centric relation (CR) bite registration and adjust the appliance in CR?

A: Obtaining a bite registration and adjusting the appliance in CR provides the practitioner with a more reproducible maxillomandibular relationship, requires less effort to obtain a well-adjusted appliance, and provides the patient with an appliance that maintains its stable occlusal environment. Unfortunately many TMD patients cannot tolerate the TMJs being seated in CR and/or cannot relax the muscles satisfactorily so CR can be attained.

Q: Do you ever provide patients with appliances that do not cover all of the teeth in the arch?

A: It is rare for me to provide an appliance that does not cover all of the teeth in the arch, because full-coverage appliances reduce the probability of teeth moving while the patient uses it.

Q: Over the years, I have received advertisements about appliances that cover only a few teeth. What are your feelings about such appliances?

A: Several prefabricated partial coverage appliances on the market may induce tooth movement and not be as effective as a full-coverage appliance.

Q: Is a maxillary appliance or mandibular appliance more effective?

A: Both maxillary and mandibular appliances can be fabricated to provide virtually a perfect gnathologic articulation, and they appear to have comparable efficacy.

Q: Do you adjust the occlusion of athletic mouthpieces that you deliver?

A: I always adjust the occlusion of the athletic mouthpiece, because it makes the mouthpiece more comfortable, less likely to cause occlusal changes, and less likely to cause patients to develop TMD symptoms.

Stabilization appliances provide a gnathologically stable occlusal environment in which the mandible can slide freely from maximum intercuspation. Numerous practitioners use these appliances for many non-TMD purposes. Their use is advocated when nocturnal parafunctional habits are believed to be contributing to tooth attrition, tooth pain, tooth mobility, abfractions, recurrent tooth fractures, and periodontal disease. Additionally these appliances are used for deprogramming proprioception prior to . dental treatment and observing a patient's tolerance to an increased vertical dimension.[1-4]

❂ FOCAL POINT
Stabilization appliances are advocated when nocturnal parafunctional habits are believed to be contributing to tooth attrition, tooth pain, tooth mobility, abfractions, recurrent tooth fractures, and periodontal disease. Additionally these appliances are used for deprogramming proprioception prior to dental treatment and observing a patient's tolerance to an increased vertical dimension.

TMD patients generally report a decrease in morning symptoms with the use of a nocturnal appliance.[5] Nocturnal muscle activity has been generally shown to decrease with nighttime appliance wear, but parafunctional activities (e.g., bruxing or clenching) do not stop.[6,7] One study found that even patients whose nocturnal muscle activity increased with nighttime appliance wear reported a decrease in TMD symptoms.[6]

❂ FOCAL POINT
TMD patients generally report a decrease in morning symptoms with the use of a nocturnal appliance.

Why stabilization appliances benefit many TMD patients is not well understood, but several hypotheses have been proposed. It appears more than one may apply simultaneously, and the impact of each varies for every individual.

The most common hypothesis is that stabilization appliances can replace a patient's occlusal disharmonies with virtually a perfect gnathologic articulation.[1,8-10] It is frequently observed that TMD symptoms improve among new patients who bring a poorly adjusted appliance with an occlusion that is significantly improved.

A second hypothesis is that wearing the appliance causes patients to be more attuned continually to their oral cavity and parafunctional habits, thereby enabling them to catch and alter these habits.[1,8,11] A few studies provided acrylic appliances that covered only a portion of the hard palate (they did not occlude with the opposing dentition) and found that these appliances improved TMD symptoms.[12-14] It is postulated the symptom improvement is primarily due to a change in the patient's cognitive awareness from wearing the nonoccluding appliance.[1,11] When, out of curiosity, nonoccluding palatal appliances were fabricated for two patients with daytime TMD symptoms, both reported symptom reduction. One related that the appliance shifted every time she started to clench, making her aware of what she was doing, so she stopped. The other reported that the appliance made her very cognizant of her mouth, and thus she noticed and reduced her daytime habits.

A third hypothesis for the TMD symptom improvement observed with the use of stabilization appliances is related to the increase in vertical dimension that occurs from their wear. An increase in vertical dimension is speculated to benefit both the TMJ and the musculature.[9] The nonoccluding palatal appliance has also been shown to increase the resting vertical dimension.[15]

A fourth hypothesis is that stabilization appliances can be fabricated so they decrease the load on the TMJ during different oral activities.[1,8,16,17] The appliance can be designed with a mandibular position (presented in the next section) that aids in minimizing the loading of the TMJs. Decreasing the load placed on the TMJ reduces the continual TMJ aggravation that occurs from parafunctional habits, thereby promoting healing of the TMJ.[16,17]

MANDIBULAR POSITIONS AND BITE REGISTRATION

Centric relation (CR) appears to be the most musculoskeletally stable position for the mandible. In CR, the condyles are seated in their most anterior-superior location against the disc's intermediate zone (the thinnest avascular portion of the disc) and the posterior slopes of the articular eminences. Theoretically a stabilization appliance appropriately adjusted using CR would be optimally effective.[10,18,19]

⊙ **QUICK CONSULT**
Using Centric Relation

Centric relation (CR) appears to be the most musculoskeletally stable position for the mandible.

CR is a very reproducible position; if the bite registration is made using CR, the resulting appliance occlusion in the mouth will be very similar to the occlusion developed on the articulator. Therefore, obtaining a bite registration and adjusting the appliance using CR should require the least amount of effort for practitioners.

If the bite registration is made and the appliance adjusted in a position anterior to CR, the patient can retrude the mandible from this position. When the patient retrudes, the condyles slide superior along the articular eminence, causing the posterior portion of the mandibular occlusal plane to move superior. As the patient then occludes onto the appliance, only the most posterior tooth or teeth would occlude on it, as demonstrated in Figures 12-1 and 12-2.

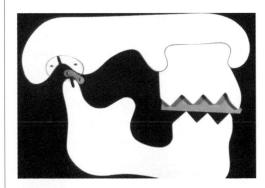

Figure 12-1. A model simulating occlusion on a stabilization appliance adjusted with the mandible in a position anterior to centric relation (CR).

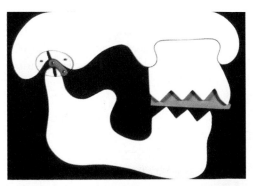

Figure 12-2. A model simulating occlusion on the adjusted stabilization appliance in Figure 12-1, with the mandible in centric relation.

Consequently, adjusting an appliance in a protruded position furnishes an appliance that may provide the patient with an unstable occlusal environment.

Obtaining a bite registration and adjusting the appliance in CR provide practitioners with a more reproducible maxillomandibular relationship, requires less effort to obtain a well-adjusted appliance, and provides patients with an appliance that maintains its stable occlusal environment. Unfortunately many TMD patients cannot tolerate the TMJs being seated in CR and/or cannot relax the muscles satisfactorily so CR can be attained.[18,20] Hence, when non-TMD patients need a stabilization appliance, it is recommended that their bite registration and adjustments be made using CR.

Many TMD patients who have TMJ inflammation find it painful to have their condyles seated into CR.[18,21] If the practitioner were to adjust these appliances so maximum intercuspation coincided with the condyles being seated in CR, one would anticipate that, whenever these patients clenched on the appliance in maximum intercuspation, the condyles would seat in CR, reproducing this pain and aggravating their TMD.

Some patients have TMJ noises (clicking, popping, or crepitus) caused by mechanical interference within the TMJ. This interference may be caused by the disc, the retrodiscal tissue, or irregularities on the head of the condyle and/or the articular eminence, as discussed in "TMJ Noise" in Chapter 3. If the condyles are seated firmly into CR, the TMJ mechanical interference often becomes more pronounced, which tends to aggravate the TMJ.

Early in my TMD training, a patient reported that about once a month her right TMJ locked and did not allow her to open wide (an intermittent acute TMJ disc displacement without reduction). No TMJ inflammation was detected, so I bilaterally manipulated her mandible to seat the condyles into CR.[22] Her right TMJ locked as the condyles were seated in CR; she telephoned me later that day to let me know that her TMJ had finally unlocked for her.

Based on clinical experiences and my understanding of the TMJ's biomechanics, it is recommended that CR be used only for TMD patients who have no detectable TMJ inflammation, TMJ noise, or history of TMJ locking. It is also recommended that CR not be used if patients have any discomfort when attempting to seat the condyles into CR.[18] Therefore, the vast majority of my TMD patients do not have their bite registrations made or appliances adjusted using CR.

▼ **TECHNICAL TIP**
Using Centric Relation

It is recommended that CR be used only for TMD patients who have no detectable TMJ inflammation, TMJ noise, or history of TMJ locking.

Instead of using CR, it is recommended that an unrestrained condylar position that approaches CR, but does not encroach upon inflamed retrodiscal tissue nor firmly seat the condyles be used. Therefore, if a patient were to have his or her appliance adjusted to this position and clench on the appliance in maximum intercuspation, the condyles would tend not to forcibly seat or load against any structure. I refer to this unrestrained condylar position as the *neutral position*.

To obtain the condyle's **neutral position**, adjust the back of the dental chair so it is approximately 10° above the horizontal plane of the floor. Ask the patient to tilt his or her head back as far as possible, place the tongue on the roof the mouth, and slide it back as far as possible. Lightly place a finger on the inferior portion of the patient's chin and repeatedly ask the patient to close and open his or her mouth (Figure 12-3). After a few arching movements, the patient develops a consistent arching of the mandible.[1]

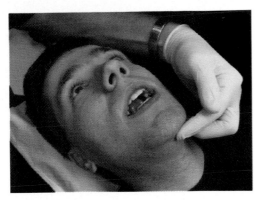

Figure 12-3. The condyle's neutral position is obtained by the back of the dental chair being approximately 10° above the horizontal plane of the floor; asking the patient to tilt his head back as far as possible and place his tongue on the roof of his mouth and slide it back as far as possible; lightly touching the inferior portion of the patient's chin; and asking the patient to close and open his mouth repeatedly.

Each of the recommended positions helps to retrude the mandible and prevent the tendency of some patients to protrude the mandible inadvertently.[10,22,23] The reader can easily observe how these positions tend to retrude the mandible on himself or herself. Sitting in your normal posture, close your teeth lightly and observe your first tooth contact. Then, tilt your head back as far as possible and again close your teeth lightly and observe your first tooth contact; most people notice that the mandible is more retruded. Continuing to hold your head back, place your tongue on the roof of your mouth and slide it back as far as possible. Once again, close your teeth lightly and observe your first tooth contact; most people notice that the mandible is further retruded.

Placing a finger on the inferior portion of a patient's chin helps to steady the mandible so he or she more easily develops a consistent arching of the mandible. Based on these recommendations, most TMD patients will have their bite registrations and appliances adjusted in the neutral position. It is not as repeatable as CR, but, as the appliance is adjusted, the patient establishes a consistent contact position.

Prior to making a bite registration, position the patient, review the procedure with the patient, and manipulate the mandible into the planned condylar position (CR or neutral position). Discuss the bite registration procedure planned with the patient. I let the patient know I will place warm wax in his or her mouth, manipulate the mandible as performed earlier, and ask the patient to bite into it slowly.

Pink baseplate wax is preferred for the bite registration. It can be warmed over a flame, under running hot water, or in a waterbath. I fold it in fourths and cut it with a pair of scissors in the shape of a trapezoid (Figure 12-4). The wax should be soft enough that it does not provide any resistance as the patient closes into it.

If a practitioner would like the wax to adhere temporarily to the maxillary teeth during the bite registration, the teeth can be dried with gauze. Manipulate the mandible into the planned condylar position. Ask the patient to open approximately 10 mm, align the trimmed baseplate wax, and ask the patient to close slowly into the wax. Ask the patient to stop closing as soon as indentations are satisfactory to provide a stable mounting for the casts (Figure 12-5).

Attempt to remove the wax without distorting it. If the teeth were dried prior to placing the wax in the mouth, the wax is more difficult to remove without deforming. Wax that has a minor amount of distortion

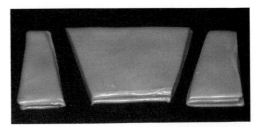

Figure 12-4. Pink baseplate wax for the bite registration: warmed, folded in fourths, and cut with a pair of scissors in the shape of a trapezoid.

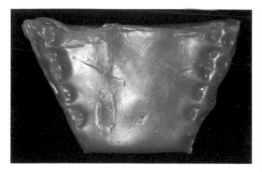

Figure 12-5. Wax bite registration.

can be straightened on the cast. Check to ensure the patient did not perforate the wax. A perforation of the wax suggests the teeth contacted and the mandible probably shifted along this contact. If a wax perforation is available, I generally retake the bite registration.

I do not use a facebow for occlusal appliance records because (a) my bite registration is approximately as thick as the desired appliance thickness, (b) acrylic is easily adjusted and inexpensive compared with gold or porcelain, and (c) the excursive movements will need to be adjusted in the mouth, and a facebow would probably not minimize these adjustments. Additionally many TMD patients have preauricular tenderness, and a facebow would almost certainly be quite painful.

If an acrylic stabilization appliance is being requested, the laboratory technician should be asked to adjust the articulator's pin so the closest opposing posterior tooth contact is 3 mm once the casts have been mounted.

PHYSICAL VARIABLES

Practitioners can choose among many physical alternatives when designing a stabilization appliance. The typical appliance covers all of the teeth in the arch, is made for the maxillary arch, is fabricated entirely with acrylic, is approximately 2 mm thick, and uses acrylic in undercuts to provide its retention.

This typical stabilization appliance may be altered for many specific situations. The following section should help practitioners better understand their choices and decide which ones to use for different patients and situations.

Full or Partial Coverage

A *full-coverage appliance* (which covers all of the teeth in the arch) reduces the probability of the teeth moving when the patient uses it.[24,25] Therefore, a full-coverage appliance is recommended except in rare situations.

A *partial coverage appliance* may cause teeth it covers to intrude and/or teeth not included in it to extrude.[1,3] Patients with heavy nocturnal parafunctional habits may be more at risk of intruding the teeth covered by a partial coverage appliance.

Generally practitioners who provide patients with partial coverage appliances instruct their patients to wear the appliance only at night, but occlusal appliances tend to improve TMD symptoms, so some patients may choose to wear it 24 hours a day to obtain additional relief despite the instructions.

Mandibular appliances that cover only the posterior teeth can be made to be quite esthetic and have minimal speech interference. Some patients who have worn this partial coverage appliance 24 hours a day have experienced occlusal changes to the degree that the anterior teeth now contact when the appliance is worn and the posterior teeth have an open bite the thickness of the appliance when it is out of the mouth.[3] Some practitioners provide this appliance for patients to wear during the day and a full-coverage appliance to wear during the night.

Similarly there is a case report of a patient who was provided an appliance that did not cover his erupted third molars. He wore the appliance 24 hours a day and, by 5 weeks later, had developed an open bite in which only his third molars occluded when the appliance was not worn.[26]

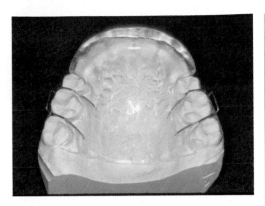

Figure 12-6. An example of a partial coverage appliance. This appliance occludes only with the mandible anterior teeth and would enable the practitioner to orthodontically move or restore the mandibular posterior teeth.

Not only do practitioners need to be concerned about tooth movement with partial coverage appliances, but they may not be as effective as full-coverage appliances.[27,28] One study provided patients with maxillary appliances that only occluded with the mandibular anterior teeth (Figure 12-6). Patients who received little or no relief from the appliance had it modified into a full-coverage appliance, and 66 percent reported their TMD symptoms were greatly or completely improved by use of the full-coverage appliance.[28]

This type of partial coverage appliance has also been shown to compress the structures within the TMJ.[29] This is a concern for any partial coverage appliance in which only anterior teeth occlude on the appliance.

Several prefabricated partial coverage appliances on the market may similarly induce tooth movement and not be as effective as a full-coverage appliance. Additionally some prefabricated partial coverage appliances cannot be molded adequately into the arch's undercuts to provide satisfactory retention. If a nonretentive appliance is worn during the day, the patient would most likely have to keep the teeth closed on the appliance to hold it in place. If the appliance is worn at night, it would slide around during sleep,

and the patient would probably unconsciously remove it. For these reasons, no prefabricated partial coverage appliances are recommended.

Partial coverage appliances do enable practitioners to avoid specific areas of the mouth. For instance, a patient may develop TMD symptoms while having a mandibular molar uprighted for the eventual fabrication of a bridge. If an occlusal appliance is needed, the patient could temporarily wear a maxillary appliance at night that only occludes with the mandibular anterior teeth (Figure 12-6).

A partial coverage appliances in recommended in only very rare circumstances, because the full-arch appliances have less iatrogenic risk and are probably more effective.

Maxillary or Mandibular

Both maxillary and mandibular appliances can be fabricated to provide virtually a perfect gnathologic articulation, and they appear to have comparable efficacy.[10] They each have specific advantages, so my choice will vary with a patient's conditions and planned wear schedule.

Mandibular appliances generally cause less speech interference and are less visible when speaking.[9,10] It would be preferable to fabricate a mandibular appliance for a patient who is to wear an appliance during the day.[1,21] For a patient to obtain immediate disocclusion of the posterior teeth with a mandibular appliance, the maxillary anterior teeth must guide along an anterior ramp. This guidance ramp generally extends anterior to the mandibular anterior teeth (Figure 12-7) and, if the patient has a large overjet, this ramp is often unacceptably long.[9]

Maxillary appliances provide stability for the maxillary anterior teeth. Patients with periodontal disease of the maxillary anterior teeth tend to develop flaring of the anterior teeth. Thus, if a patient has compromised bony support of the maxillary anterior teeth,

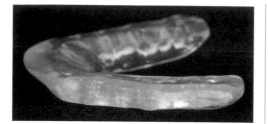

Figure 12-7. A mandibular appliance depicting the guidance ramp extending anterior to the anterior teeth, enabling the maxillary anterior teeth to provide immediate disocclusion of the posterior teeth. Notice that the angle of the anterior guidance ramp is only about 5° steeper than the appliance's occlusal plane.

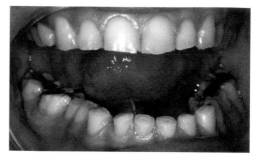

Figure 12-8. An example of patient with severe tooth attrition, for which a maxillary appliance is recommended.

it is recommended that a maxillary appliance be fabricated to prevent this flaring.

If a patient has very strong parafunctional habits (primarily identified by the degree of tooth attrition), the mandibular appliance's anterior guidance ramp will transfer more lateral force to the maxillary anterior teeth than usual. Out of fear that excessive parafunctional forces may similarly cause flaring of the anterior teeth even for patients with normal bony support, if a patient has severe tooth attrition (Figure 12-8) it is recommended that a maxillary appliance be fabricated so as not to risk the possibility of contributing to the maxillary anterior teeth flaring.

If a patient has missing teeth, an occlusal appliance can bridge over the edentulous areas and provide occlusal contacts for the opposing teeth. The appliance can also be fabricated to provide posterior edentulous extensions (Figure 12-9).[3] It would be preferable to fabricate the appliance for the arch that will provide greater occlusal stability; this is generally the arch with more missing teeth (Figures 12-10 and 12-11).[1,3] Occlusal appliances can also be fabricated to be worn over complete or partial dentures.

Hence, if a patient has compromised bony support of the maxillary anterior teeth, severe tooth attrition, or a large overjet, a maxillary appliance is recommended. If none of these apply, it is recommended that the practitioner observe for missing teeth and

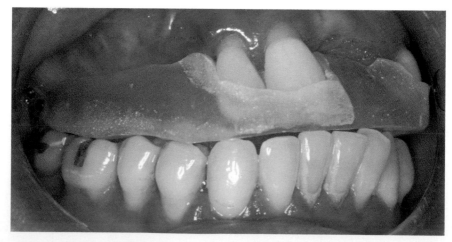

Figure 12-9. An appliance with a posterior edentulous extension enables the patient to obtain occlusal contacts over this area. The lighter-colored portion of the appliance is due to its recent repair.

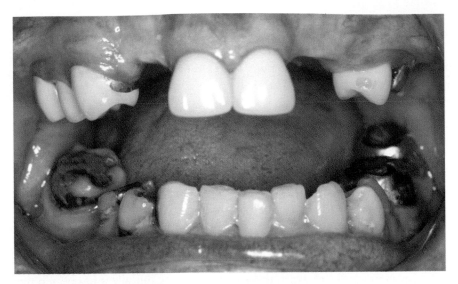

Figure 12-10. Because of this patient's missing teeth, fabricating a maxillary rather than a mandibular appliance for this patient would provide greater occlusal stability.

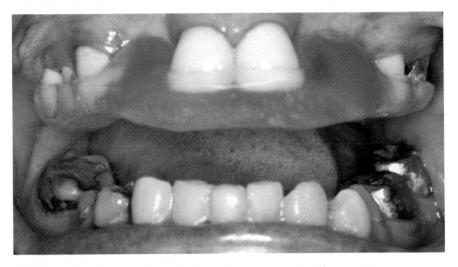

Figure 12-11. The maxillary appliance fabricated for the patient in Figure 12-10.

seek to fabricate the appliance for the arch that will provide greater occlusal stability. If the practitioner plans for the appliance to be worn during the day, the patient would probably prefer a mandibular appliance. If greater occlusal stability could be obtained with a maxillary appliance, but the practitioner plans for the appliance to be worn during the day, it is recommended the practitioner attempt to balance the difference in occlusal stability with improved esthetics and speech to determine the better arch on which to fabricate the appliance. One can also choose to fabricate a maxillary appliance for nighttime wear and a mandibular appliance for daytime wear.[21]

Hard or Soft

A wide variety of materials can be used to fabricate occlusal appliances. If one reviews the hypotheses for why stabilization appliances benefit many TMD patients (discussed at the beginning of this chapter), one will notice that probably the only variation a different material would have is if it alters the appliance's ability to provide an ideal occlusal environment.

⊙ **QUICK CONSULT**

Varying Appliance Material

Probably the only variation that appliance material would have on an appliance's efficacy would be related to its ability to provide an ideal occlusal environment.

The traditional stabilization appliance is fabricated using clear acrylic, of which there are many brands and processing methods, providing varying rates of attrition.[30] Some practitioners prefer to fabricate the appliance in the mouth, using a hard thermoplastic sheet molded over the patient's cast as the base and adding self-curing acrylic.[10] Most stabilization appliance studies have used acrylic appliances, thereby providing well-documented scientific support for their efficacy.

Soft stabilization appliances are typically fabricated from a soft thermoplastic sheet that is warmed and formed over the cast. Since the author is not aware of a clinically feasible method to add additional material to these appliances, it is recommended the 0.15-inch (3.8 mm)-thick material be used. This and the 4.0-mm-thick material are the maximum thicknesses commercially available that provide the greatest opportunity to perfect a patient's occlusion. These appliances are fast and easy to fabricate; it would be relatively simple for a dental staff member to fabricate these in the practitioner's office.

For many years, the findings of studies evaluating the efficacy of soft stabilization appliances were contradictory. Since the material is resilient, some investigators did *not* adjust or adequately adjust these appliances. This resulted in findings one would expect from providing TMD patients with inade-

quately adjusted appliances—many patients had symptom aggravation.[31,32]

More recently, studies have found that TMD patients obtain comparable symptom improvement with soft and hard appliances.[33,34] The different results appear to be due to the soft appliances being adequately adjusted. This is also supported by clinical experience that the occlusion on soft appliances must be meticulously adjusted, just as a practitioner would adjust an acrylic appliance.[3,35,36]

Some practitioners find that patients tend to play with soft appliances and believe that soft appliances may trigger parafunctional habits.[1,37] Clinically it has been observed that patients tend to play with a soft appliance that is not well adjusted. Patients given an unadjusted soft appliance often occlude against only one or two opposing teeth and tend to clench on the appliance to produce more occlusal contacts, thereby increasing its occlusal stability. Conversely patients provided a well-adjusted appliance with even posterior contacts do not find their stability is improved by clenching and thus do not have the tendency to play with the appliance.

A study was once conducted to evaluate the speed at which occlusal changes can take place. The investigators induced these changes by having patients wear unadjusted soft appliances.[38] This study appeared to create concern that soft appliances may cause occlusal changes. To determine whether this occurs for patients wearing adjusted soft appliances, another study used shim stock to follow the occlusion in patients wearing adjusted soft appliances and determined that they do not cause the occlusion to change.[39]

If a practitioner were to provide soft appliances to TMD patients without adjusting the occlusion, it is anticipated that their symptom response would be similar to the findings obtained by Nevarro and colleagues.[32] After providing unadjusted soft appliances, they found the numbers of patients who reported TMD symptom improvement, no change, and aggravation were one, two, and six, respectively. Clinically, similar patient responses have been observed from working with practitioners who routinely did not adjust the occlusion on their soft appliances.

Soft appliances can be fabricated for either the maxillary arch or the mandibular arch. An appliance to be used as an athletic mouthpiece should be fabricated for the maxillary arch. I always adjust the occlusion of athletic mouthpieces, because it makes a mouthpiece more comfortable, less likely to cause occlusal changes, and less likely to cause a patient to develop TMD symptoms.

Acrylic appliances have several advantages in comparison with soft thermoplastic appliances. Acrylic appliances (a) provide a precise occlusal mark, allowing practitioners to obtain a very accurate adjustment of the appliance; (b) can be fabricated with additional material in specific locations, so these areas (i.e., edentulous areas, crossbites, and other large discrepancies) can attain contact with the opposing dentition; and (c) bond with self-curing acrylic, enabling practitioners to add missing contacts, add retention (by internally relining the appliances), and repair fractured appliances.

One would anticipate that these acrylic appliance advantages would enable practitioners to develop greater occlusal harmony for some patients, thereby providing a better average treatment effect. In a large study comparing the two appliances over a 12-month period, even though there was no significant difference between the two appliances, on average the acrylic appliance did have a better average treatment effect.[34]

Since *soft appliances* are easily fabricated, are inexpensive, and may be inserted at an initial appointment, practitioners may desire to use soft appliances in many situations:

1. In emergencies. For example, a patient is in acute distress (especially if an acrylic appliance may not be available for some time) or presents with a nonrepairable appliance that the patient depends on.

2. When the soft appliance will serve as a prognostic tool to evaluate whether an occlusal appliance would be beneficial. A practitioner may be unsure whether a patient has TMD or whether appliance therapy will improve the patient's complaint (e.g., tinnitus or headaches). Patients who obtain symptom reduction with the use of a soft appliance generally also benefit from the use of an acrylic appliance.[1,40]

3. When a practitioner desires an easily adjustable interim appliance. For example, a patient has a lateral pterygoid myospasm, the practitioner knows the patient will have significant occlusal changes as symptoms improve, and during this transition a soft appliance would be easy to adjust whereas the acrylic appliance may need to be relined.

4. For TMD management of children during their mixed dentition. It has been speculated that a soft appliance will not significantly affect the development of the dentition[41] and will not need the number of adjustments that an acrylic appliance may require to accommodate minor tooth movements.

5. When a patient's financial situation is an overwhelming concern.

Conversely there are situations in which it is recommended that a soft appliance not be used:

1. When a patient has such a significant occlusal discrepancy that the soft appliance material would not be thick enough to accommodate for the discrepancy.

2. When a patient has missing teeth in which the thermoplastic soft appliance will not be able to provide occlusal contacts for the opposing teeth.

3. When a patient has moderately severe or severe tooth attrition from nocturnal parafunctional habits. Soft appliances appear

to wear more rapidly than acrylic appliances, so patients with excessively heavy parafunctional habits may wear through the soft appliance in a relatively short time.

Many other materials on the market have resiliency and flexibility between that of the hard acrylic and soft thermoplastic materials. There are several advantages in using an *intermediate material for occlusal appliances*: (a) Patients generally find the softer material more comfortable, and it better dissipates heavy parafunctional loading.[9,42,43] (b) The softer materials can compensate for minor errors that might cause an acrylic appliance to rock or cause pressure on the supporting teeth. (c) Laboratory technicians can compensate for missing teeth and occlusal discrepancies when fabricating these appliances, thereby overcoming the problems associated with the soft thermoplastic material's limited thickness. (d) Many intermediate materials can also bond with self-curing acrylic, providing an avenue to deal with problems that may occur after appliance fabrication.

These materials appear to be a reasonable alternative to acrylic appliances. If a practitioner decides to use an appliance fabricated with an intermediate material, it is recommended that the practitioner ensure the appliance can be well adjusted and the material does not wear excessively.

There are also *dual laminate thermoplastic materials* that can be used for occlusal appliances. Such material provides a soft internal surface and a hard thermoplastic external surface (discussed in "Appliance Examples" in this chapter). Once the material is molded over the cast, self-curing acrylic is added to its external surface by the laboratory technician or intraorally by the practitioner. Occlusal appliances fabricated with dual laminate thermoplastic material have the following advantages: (a) they are comfortable to the supporting teeth, (b) the soft internal material can compensate for minor errors that might cause an acrylic appliance to rock or cause pressure on teeth, (c) they can compensate for missing teeth and occlusal discrepancies; and (d) self-curing acrylic will bond to the external surface.

Two disadvantages with this material have been observed. First, the appliance needs to be fabricated approximately 1 mm thicker than the acrylic appliance in order to allow for the soft layer that overlays the teeth. Second, the internal surface more readily discolors over time than does the external acrylic.

The dual laminate thermoplastic material also appears to be a reasonable alternative to the acrylic appliances. If a practitioner decides to use appliances fabricated with this material, it is recommended the 2.5-mm-thick or thicker material be used. It is felt that the flanges from the 1.8-mm material are too fragile, because once one of my patients given an appliance made of this material fractured the flange after he put the appliance in his shirt pocket and someone bumped into him. This problem has not occurred for me with the thicker dual laminate materials.

Another material that is occasionally used by people who have TMD symptoms, but are trying to avoid seeing a dentist for treatment, is a *commercial athletic mouthpiece*. It has been observed that patients have mixed results with such appliances and believed a poor response may be related to (a) the opposing occlusal indentations having been made with the condyles in an inappropriate positions, (b) the occlusal indentations not allowing the patient to move the mandible freely, or (c) the mouthpiece not providing adequate retention, requiring the patient to hold it in place by keeping the teeth together. It is strongly recommended that patients do not attempt to use a commercial athletic mouthpiece, because of fear that it may cause occlusal changes if it does not cover or evenly occlude with all of the teeth.

Thick or Thin

Muscle contraction is achieved by actin and myosin sliding along each other; its efficiency is related to the degree the actin and myosin overlap, which varies with a muscle's length.[44,45] The optimum physiological muscle length is speculated to be at the location the muscle has its minimal surface electromyelographic (EMG) activity. The vertical opening at which the masseter and temporalis muscles produce their minimal surface EMG activity varies from patient to patient, but falls within the range of 4.5 to 18 mm.[46,47]

It has been postulated that a stabilization appliance would be more effective if it were fabricated at the vertical opening where the muscle has its minimal surface EMG activity. To test this hypothesis, TMD patients were randomized into three groups. One group was provided stabilization appliances that increased the vertical dimension by 1 mm, the second group was provided appliances with the thickness of one-half the opening that produced minimal masseter muscle surface EMG activity (average, 4.4 mm), and the third group was provided appliances with the thickness of the opening that produced minimal EMG activity (average, 8.2 mm). The third group experienced the most rapid reduction in TMD symptoms, the second group's symptom reduction took slightly longer, and the first group's symptom reduction took the longest time. The findings of this study suggest that *thicker appliances* (up to the minimal EMG activity) may resolve TMD symptoms more quickly.[48]

Through my teaching experience, it has been observed that many dentists believe an occlusal appliance cannot be thicker than a patient's freeway space. They fear that, if the appliance is thicker than 2 or 3 mm, the patient may clench on it uncontrollably and increase the TMD symptoms. Patients also tend to find thicker appliances more ob-trusive and prefer to have a thinner appliance, especially if they previously had a thin appliance.

It is not advocated that 8-mm-thick stabilization appliances be fabricated for patients, because *thinner appliances* appear to be reasonably effective and have a high degree of patient acceptance. It is important for dentists to realize stabilization appliances can be more than 2 or 3 mm thick without causing detrimental consequences. Therefore, the additional millimeters needed for the dual laminate thermoplastic appliance's thickness should not present a problem, nor should it be a problem if the practitioner's laboratory accidentally fabricated an appliance a little thicker than requested.

It is generally recommended that appliances be fabricated between 1 and 4 mm thick.[1,2,10] As mentioned in "Mandibular Positions and Bite Registration" in this chapter, when requesting an acrylic stabilization appliance, I ask the laboratory technician to adjust the articulator's pin so the closest opposing posterior tooth contact is 3 mm. Requesting stabilization appliances be fabricated at this thickness generally enables me to provide the patient with an appliance that does not have perforations and has sufficient thickness for attrition.

Appliance or Wire Retention

Appliance retention is achieved by portions of the appliance acting as guide planes while other sections flex and engage into undercuts. The undercuts are primarily in the interproximal sites of the posterior teeth, and the portion that flexes into the undercut can be the appliance itself or wires added to it.

The appliance should have a similar degree of retention as a removable partial denture. The retention should not be so strong that it might cause the patient to break a fingernail, but not so weak that he or she can dislodge the appliance with the tongue.

Clinically it has been observed that

patients given appliances with insufficient retention report their TMD symptoms were aggravated by their appliances. It is speculated the symptom aggravation may be from patients holding their opposing teeth on the appliance to stabilize it or from playing with it. It has also been observed that patients given appliances with insufficient retention report they unconsciously remove them at night while they sleep.

If the appliance does not have enough retention, for appliances with wire retention, the wires need to be adjusted to further engage the undercuts. For appliances without wires and an internal surface that can bind with self-curing or light-cured acrylic, the internal surface needs to be relined. Relining the internal surface as described in "Appliance Adjustments" in this chapter generally provides an ideal amount of retention.

There are many reasons an appliance is too retentive. A very common reason a new appliance has too much retention is that it fits too tightly, thereby causing excessive frictional retention. The appliance needs first to be adjusted so it is comfortable (a technique explained in "Appliance Adjustments" in this chapter); then the retention should be reevaluated.

Generally an appliance that fits comfortably and is too retentive has excessive retention in the posterior due to the appliance engaging too deeply into the posterior interproximal undercuts. In this situation, if wires provide the retention, they need to be adjusted to decrease it. If the inner portion of the appliance provides the retention, the sites engaging the posterior undercuts should be reduced. This is the portion that protrudes into the dental embrasures and can be reduced by lightly running an acrylic bur over them. When adjusting this, it is recommended that practitioners err on the side of reducing the retention too little rather than too much and that these sites be repeatedly reduced until the proper retention is achieved.

My personal preference is to have the appliance's internal material engage the undercuts rather than wires added to the appliance.

APPLIANCE ADJUSTMENTS

The stabilization adjustments are the most critical phase for providing an effective appliance. It is common for me to hear new patients report they previously received an appliance that was too tight, causing them pain, so they stopped wearing it. Delivering a well-adjusted appliance is challenging, and one fabricated entirely with acrylic takes me about 45 minutes to deliver.

> ✪ **FOCAL POINT**
> The stabilization adjustments are the most critical phase for providing an effective appliance.

After completing my appliance adjustments, I ask the patient to insert the appliance, to tell me whether the posterior occlusion is hitting as evenly as possible, and to tell me whether he or she knows of anything that can be done to improve the appliance. Sometimes I am unaware of a minor problem that may annoy a patient (e.g., a rough spot on the lingual flange, a rough excursive movement, excessive bulk, or a tendency for the appliance to cause gagging) and cause the patient to play with the annoyance, which could lead to aggravation of the TMD symptoms.

Occasionally patients report they unconsciously remove their appliance during sleep. It is my clinical experience that, in this situation, the appliance appears to bother patients in some manner while they sleep and, once this problem is corrected, they usually stop removing it. Four approaches have been found that commonly correct this problem: (a) tighten a loose appliance, (b) loosen a tight appliance, (b) perfect the appliance's occlusion, or (d) thin a bulky appliance.

Internal Adjustments

The majority of new appliances with a hard inner surface that I receive from the laboratory are too tight and need internal adjustments. This section primarily pertains to appliances fabricated with a hard inner surface, because clinical experience has shown that appliances with a soft inner surface rarely need internal adjustments.

Prior to attempting to insert an appliance in a patient's mouth, ensure the appliance appears appropriate and determine whether any adjustments are indicated prior to insertion; e.g., whether it is overly bulky or whether there are sharp areas that could hurt the patient. Also observe to ensure the appliance is not overextended beyond the most posterior teeth, unless this extension is to obtain the contact of a more posterior opposing tooth.

As the appliance is initially inserted, do not use a tremendous amount of force. Occasionally residents who insert an appliance with too much force will have great difficulty or be unable to remove it. In these situations, the end of the mouth-mirror handle can be placed interproximally on the edge of the appliance flange in an attempt to forcibly work the appliance loose.

▼ **TECHNICAL TIP**
Inserting an Appliance
As the appliance is initially inserted, do not use a tremendous amount of force or it may be difficult to remove.

If the appliance will not seat by using a moderate amount of force, ask the patient where the appliance feels tight. Generally the restriction is located along the anterior teeth, and my experience in this situation is that the labial extension is often overextended. Laboratory technicians fabricating appliances with hard inner surfaces (instructions are provided in Appendix 7, "Laboratory Occlusal Appliance Instructions") are in-

structed to extend the appliance only 1 to $1^1/_2$ mm below the incisal edge of the anterior teeth. When the appliance is too tight over the anterior teeth and the labial extension is longer than requested, it is generally most productive to first shorten the extension to the requested length.

If the appliance is too tight for it to seat and the labial extension is the correct length, clinical experience has shown the best manner for marking tight internal areas is using Accufilm (Parkell, Farmingdale, NY, USA). Place a piece of Accufilm (the black color best marks an appliance) between the appliance and the teeth, in the area of the restriction, and firmly seat and remove the appliance (Figure 12-12).

▼ **TECHNICAL TIP**
Identifying Internal Tight Areas
The internal splint locations that need to be relieved can be identified by placing a piece of Accufilm (the black color best marks an appliance) between the appliance and the teeth, and firmly seating and removing the appliance.

The appliance's retention is usually provided by the portion of the appliance that fits into the interproximal embrasures, so at first attempt to remove the restriction by adjusting only nonretentive areas. In addition to adjusting the areas that mark with Accufilm, there are often interproximal fins of material that do not provide a benefit and can also restrict appliance seating. These fins run faciolingual as formed by the occlusal or incisal embrasures of the teeth (Figure 12-13). While adjusting the Accufilm marks, it is recommended that these fins also be reduced.

This procedure may take repeated markings and adjustments. With a clear appliance, the practitioner can see whether the appliance is seated, and it is seated when there is no observable space between the appliance and the incisal edges or cusp tips. When adjusting the internal Accufilm

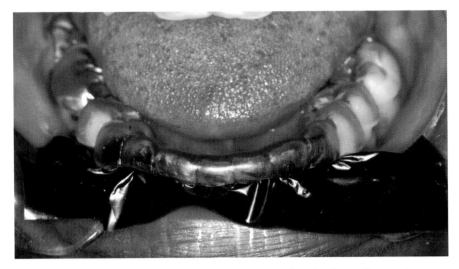

Figure 12-12. The black side of an Accufilm sheet marks the heaviest internal contacts on an appliance.

markings, I tend to be fairly conservative in the beginning and become more aggressive with each successive adjustment. After five to ten adjustments, if the appliance does not appear to be seating, I remove about 1/4 mm from the buccal and lingual surfaces, ensure the appliance is not tight, and reline its internal surface. This generally provides a well-fitting appliance more rapidly than continuing to adjust the appliance.

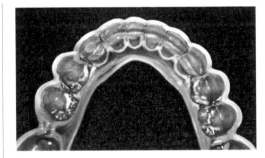

Figure 12-13. Black Accufilm marks on the internal surface of an appliance. Note the interproximal fins of material that run faciolingual, which fill in the occlusal and incisal embrasures of the teeth. These can also restrict appliance seating.

▼ TECHNICAL TIP

Adjusting Conservatively or Aggressively

When adjusting the internal Accufilm markings, I tend to be fairly conservative in the beginning and become more aggressive with each successive adjustment.

Another common problem that occurs when attempting to seat an appliance fully is that it rocks. In this situation, rock the appliance back and forth to locate the fulcrum. Place Accufilm between the appliance and the area of the fulcrum and apply firm pressure over the fulcrum to create a definitive mark. Aggressively adjust the fulcrum area and err on the side of removing excess material. If several attempts to remove the rock

are unsuccessful, the appliance's internal surface can be relieved and relined. To do this, remove about 1/4 mm of acrylic from all surfaces (including the occlusal or incisal surface) in the area of the rock, relieve retentive areas to ensure the appliance is not tight, and reline its internal surface.

Once the appliance's internal surface is adjusted so the appliance fully seats, ask the patient whether it feels too tight in the fully seated position. If it is too tight, mark the appliance with Accufilm and adjust the nonretentive surfaces accordingly.

Clinically it has been observed that the anterior teeth cannot tolerate as much pressure as the posterior teeth. If a patient is un-sure whether the pressure is excessive, I ex-plain to the patient that an appliance is like a new pair of shoes: you will notice it is there, but over time (minutes to hours) the pres-sure sensation worsens if it is too tight. If the patient continues to be unsure, I often rec-ommend the other appliance adjustments be performed to give the patient more time to determine whether it is too tight.

Accufilm nicely marks hard internal appli-ance surfaces where a tooth firmly contacts the appliance, but it will not mark soft inter-nal appliance surfaces nor a soft-tissue im-pingement. For soft internal appliance sur-faces, adjust the areas as the patient directs and, for discomfort from the soft tissue, if needed, use pressure-indicator paste or spray.

Once the appliance fits comfortably, check its retention. The appliance should have a similar degree of retention as a remov-able partial denture. The retention should not be so strong that the patient has unwar-ranted difficulty removing it, but be suffi-cient so the patient cannot dislodge it with the tongue. An appliance being too retentive is generally due to it engaging the posterior undercuts too deeply, and the depth of en-gagement should be reduced.

Evaluating an Appliance's Retention
Once the appliance fits comfortably, check its retention. The appliance should have a similar degree of retention as a removable partial denture.

If the appliance does not have enough re-tention, and the internal surface provides the retention and can bind with self-curing or light-cured acrylic, reline the internal surface. For appliances with wire retention, the wires need to be adjusted to engage the undercuts further.

Internal Reline

The appliance's internal surface can be re-lined with self-curing or light-cured acrylic. Self-curing acrylic has a bad taste, but I con-tinue to teach this technique out of fear that the residents may not have access to light-cured acrylic in their future dental practices. When only part of the appliance is being re-lined, it generally does not fully seat, creating a gap where the reline material was not added (Figure 12-14). Therefore, I generally

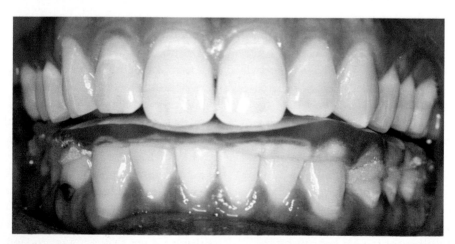

Figure 12-14. This appliance lacked retention posteriorly, so acrylic was added to the internal portion of its posterior area. The appliance was seated in the mouth, and the patient was asked to squeeze on the appliance to seat it further. Note the gap between the anterior teeth and the appliance due to the in-complete seating of the appliance.

reline the entire internal surface so there are no internal gaps or junctions.

▼ TECHNICAL TIP
Relining the Internal Portion of an Appliance
When relining the internal portion of an appliance, I generally reline the entire internal surface so there are no internal gaps or junctions.

Prior to providing the internal reline, remove any Accufilm marks on the internal surface; otherwise, the marks will be buried below the clear reline and may visually bother the patient. It is recommended that the procedure be discussed and the mandibular manipulation demonstrated to patients so they will not be startled during the procedure and disrupt its progress.

To reline an appliance with self-curing acrylic, first moisten the entire internal portion of the appliance with monomer (which makes the appliance's surface tacky) and shake out the excess. Pour approximately a teaspoon of powder in a paper cup, add a little more monomer than is required to moisten all of the powder granules, and mix with a wooden tongue depressor. While mixing the acrylic, have the patient swish with mouthwash to help lubricate the teeth and desensitize the taste buds.

Put the acrylic into the appliance with the tongue depressor, ensuring that about 1 mm of the mixed acrylic covers all of the internal surfaces, and scoop out the excess material with a gloved finger (Figure 12-15). Place the appliance into the patient's mouth, manipulate the mandible to the position that will be used to adjust the appliance, and ask the patient to squeeze the appliance into place. Using this mandibular position will enhance the speed of adjusting the occlusal portion of the appliance.

Ask the patient to hold pressure on the appliance for 1 to 1½ minutes, during which a periodontal probe can be used to remove the excess acrylic that has squeezed fa-

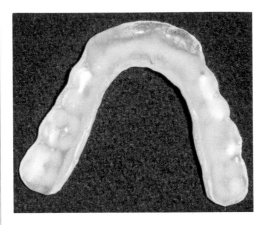

Figure 12-15. Internal appliance reline: moist acrylic is added to the internal surface of the appliance.

cially from the appliance. If the buccal flanges are short of the undercuts, the flanges will probably need to be extended to engage the undercuts, so the excess acrylic should probably not be removed from these areas. Some practitioners wait and remove this excess with a pair of scissors during one of the intermediate occasions when the appliance is removed and the material has a rubber consistency.

At 1½ minutes after placing the appliance in the mouth, dislodge it from the supporting teeth (not from the mouth) and reinsert it. Continue this every 30 seconds until the acrylic reaches its final set (Figure 12-16). It has been observed that the acrylic's setting shrinkage will usually cause the appliance to fit too tightly if one stops prior to the acrylic's final set.

Inserting and removing the appliance every 30 seconds appears to compress the acrylic in the undercut areas properly so they are not too deeply engaged. There appears to be a critical time (approximately 3 to 4 minutes into the procedure) in which the appliance suddenly takes a little more force to dislodge. I have had two incidents in which residents did not follow my instructions (e.g., "I just turned and did a little paperwork"), and the appliance had to be removed in pieces.

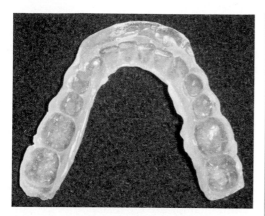

Figure 12-16. Internal appliance reline: once the acrylic hardened, the appliance was removed from mouth.

At the end of this procedure, patients generally like to swish with mouthwash. Trim the reline material back to the original flanges, unless the buccal flanges should be lengthened (Figure 12-17). If lengthening the buccal flanges, trim and smooth the area, leaving approximately 2 mm of the interproximal material to engage the undercuts. Reevaluate the appliance's retention and make any adjustments that are needed.

The light-cured acrylic can be used to reline the appliance's internal surface in a similar manner. Once the light-cured acrylic has been added to the internal portion of the appliance and seated in the mouth, ask the pa-

tient to squeeze the appliance into place with the mandibular position that will be used to adjust the appliance. A periodontal probe can be used to remove the excess acrylic that has facially expressed from the appliance.

With the appliance seated, use the light wand intraorally to partially cure the acrylic (for less than 1 minute). Remove the appliance, trim the excess acrylic, replace the appliance, and use the light wand to continue curing the acrylic.[49] Multiple partial curing procedures followed by dislodging the appliance may provide the best results.

Occasionally patients will need a restoration placed on a tooth that is covered by an occlusal appliance. Whenever a filling or crown is placed on one of these teeth, the new restoration's contours are different, which generally keeps the appliance from seating fully. Clinical experience has shown that, if the patient had a small to medium-sized filling placed, a few internal appliance adjustments are often sufficient to allow the appliance to accommodate for the new restoration, and sufficient appliance-tooth contacts will remain so the tooth will not shift under the appliance.

If an appliance does not seat fully after the placement of a small to medium-sized filling, mark the appliance's internal surface by attempting to seat the appliance with Accufilm between the new restoration and the appliance. Aggressively remove the areas of the appliance that were marked by the new restoration and err on the side of removing too much acrylic. Generally, after a few adjustments, the appliance can seat as it did prior to the restoration.

If the patient had a crown or an extensive filling placed, it is probably more efficient to relieve and reline the internal portion of the appliance where the restoration is located. To do this, remove about 1/4 to 1/2 mm of acrylic from all aspects of the appliance where the restoration may touch. Insert the appliance and, if the new restoration causes pressure on or restricts seating of the appli-

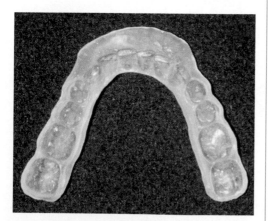

Figure 12-17. Internal appliance reline: excessive reline material is reduced and the edges smoothed.

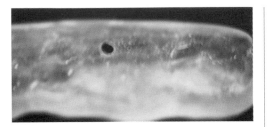

Figure 12-18. Internal appliance reline for a single tooth: a vent hole has been placed in the appliance.

ance, relieve the appliance until it seats fully and comfortably. Accufilm can be used to identify the areas of pressure or restriction.

Various techniques can be used to reline an appliance for a single tooth, and this is one of the few situations in which I perform a partial appliance reline. It is important when performing this reline that the added acrylic does not keep the appliance from seating fully. If this occurs, there will be a gap between the appliance's internal surface and the adjacent teeth, and the appliance's occlusion will have shifted. To prevent this, I often place a vent hole in the appliance (Figure 12-18) and mix the acrylic so it is a little more moist than used in the previously discussed reline.

Prior to performing the internal reline, remove any Accufilm marks that may be in

the area. Moisten the portion of the appliance that will be relined with monomer and shake out the excess. Pour the estimated amount of acrylic powder into a paper cup, add the monomer, and mix with a wooden tongue depressor. Put the acrylic into the appliance so approximately 1 mm of acrylic covers the surfaces to be relined and it is a little short of the desired gingival extent. (The acrylic generally flows gingivally 1 or 2 mm.) Place the appliance into the patient's mouth, manipulate the mandible to the position in which the appliance was adjusted, and ask the patient to squeeze the appliance into place, ensuring the appliance is fully seated (Figure 12-19).

After the patient has held pressure on the appliance for 2 minutes, dislodge and reinsert it. Continue this every 30 seconds until the acrylic reaches its final set (Figure 12-20). Some patients like to swish with mouthwash before and after this procedure. Trim the added acrylic and adjust the appliance's occlusion as needed.

External Adjustments

If the appliance stimulates the gag reflex, reduce the appliance when adjusting the internal surfaces. The degree of reduction is bal-

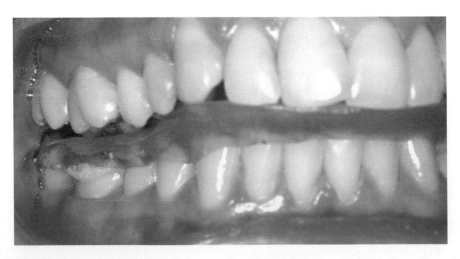

Figure 12-19. Internal appliance reline for a single tooth: the patient is squeezing on appliance to seat it fully.

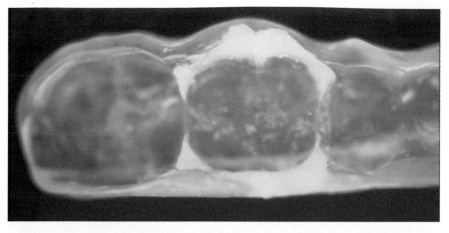

Figure 12-20. Internal appliance reline for a single tooth: the appliance with hardened acrylic has been removed from mouth; excess material needs to be removed and the edges smoothed.

anced between making the appliance too fragile and making it comfortable; it has to be acceptably comfortable or the patient will not wear it. Clinical experience has shown that mandibular appliances tend to stimulate the gag reflex less, but some patients suffer less gagging with a maxillary appliance.

Any lingual portion of the appliance has been observed to elicit a patient's gag reflex. Unless the patient directs certain areas be reduced, it is recommended that the posterior lingual flange first be thinned to 1/2 to 1 mm thick. If this is not satisfactory, shorten the lingual flange as needed; I rarely have to reduce it beyond the cervical margins of the teeth. If necessary, cut the posterior lingual portion so it overlaps the lingual cusps only by 1 mm and the anterior lingual flange to the cervical margins of the anterior teeth.

Once the appliance fits comfortably and has appropriate retention, adjust its occlusion by using the traditional gnathologic principles used by dentists for many years.

▼ TECHNICAL TIP

Adjusting Appliance's Occlusion

Once the appliance fits comfortably and has appropriate retention, adjust its occlusion.

If a patient plans to wear an orthodontic retainer or partial denture opposing the ap-

pliance, adjust the appliance with it in place. This ensures the appliance will not occlude too hard on the retainer or denture.

The appliance's occlusal surface should be flat so the anterior teeth can slide smoothly along the appliance surface from the centric position and provide immediate disocclusion of the posterior teeth.[9,21] If the occlusal surface has cuspal indentations, as the mandible begins to move excursively, the cusp tip may bump the indentation's edge, disrupting this smooth flow. Therefore, the laboratory technician should not leave indentations and, if they are present, remove them as the appliance's occlusal surface is adjusted.

Instruct the patient to insert and remove the appliance for each adjustment. This ensures the patient can insert the appliance, ensures the appliance does not have too much retention, frees the practitioner to do other things (e.g., pick up the articulating forceps while the patient seats the appliance) and, if the cheek is caught during insertion, the practitioner would not be aware of this and continue to attempt to seat the appliance.

Mark the opposing tooth contacts on the appliance with two sheets of Accufilm in the articulating forceps, using black to mark the centric contacts. Hold the forceps at a slight angle in the mouth so the patient can mark the third molar as well as the central

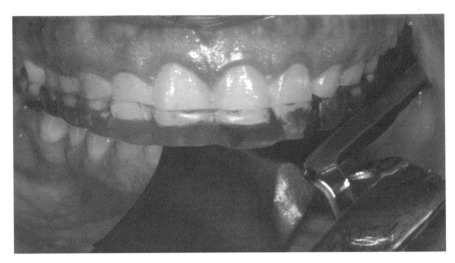

Figure 12-21. Accufilm held in this position can mark contacts from central incisors to third molars.

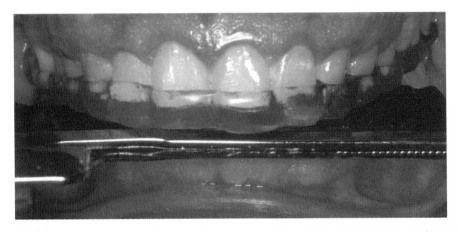

Figure 12-22. It is recommended that Accufilm never be held in this position because patients tend to protrude the mandible in this situation.

incisor at the same time (Figure 12-21). It has been observed that, if the anterior teeth are marked independently (Figure 12-22), patients tend to protrude the mandible for these markings.

With the mandible in the desired position (neutral position or centric relation, as discussed in "Mandibular Positions and Bite Registration" in this chapter) and the Accufilm in place, ask the patient to tap on the appliance. As the patient does so, ensure the patient does not deviate from his or her normal closing arch. Some patients shift their mandible to the side that is being marked. If this occurs, request the patient to "tap straight up and down with your jaw in the center." If the patient cannot stop shifting the mandible, simultaneously place Accufilm on both sides of the appliance, which usually eliminates this problem. It is also important that the patient does not have his or her head tilted to the side when the appliance is marked; this causes the mandible to shift to the side, and the markings will also be incorrectly positioned.

It is important to realize that only the supporting cusps provide the centric contacts from the opposing posterior teeth. There-

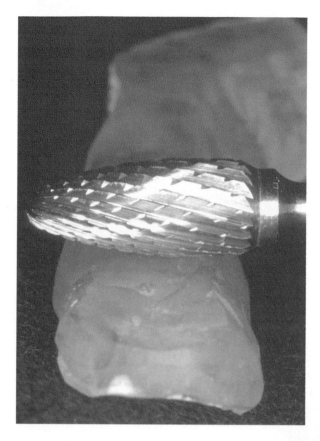

Figure 12-23. If an appliance is adjusted with the flat side of an acrylic bur, the adjustment tends also to remove potential excursive contacts, increasing the speed with which the practitioner can perform the adjustment.

fore, the maxillary appliance occludes with the mandibular buccal cusps, whereas the mandibular appliance occludes with the maxillary lingual cusps. The nonsupporting cusps never touch the appliance, except when a tooth is rotated to the degree that the supporting cusp cannot harmoniously occlude with the appliance, in which case one can attempt to occlude the nonsupporting cusp with the appliance.

To enhance the appliance adjustment, adjust the centric marks with the acrylic bur's flat side rather than its point (Figures 12-23 and 12-24). This helps to provide a flat occlusal surface and reduces the probability of posterior excursive interferences.

As the practitioner repeatedly marks and adjusts the appliance, he or she should slowly develop even, centric marks from the opposing posterior teeth. At least one contact from each posterior tooth should evenly occlude with the appliance, unless the tooth

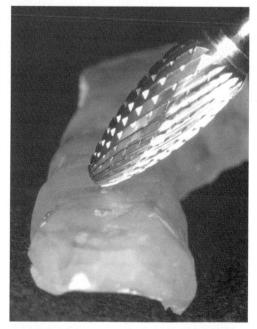

Figure 12-24. If an appliance is adjusted with the point of an acrylic bur, the adjustment tends to leave areas that will be excursive interferences that will need to be removed later.

is malposed, e.g., not within the arch's occlusal plane, and does not occlude with the opposing dentition. The centric marks from the anterior teeth should be light or none in comparison with the posterior marks.[8] The cuspid marks may be in harmony with the marks from the anterior or posterior teeth.

The appliance should allow the patient to slide into excursive positions easily. Therefore, adjust the appliance so it has minimal disocclusion of the posterior teeth.[50] For efficiency, as I adjust the anterior centric contacts, I generally also adjust the angle of the anterior guidance ramp so it is only about 5° steeper than the appliance's occlusal plane (Figure 12-7).

▼ **TECHNICAL TIP**

Occluding Cusps

Only supporting cusps provide an appliance's centric contacts. Therefore, the maxillary appliance occludes with the mandibular buccal cusps, whereas the mandibular appliance occludes with the maxillary lingual cusps.

As the appliance is being adjusted, periodically observe the distance the various cusp tips are from occluding with the appliance. If most of the cusp tips are a significant distance from occluding, it may be faster to reline the entire occlusal surface than removing acrylic to obtain the desired occlusion. If all of the cusp tips except one or two are hitting evenly on the appliance, and the cusp tips are 1/2 mm or more from occluding with the appliance, it may be faster to add acrylic to that portion of the appliance. Occasionally a cusp tip is buccal or lingual to the appliance's occlusal surface, and the occlusal surface needs to be extended. Adding acrylic to an appliance's external surface is discussed in the next section, "External Reline."

The amount of acrylic to remove with each adjustment varies with how much each contact should be reduced. This changes with the number of centric marks obtained

and how far the other cusp tips are from occluding with the appliance. If only one or two contacts are marking the appliance and the other cusp tips are a sufficient distance from marking, reduce each mark several times the amount that it takes to remove the mark; this more rapidly allows the other cusp tips to come into contact. When most of the cusp tips are marking and the other cusp tips are close to marking, I usually grind just enough to remove each mark plus a little extra on the heavier marks. When all of the desired cusp tips are marking and the practitioner is attempting to create uniform centric marks, he or she should lighten the heavier marks by only about 50 percent. With experience, these various degrees of adjustments become second nature.

Occasionally patients have less biting strength on one side of their mouth and consistently tap lighter on that side. As the practitioner attempts to develop uniform bilateral marks of equal intensity, generally the appliance is inadvertently adjusted so the weaker side hits harder than the stronger side. Therefore, as adjusting the appliance for centric contacts nears completion, periodically ask the patient to close on the appliance (without Accufilm in the mouth) and to say whether the left or right side hits first or harder. Adjust the appliance so the patient feels that both sides hit evenly and each side of the appliance has marks of equal intensity independent of the other side.

Since crowns supported by dental implants do not have periodontal ligaments, they do not compress when patients clench on them. To ensure these crowns are not overloaded against the appliance, adjust the opposing appliance so anterior teeth supported by dental implants are just out of occlusion and posterior teeth supported by dental implants produce significantly lighter marks on the appliance. If the implant is a single tooth, the practitioner may make the contact so it is just out of occlusion, because there is no fear that these teeth will extrude.[51]

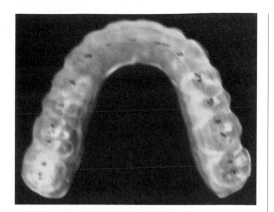

Figure 12-25. Accufilm marks of centric contacts on an adjusted appliance.

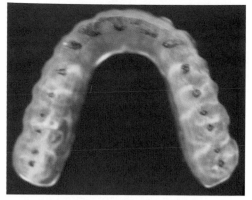

Figure 12-26. Red Accufilm marks of excursive contacts and black Accufilm marks of centric contacts on an adjusted appliance.

Occasionally patients cannot repeatedly close to the same position on the appliance, even though the practitioner uses the mandibular positioning technique previously described. In this situation, I adjust the appliance to the degree I am able, allow the patient to use the appliance and, when the patient returns, he or she can generally provide repeatable centric contacts.

Once the desired centric contacts are obtained (Figure 12-25), begin adjusting the excursive movements. First observe the distance the posterior teeth separate as the patient slides the mandible into the excursive positions. This gives a feel for how much and in which direction(s) the anterior guidance needs to be lowered.

Place two sheets of red Accufilm in the patient's mouth as previously described and ask the patient to grind his or her teeth side to side, and forward and backward; do this for both sides of the mouth. Then place the black Accufilm in the patient's mouth and ask the patient to tap on the appliance to remark the centric contacts. This provides the appliance with black centric contacts on top of the red excursive marks.

Repeatedly adjust the posterior portion of the appliance so no red posterior excursive marks are produced and the anterior portion of the appliance so the amount of separation between the closest posterior contact and the

appliance is only 1/2 to 1 mm.[50] I prefer to have the anterior guidance distributed among as many anterior teeth as possible (Figure 12-26). Some practitioners prefer to have the anterior guidance provided only by the canines, which is also an acceptable technique.[10]

If it is planned for the patient to wear the appliance during the day, after the appliance is adjusted in the reclined position, reposition the dental chair into the sitting position and ask the patient to sit with feet to the side so they are on the floor. Adjust the appliance in this position because it simulates the patient's normal upright position.[1] Adjusting the appliance in this position generally takes only a few additional adjustments.

▼ **TECHNICAL TIP**

Adjusting Appliance for Daytime Wear

If it is planned for a patient to wear an appliance during the day, after the appliance is adjusted in the reclined position, reposition the dental chair into the sitting position, ask the patient to sit with feet to the side, and adjust the appliance with the patient in this sitting position.

Clinical experience has demonstrated the appliance's occlusion should be well adjusted to provide its maximal effect. Patients referred to me with a poorly adjusted appliance sometimes obtain considerable symptom improvement after having its occlusion improved.

Sometimes the appliance is perforated during adjustments. These perforations are generally over the cusp tips of teeth underlying the appliance, so perforations would rarely compromise its ability to support the occlusal contacts of the opposing teeth and would not have a detrimental effect on its efficacy. If I perforate the appliance, I always show the perforations to the patient, who otherwise may think the appliance is breaking. Once I explain that the perforations are not a concern and the appliance would need to be thicker for it to not have them, I have never had a patient request the appliance be thickened to eliminate them.

▼ TECHNICAL TIP
Observing Perforations
Appliance perforations are generally over the cusp tips of teeth underlying the appliance, so perforations would rarely compromise the appliance's ability to support the occlusal contacts of the opposing teeth and would not have a detrimental effect on the appliance's efficacy.

Once the appliance's occlusion is adjusted and the markings demonstrate the portion of the occlusal surface that is needed to support the opposing teeth, contour the sides of the appliance. Clinically most patients appear to need only about 7 mm for anterior guidance, so any unnecessary portion of the guidance ramp can be removed. Clinically most patients appear to prefer to have the appliance's occlusal surface line angles rounded so they have a similar occlusal gingival curvature to the teeth they cover. In some cases, an occlusal contact may be near the appliance's line angle, so this portion of the appliance may be able to have only minimal contouring.

Thin the flanges and the portions that overlay the side of the teeth so they are approximately 1 mm thick. If the appliance will be worn only at night, one may desire to leave these thicker so there is less chance of fracturing the appliance. The external surface needs to flow smoothly and have a relatively smooth surface; otherwise, patients tend to play with areas of disharmony, which may cause an increase in TMD symptoms.

If the appliance will be worn during the day, patients generally prefer a mandibular appliance with the lingual surface as thin as possible. Make the entire lingual surface of the mandibular appliance 1 mm thick and carry the flange below the tongue's resting position so patients do not continually rub across its border as they speak. If a patient has mandibular tori, trim the lingual flange so it blends into the superior portion of the tori.

Patients who will wear a maxillary appliance during the day generally prefer shorter lingual flanges that are no thicker than 1 mm.[21] For most patients to obtain immediate disocclusion of the posterior teeth, a guidance ramp generally needs to extend lingual to the maxillary anterior teeth. Patients usually prefer the area gingival to this ramp to be concave, so the appliance's bulk is minimized.

After my appliance adjustments are completed, I ask the patient to insert the appliance, to tell me whether the posterior occlusion hits as evenly as possible, and to tell me whether he or she knows of anything that I can do to improve the appliance. Sometimes a minor problem may annoy a patient (e.g., a rough spot on the lingual flange, a rough excursive movement, excessive bulk, or a tendency for the appliance to cause gagging) and cause the patient to play with the annoyance, which could lead to aggravation of the TMD symptoms.

Clinical experience has shown that it is not necessary to provide the patient with a highly polished occlusal appliance. For appliances with an outer acrylic surface, smooth the flanges and edges along the occlusal surface with coarse pumice. I do not pumice the occlusal portion where the opposing teeth mark, for fear that this may disrupt the occlusal patterns. I have found there is no need to pumice with finer polishing agents and have never had a patient request that the appliance's surface be more highly polished.

External Reline

There are numerous reasons for adding clear acrylic to the external surface of an appliance, and it is most commonly done when a practitioner is inserting an appliance. For instance, while adjusting the appliance, the practitioner may observe that all of the cusp tips except one or two occlude evenly on the appliance and the nonmarking cusp tips are a 1/2 mm or more from occluding with it. In this situation, it is generally faster to add acrylic to the nonmarking portion of the appliance rather than thin the appliance until all of the cusp tips eventually occlude.

A second situation can occur after an appliance is seated and the practitioner observes the occlusion with the opposing arch is quite different than the occlusion that was fabricated for the appliance. Occlusal discrepancies during appliance insertion routinely occur with TMD patients because the condyle's neutral position tends to change with a patient's normal TMD symptom pattern flucuation.[52,53] If the occlusal discrepancy is quite large, the practitioner may prefer to add acrylic to the entire occlusal surface because the appliance may not be thick enough to accommodate the large occlusal discrepancy and the practitioner would probably find it faster.

In this situation, I generally mark and aggressively adjust the appliance contacts several times to minimize the amount of acrylic that will need to be added to the occlusal surface. After the aggressive adjustments, the opposing dentition may occlude facial or lingual to the appliance's occlusal surface, and

acrylic may also need to be added to move the appliance's occlusal surface. At other times, the aggressive adjustments may have improved the occlusion to the degree that only a portion of the occlusal surface needs acrylic added.

If the practitioner routinely finds a large occlusal discrepancy, improvements can probably be made in the bite registration technique, e.g., using softer wax or ensuring the patient's head is maximally rotated back. For possible technique improvements, practitioners may wish to review "Mandibular Positions and Bite Registration" in this chapter.

◉ **QUICK CONSULT**

Observing Bite Registration Errors

If a practitioner routinely finds a large occlusal discrepancy, improvements can probably be made in the bite registration technique, e.g., using softer wax or ensuring the patient's head is maximally rotated back.

Some practitioners routinely add acrylic to the entire occlusal surface of certain appliances. This is most commonly done when fabricating an appliance by using a 2-mm hard thermoplastic shell in which the occlusal contacts may routinely be obtained by adding acrylic to the appliance's occlusal surface.[10] An example of this appliance is presented in "Hard Thermoplastic Stabilization Appliance" in this chapter.

The entire occlusal surface may also need to be relined for patients who heavily grind on their appliance at night. The appliance may wear thin, and the patient may periodically return to have acrylic added to the entire occlusal surface.

The reline technique is similar for each of these situations and can be performed with either self-curing or light-curing material. For simplicity, the self-curing technique is explained, but can be similarly used with the light-curing material.

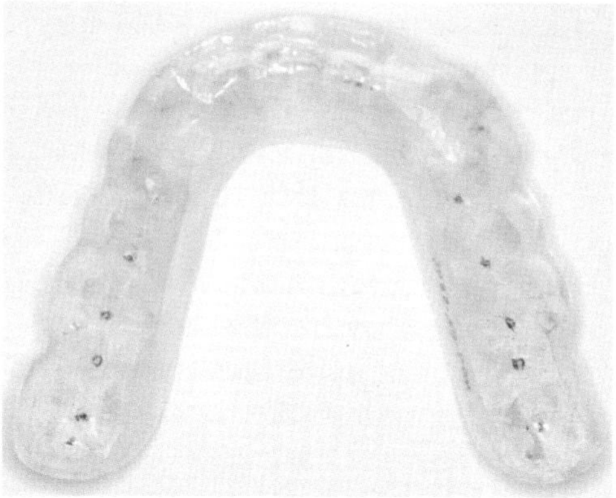

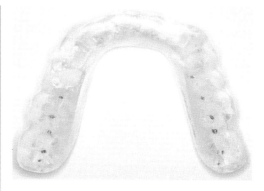

Figure 12-27. Adding a single contact to an appliance, which is missing a contact mark from the right first bicuspid.

Begin by removing any marks on the surface that will be covered by acrylic; moisten the area with monomer and shake off the excess. For one or two cusp tips (Figure 12-27), only a drop of monomer may be necessary. Pour the estimated needed acrylic powder into a paper cup, add only enough monomer to moisten all of the powder granules, and mix with a wooden tongue depressor.

If adding acrylic only so one or two non-marking cusp tips occlude with the appliance, place a piece of acrylic about 5 mm in diameter and 3 mm high onto the desired location(s) (Figure 12-28). If desired, the buccal portion of the appliance may be marked with a pencil to delineate the location where the acrylic is to be added. Wait until the acrylic firms to the consistency of clay before placing the appliance into the mouth. Sometimes, while waiting, the acrylic slumps or flows and needs to be re-molded. Once the appliance is in the mouth, manipulate the mandible to the position used to adjust the appliance and ask the patient to close and tap onto the appliance (similar to tapping on Accufilm). Some patients tend not to close fully onto the appliance, resulting in the added acrylic being too thick.

Remove the appliance and place it in

Figure 12-28. Adding a single contact to an appliance: acrylic in clay consistency.

warm water so the acrylic will cure faster. A few patients wish to rinse their mouth with mouthwash at this time. Once the acrylic is hard (Figure 12-29), mark the cuspal indentation depth(s) with a pencil and use the flat side of the acrylic bur to reduce the added acrylic. It has been observed that, if the acrylic is reduced so the pencil mark(s) are lightened by about 50 percent, the Accufilm mark(s) on the added acrylic will be very close to the other marks on the appliance (Figure 12-30).

When relining a larger portion of the occlusal surface, this area can be delineated by marking the appliance's buccal area with a pencil. Place the acrylic onto the desired area(s) of the appliance and use gloved fingers to position it, slightly overestimating the

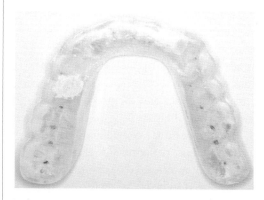

Figure 12-29. Adding a single contact to an appliance: hardened acrylic removed from a patient's mouth.

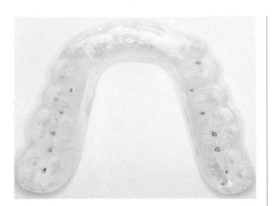

Figure 12-30. Adding single contact to appliance: contact added to an appliance.

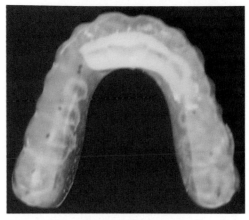

Figure 12-31. Adding acrylic to an anterior appliance segment: hardened acrylic removed from a patient's mouth.

amount of acrylic needed. Wait for the acrylic to firm into the clay consistency before placing the appliance into the patient's mouth. The acrylic may slump or flow while we are waiting, and it is important to ensure the acrylic does not flow into the internal area of the appliance. Therefore, the appliance is generally held with the added acrylic toward the floor, and I generally have to remold the acrylic once or twice during this wait.

Once the acrylic is the consistency of clay, place the appliance in the mouth, manipulate the mandible to the position where the appliance will be adjusted, and ask the patient to close slowly into the soft acrylic. As the patient does so, observe whether the soft acrylic needs to be repositioned. This can be done by asking the patient to open and molding the soft acrylic into the proper position. Again manipulate the mandible and ask the patient to close slowly into the soft acrylic and stop when he or she hits the hard acrylic. Patients tend not to close fully onto the appliance, resulting in the added acrylic being too thick. Therefore, while the patient is closed, look at the portions of the appliance where acrylic was not added to ensure he or she has completely closed. If adding acrylic only to a relatively small area, ask the patient to tap onto the appliance.

The appliance is removed, placed in

warm water to speed the curing process, and/or placed in a pressure-curing unit to decrease the added acrylic's porosity. Some patients wish to rinse their mouth with mouthwash at this time. Once the acrylic is hard (Figure 12-31), mark the cuspal depths with a pencil and use the flat side of the acrylic bur to reduce the added acrylic. It has been observed that, if the acrylic is reduced so the pencil mark is lightened by about 50 percent, the Accufilm marks on the added acrylic will be very close to the other marks on the appliance.

If acrylic is to be added to the entire occlusal surface, place the acrylic onto the occlusal surface with the tongue depressor and mold it with gloved fingers. As with the other techniques, wait for the acrylic to firm into the clay consistency before placing the appliance into the patient's mouth. The acrylic may tend to flow into the internal area of the appliance, so the appliance is generally held with the occlusal surface toward the floor and the new acrylic is remolded as needed. Once the acrylic is the consistency of clay, place the appliance in the mouth, manipulate the mandible to the position where the appliance will be adjusted, and ask the patient to close slowly onto the soft acrylic. As the patient closes, observe

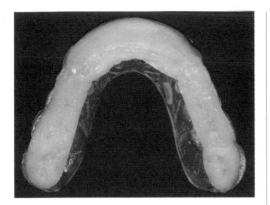

Figure 12-32. Adding acrylic to an entire occlusal surface: acrylic in clay consistency.

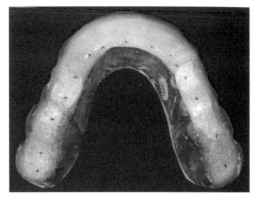

Figure 12-34. Adding acrylic to an entire occlusal surface: Accufilm marks of centric contacts on an adjusted appliance.

whether the soft acrylic needs to be repositioned. If so, ask the patient to open while the soft acrylic is shaped into the proper position. Again manipulate the mandible and ask the patient to close slowly into the soft acrylic and to stop when the jaw is at the desired vertical dimension.

The appliance is removed, placed in warm water to speed the curing process, and/or placed in a pressure-curing unit to decrease the added acrylic's porosity. Many patients wish to rinse their mouth with mouthwash at this time. Once the acrylic is hard (Figure 12-32), mark the cuspal depths with a pencil (Figure 12-33) and use the flat side of the acrylic bur to reduce the added acrylic so that all of the indentations are removed and the pencil marks are lightened.

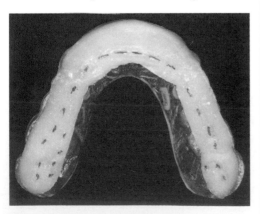

Figure 12-33. Adding acrylic to an entire occlusal surface: cusp depths marked with pencils.

The external surface of the splint is adjusted as previously described (Figures 12-34 to 12-36).

Adding acrylic to the occlusal surface sometimes causes undesirable concavities along the side of the appliance. These are easily filled by moistening the area with monomer and similarly mixing the acrylic, placing it in the concavity, and contouring it with a gloved finger. A smooth finish can be achieved by applying a little monomer over the surface and further smoothing with a gloved finger.

Appliance Repair

Fractured acrylic occlusal appliances can be repaired by the laboratory. If no portion of the appliance is missing and the fractured pieces can be aligned by hand the appliance can be given to the laboratory in this state for repair. If a portion of the appliance is missing and the practitioner wants the laboratory fix it, the appliance needs to be seated on the teeth and an impression made over it. The stone cast is poured with the appliance seated in the impression material. If the opposing dentition occludes with the missing piece, the practitioner may want the laboratory also to adjust the occlusion with the added section. This would require that the practitioner also make an impression of the

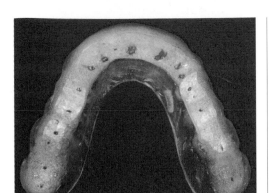

Figure 12-35. Adding acrylic to an entire occlusal surface: red Accufilm marks of excursive contacts and black Accufilm marks of centric contacts on an adjusted appliance.

opposing teeth and provide a means to mount the opposing cast with the appliance (a bite registration or occlusal markings on the appliance).

I prefer to repair broken occlusal appliances directly in the mouth, because it is relatively quick and the patient does not have to be without the appliance. My experience is that repairs of traditional acrylic appliances do not tend to refracture in the location they previously broke, but the appliances made with the 2-mm thermoplastic material tend to refracture at that location. For this reason, I have not attempted to repair appliances made of the dual laminate thermoplastic material, and I do not know of a technique to repair soft thermoplastic appliances. There-

fore, this appliance-repair discussion is limited to the traditional acrylic appliances.

⊙ **QUICK CONSULT**

Repairing Broken Appliances

❙ prefer to repair broken occlusal appliances directly in the mouth, because it is relatively quick and the patient does not have to be without his or her appliance.

Occasionally patients develop a hairline fracture extending along an appliance's occlusal surface. It is speculated that these cracks usually occur as a result of the occlusal surface not being thick enough to withstand the patient's heavy clenching activity. Therefore, it is recommended that the fracture be repaired and the occlusal surface thickened simultaneously. I prefer to seal the crack by flowing clear acrylic into the hairline fracture, which requires opening the fracture to provide a space for the acrylic. Open the hairline fracture with a bur (e.g., a number 330 bur). If the appliance is sufficiently thick along the fractured area, provide a slight bevel to the external margins of the cut made. Then reline the entire occlusal surface of the appliance as described in the previous section ("External Reline") so an additional 1 to 2 mm of acrylic is added over this area. This simultaneously seals the hairline fracture and thickens the appliance's occlusal surface.

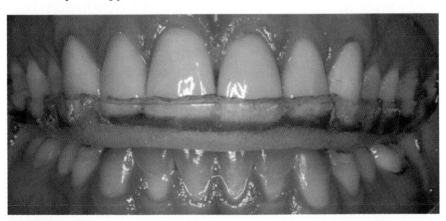

Figure 12-36. Adding acrylic to an entire occlusal surface: relined appliance in the mouth.

The most common occlusal appliance fracture I see is the appliance that has broken into two pieces with the fracture in the anterior region. In this situation, increase the cross-sectional area of the fractured surface and provide approximately 1 mm of space between the two halves by slightly overbeveling the internal and external edges of the fracture (Figure 12-37).

After beveling the edges, insert both halves onto the teeth to ensure both halves fit properly and there is a space between the beveled edges for the acrylic. The halves are removed, and the beveled edges are moistened with monomer. Pour the estimated needed acrylic powder into a paper cup, add only enough monomer to moisten all of the powder granules, and mix with a wooden tongue depressor. Independently place acrylic on the beveled edges of each half, place both halves onto the teeth, and press the soft acrylic to join the two portions. If necessary, a gloved finger can be used to add acrylic to overbulk the area slightly (Figure 12-38).

A portion of the acrylic often flows or is pressed into an interproximal undercut. Therefore, the appliance needs to be raised off the supporting teeth periodically or the acrylic residing in the undercut will harden and may not allow the appliance to be re-

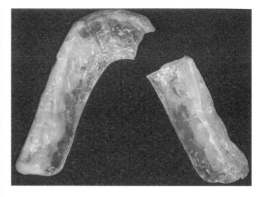

Figure 12-37. Intraoral appliance repair: fractured edges are beveled.

moved. Approximately 2 to 3 minutes after placing the two halves in the mouth, raise the fractured portion of the appliance off the teeth (not from the mouth) and reinsert the appliance. Continue this every 30 seconds until the acrylic reaches its final set. Then remove the appliance, trim the added acrylic to the desired shape, and polish the appliance (Figure 12-39).

Occasionally patients have a portion of their appliance missing, such as one of my patients who related her dog got ahold of her appliance. After inserting the appliance to ensure it fits properly, bevel the fracture's external edge to increase its cross-sectional area. Moisten the beveled edge with monomer, similarly mix acrylic in a paper

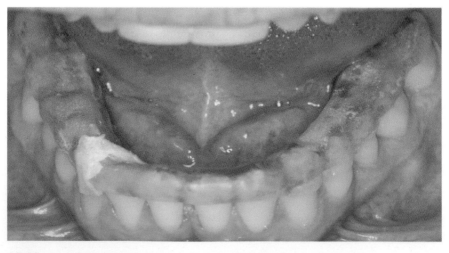

Figure 12-38. Intraoral appliance repair: added acrylic hardening in the mouth.

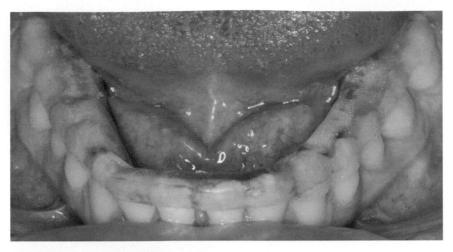

Figure 12-39. Intraoral appliance repair: repaired appliance.

cup, and place the appliance onto the patient's teeth (without acrylic on it). As the mixed acrylic loses its sheen, apply the acrylic with a gloved finger to the area where it is missing and have the patient close the opposing teeth into it. Check to ensure the added acrylic is thick enough that the supporting cups of the opposing teeth occlude into it.

Approximately 2 to 3 minutes after adding acrylic to the appliance, carefully dislodge it so the added acrylic does not lock the appliance into the undercuts. Reinsert the appliance and continue this every 30 seconds until the acrylic reaches its final set. Remove the appliance and trim the acrylic to the desired shape. If the missing portion occludes with the opposing teeth, mark the cuspal depths with a pencil, use the flat side of the acrylic bur to reduce the added acrylic so the pencil marks are lightened by about 50 percent, and adjust the appliance's occlusion in the usual manner.

If there does not appear to be a cause for the appliance breaking (e.g., a dog chewing it), the occlusal surface may be too thin for the patient's heavy clenching activity and the occlusal surface may also need to be thickened. The entire occlusal surface can be thickened in combination with replacing the missing portion of the appliance.

⊙ **QUICK CONSULT**
Observing Broken Appliances

If there does not appear to be a cause for the appliance breaking, the occlusal surface may be too thin for the patient's heavy clenching activity and the occlusal surface may also need to be thickened.

If the appliance is fractured in addition to missing a piece, the practitioner may desire to separate these into two procedures, repairing the fracture first and then replacing the missing portion. If multiple steps will be needed to repair an appliance, there comes a point at which it would be better to fabricate a new one.

APPLIANCE EXAMPLES

The following examples are provided to help readers better apply the principles discussed for stabilization appliances. These examples were chosen because of the various procedures they demonstrate, rather than recommending any certain appliance form or technique. These procedures can be used in many combinations to fabricate various appliances.

The first two examples are fabricated with clear acrylic, whereas the next three use thermoplastic materials, which are typically warmed by a heat lamp and formed over a patient's cast by vacuum suction or pressurized air. Thermoplastic materials come in various thicknesses and are used in many aspects of dentistry, e.g., athletic mouthguard, bleaching tray, and tray for fabricating a temporary crown.

Some practitioners preprint their occlusal appliance laboratory prescriptions with fabrication guidelines so the laboratory technician provides an appliance that meets the practitioner's preferences. An example of my fabrication guidelines is provided in Appendix 7, "Laboratory Occlusal Appliance Instructions." The example is formulated so the practitioner can simply add the date of insertion, circle the desired appliance, and sign the prescription.

Pressure-cured Mandibular Acrylic Stabilization Appliance

Many techniques can be employed to fabricate an acrylic stabilization appliance, and the appliance's attrition rate will vary with the selected acrylic and processing method.[30] When the same acrylic is used, a pressure-cured appliance is more resistant to attrition than one that has been bench cured.[30]

The pressure-cured appliance generally takes the laboratory a little longer to fabricate, so the laboratory fee is generally higher. For this appliance, the practitioner makes impressions of the maxillary and mandibular teeth and the desired bite registration. The casts are mounted on an articulator with the bite registration (Figure 12-40), and the desired areas are blocked out on the arch for which the appliance will be fabricated. (For details, see Appendix 7, "Laboratory Occlusal Appliance Instructions.") I generally request the laboratory block out the deep grooves on the teeth and all undercuts except the buccal embrasures of posterior teeth (Figure 12-41). This leaves the buccal undercuts of the posterior teeth open, which provides an appliance that engages into these

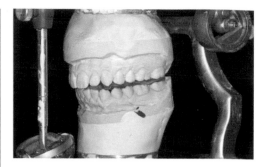

Figure 12-40. Pressure-cured mandibular acrylic stabilization appliance: casts mounted.

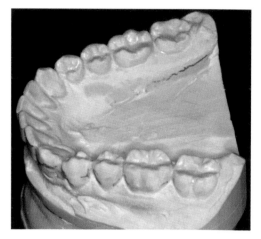

Figure 12-41. Pressure-cured mandibular acrylic stabilization appliance: blockout placed on mandibular cast.

undercuts, thereby supplying retention to this area.

Using the mounted blocked-out cast and the opposing cast, a new registration relating these casts is made. The blocked-out cast is duplicated and mounted on the articulator by using the new registration (Figure 12-42). The appliance is waxed onto the duplicate cast, and the wax pattern on the cast is placed in a flask (Figures 12-43 and 12-44). In Figure 12-43, note that an anterior guidance ramp extends anteriorly from the mandibular anterior teeth, enabling the appliance to provide immediate disocclusion of the posterior teeth. In Figure 12-44, note that the guidance ramp's guidance is only about 5° steeper than the posterior occlusal plane. This shallow guidance angle will minimize the resistance encountered when the patient attempts to move the mandible in an excursive direction.

Once the appliance is cured, it is removed from the flask. The original master cast is replaced on the articulator, and the appliance

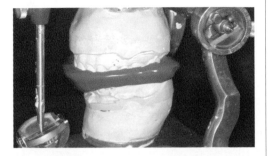

Figure 12-42. Pressure-cured mandibular acrylic stabilization appliance: duplicated cast of blocked-out model mounted with new registration.

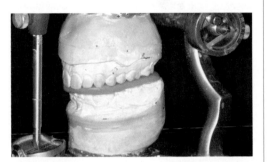

Figure 12-43. Pressure-cured mandibular acrylic stabilization appliance: waxed appliance.

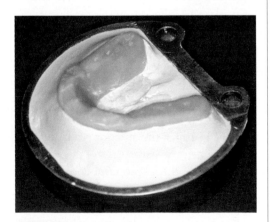

Figure 12-44. Pressure-cured mandibular acrylic stabilization appliance: wax pattern placed in a flask.

is seated on this cast. The occlusion is marked and adjusted, and the appliance is polished (Figures 12-45 to 12-47). In Figures 12-46 and 12-47, note that the entire facial and lingual portions of the appliance and the acrylic lingual to the anterior teeth are approximately 1 mm thick.

The appliance is inserted in the patient's mouth. If the appliance cannot fully seat with a moderate amount of force or causes an uncomfortable pressure, its internal surface is adjusted, as explained in "Internal Adjustments" in this chapter.

Once the appliance fits comfortably, the mandible is manipulated into the desired position, and the occlusion of the appliance is adjusted. It is recommended that two sheets of black Accufilm be placed in an articulat-

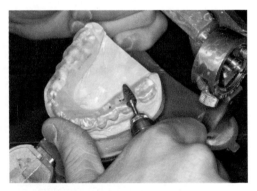

Figure 12-45. Pressure-cured mandibular acrylic stabilization appliance: adjusted on articulator.

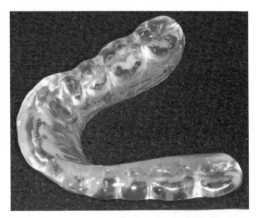

Figure 12-46. Pressure-cured mandibular acrylic stabilization appliance: completed.

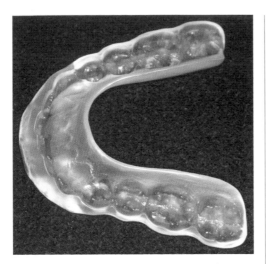

Figure 12-47. Pressure-cured mandibular acrylic stabilization appliance: note the thickness of buccal and lingual flanges, and the acrylic thickness lingual to the anterior teeth.

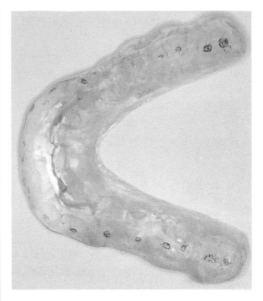

Figure 12-48. Pressure-cured mandibular acrylic stabilization appliance: centric contact Accufilm marks on adjusted appliance; it is a little heavy on one second molar, but will be lightened when adjusting the excursive movements.

ing forceps to mark the centric contacts (discussed in "External Adjustments" in this chapter). Repeatedly mark and adjust the appliance so as to obtain at least one centric mark from each posterior tooth and light to no marks from the anterior teeth in comparison with the posterior marks. The cuspid marks may be in harmony with the marks from the anterior or posterior teeth (Figure 12-48).

While adjusting the centric contacts, practitioners may find it necessary or more expedient to reline a portion of the occlusal surface (discussed in "External Reline" in this chapter). As the centric contact adjustments near completion, periodically ask the patient to close on the appliance (without Accufilm in the mouth) and tell whether the left or right side hits first or harder. Adjust the appliance so the patient feels that both sides hit evenly and each side of the appliance has uniform centric marks independent of the other side.

Once the desired centric contacts are obtained, adjust the appliance so the patient can slide easily into excursive positions, disoccluding the posterior teeth with the closest posterior contact being 1/2 to 1 mm from

the appliance. To obtain a feel for how much and in which direction(s) the anterior guidance ramp will need to be adjusted, first observe the distance the posterior teeth separate as the patient slides the mandible into these excursive positions.

Using two sheets of red Accufilm, mark the appliance in excursive positions. Ask the patient to grind the teeth side to side and forward and backward on the red Accufilm. Then ask the patient to tap in the centric position on black Accufilm to provide the appliance with black centric contact marks on top of the red excursive marks.

Adjust the posterior portion of the appliance so no red posterior excursive marks are produced. Adjust the anterior guidance ramp so that, when the patient is in the excursive positions, the closest posterior contact is only 1/2 to 1 mm from the appliance and the forces along the guidance ramp are distributed as evenly as possible among the anterior teeth (Figure 12-49), as demonstrated in Figures 12-51 to 12-53.

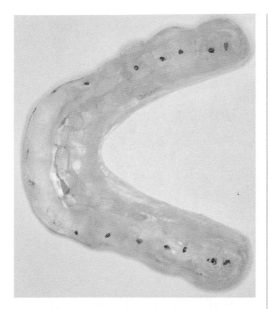

Figure 12-49. Pressure-cured mandibular acrylic stabilization appliance: red Accufilm marks of excursive contacts and black Accufilm marks of centric contacts on the adjusted appliance.

If the appliance is to be worn during the day, also adjust the appliance with the patient in an upright position. Reposition the dental chair into the sitting position and ask the patient to sit with feet to the side so they are on the floor. Mark and adjust the appliance using the same criteria; this generally takes only a few additional adjustments.

Once the appliance's occlusion is adjusted, contour the sides of the appliance. Patients generally appear not to need more than 7 mm for their anterior guidance, so remove any unnecessary portion of the guidance ramp. Most patients also seem to prefer to have the appliance's occlusal surface line angles rounded so the occlusal gingival curvature is similar to the tooth that it covers.

If any portion of the appliance's sides are thicker than 1 mm, consider thinning these areas, especially if the patient plans to wear the appliance during the day. Thinner flanges make the appliance feel less obtrusive and enable the patient to speak better when wearing the appliance.

Once the appliance is adjusted satisfactorily, ask the patient to insert it. Inform the patient that it will be smoothed further, but that you want to ensure that the posterior teeth hit the appliance as evenly as possible and determine whether the patient knows of anything that can be done to make the appliance more comfortable. Once the appliance meets with the patient's approval, smooth its sides and ask whether it feels satisfactorily smooth.

Maxillary Acrylic Stabilization Appliance

The principles for the maxillary appliance are almost identical to those for the mandibular appliance. There are two prominent differences: (a) the excursive movements are in the opposite directions on the appliance, so the anterior guidance ramp will be lingual

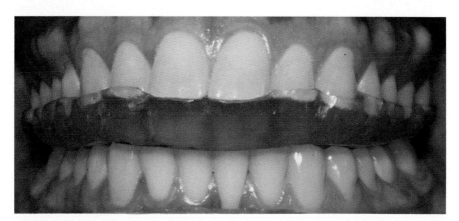

Figure 12-50. Patient occluding on appliance in the neutral position.

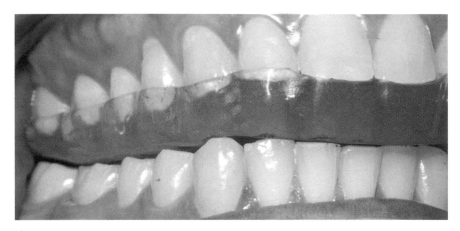

Figure 12-51. Patient occluding on appliance in right lateral: note the minimal disocclusion of the posterior teeth.

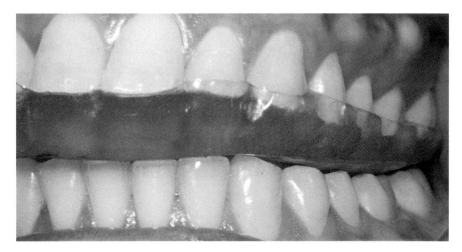

Figure 12-52. Patient occluding on appliance in left lateral: note the minimal disocclusion of the posterior teeth.

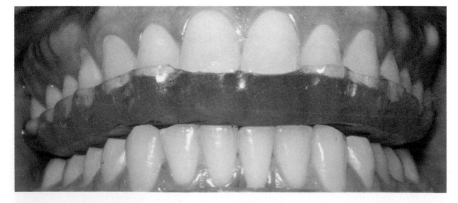

Figure 12-53. Patient occluding on appliance in protrusive: note the minimal disocclusion of the posterior teeth.

to the anterior teeth; and (b) the opposing supporting cusps that provide the appliance's posterior centric contacts are the maxillary lingual cusps for the mandibular appliance, whereas they are the mandibular buccal cusps for the maxillary appliance.

For the fabrication of this appliance, make impressions of the maxillary and mandibular teeth and a bite registration. Once the laboratory has fabricated the maxillary acrylic stabilization appliance, attempt to insert it into the patient's mouth with a moderate amount of force. If the appliance does not seat fully or causes an uncomfortable pressure, then its internal surface needs to be adjusted.

After the appliance seats fully and fits comfortably, the mandible is manipulated into the desired position and the appliance's occlusion is adjusted. Using two sheets of black Accufilm, mark the centric contacts, repeatedly adjusting the marks so at least one centric mark from each posterior tooth and light to no marks from the anterior teeth are obtained. The cuspid marks may be in harmony with the anterior or posterior marks (Figures 12-25 and 12-26).

While adjusting the occlusion, practitioners may find it necessary or more expedient to reline a portion of the occlusal surface. While obtaining the desired centric contacts, periodically ask the patient to close on the appliance and to say whether the left or right side hits first or harder. Adjust the appliance so the patient feels that both sides hit evenly and each side of the appliance has uniform centric marks independent of the other side.

After obtaining the desired centric contacts, adjust the excursive movement. The appliance should allow the patient to easily slide the mandible into the excursive positions, disoccluding the posterior teeth with the closest posterior contact being 1/2 to 1 mm from the appliance. Prior to initiating the excursive movement adjustments, observe the distance the posterior teeth separate

as the patient slides the mandible into these positions. This provides an estimate of how much the anterior guidance ramp will need to be adjusted in each direction.

Mark the excursive movements with two sheets of red Accufilm and ask the patient to grind the teeth side to side and forward and backward on the Accufilm. Using black Accufilm, ask the patient to tap in the centric position to provide the appliance with black centric contact marks on top of the red excursive marks.

The posterior portion of the appliance is adjusted so no red marks are produced with excursive movements. The anterior guidance ramp is adjusted so the closest posterior contact is only 1/2 to 1 mm from the appliance when the patient is in excursive positions and the forces along the guidance ramp are distributed as evenly as possible among the anterior teeth (Figures 12-50 to 12-53).

Sometimes I plan for a patient to wear the maxillary appliance occasionally during the day, e.g., when driving or using the computer. If the appliance is to be worn during the day, also adjust it while the patient is in an upright position. Reposition the dental chair into the sitting position, ask the patient to sit with feet to the side so they are on the floor, and adjust the appliance by using the same criteria.

Contour the appliance after its occlusion is adjusted. Patients generally do not need more than 7 mm of anterior guidance, so remove any unnecessary portion of the ramp. Patients prefer to have shorter and thinner lingual flanges,[21] so consider thinning any portion of the appliance's sides that are thicker than 1 mm, especially if the patient plans to wear the appliance during the day. To minimize unnecessary acrylic, create a smooth-flowing concavity gingival to the guidance ramp. Contour the appliance's occlusal surface line angles so the occlusal gingival curvature is similar to the tooth that it covers.

Once the appliance is satisfactory, ask the

patient to insert it. Inform the patient that the appliance will be smoothed further, but that you want to ensure that the posterior teeth hit it as evenly as possible and determine whether the patient knows of anything that can be done to make the appliance more comfortable. Once the appliance meets with the patient's approval, smooth its sides and ask the patient whether it feels smooth enough.

Hard Thermoplastic Stabilization Appliance

Hard thermoplastic materials are available in a large variety of thicknesses. Those that have a thickness of 1 mm or less will flex around the convexities of the teeth and are often used to form bleaching trays, trays used in fabricating temporary crowns, etc. Those that have a thickness of 2 mm or more are comparatively rigid and used to form items such as custom impression trays and orthodontic retainers.

The 2-mm material is typically used to fabricate occlusal appliances.[10] The 1-mm material appears to be too fragile for long-term appliance use, and material greater than 2 mm provides unnecessarily bulk for the appliance.

I use the following 2-mm hard thermoplastic appliance when an appliance is desired for the patient to wear during the day that is very esthetic and has minimal effect on speech. It is preferred that patients learn to break their daytime habits rather than rely on wearing this appliance to relieve their TMD symptoms. Clinically it is observed that some patients who are initially provided this appliance for daytime wear become unmotivated to break their daytime habits.

◉ **QUICK CONSULT**
Fabricating an Appliance for Daytime Wear
❚ use the 2-mm hard thermoplastic appliance when an appliance is desired for the patient to

wear during the day that is very esthetic and has minimal effect on speech.

Wearing an Appliance during the Day
❚t is preferred that patients learn to break their daytime habits rather than rely on wearing an appliance during the day. Clinically it is observed that some patients who are initially provided a 2-mm hard thermoplastic appliance for daytime wear become unmotivated to break their daytime habits.

Therefore, though I use this appliance infrequently, I have most often used it for (a) patients who have been working to break their daytime habits and continue to have significant daytime pain for which their occlusal appliance is beneficial, but find their appliance not esthetically acceptable or too interfering with speech [these patients are generally asked to wear their current appliance at night and this new appliance during the day (never eating with it)]; and (b) patients who have intermittent daytime pain, are not willing to treat their pain with traditional behavioral techniques, and want an esthetic appliance for intermittent daytime use.

Since the purpose of this appliance is to minimize the traditional appliance esthetic and speech problems, I make a mandibular appliance without an anterior guidance ramp for the maxillary anterior teeth.[9] Only an impression of the mandibular teeth is needed, and the laboratory is requested to fabricate a clear 2-mm hard thermoplastic appliance, as specified in Appendix 7, "Laboratory Occlusal Appliance Instructions."

Once the appliance is fabricated (Figure 12-54), insert it in the patient's mouth. If the appliance does not seat fully with a moderate amount of force or causes an uncomfortable pressure, the internal surface of the appliance is adjusted, as explained in "Internal Adjustments" in this chapter. Once the

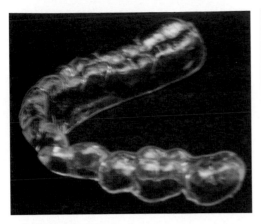

Figure 12-54. Hard thermoplastic stabilization appliance: the 2-mm shell.

appliance is comfortable, determine whether it is satisfactorily retentive. The retention should not be so strong that the patient has unwarranted difficulty removing it, but be sufficient that the patient cannot dislodge it with the tongue. An appliance that is too retentive generally engages the posterior undercuts too deeply, so the depth of engagement should be reduced. If there is insufficient retention, the internal surface of the appliance should be relined, as explained in "Internal Reline" in this chapter.

The thermoplastic material is 2 mm thick prior to appliance fabrication, but thins to approximately 1 mm once it is warmed and stretched across the patient's cast. Clinical experience has shown that this is rarely thick enough to develop the desired maxillary occlusal contacts without creating multiple perforations of the appliance's occlusal surface. Therefore, once the appliance fits comfortably, it routinely needs to have clear orthodontic acrylic added to obtain the appliance's occlusal scheme from the maxillary first bicuspid's lingual cusp to the most posterior tooth.

A grease pencil is often used on the appliance to delineate the anterior extent to which acrylic needs to be added. Using monomer, moisten the area of the appliance where acrylic is to be added. Pour approximately a teaspoon of acrylic powder into a

paper cup, add only enough monomer to moisten all of the powder granules, and mix with a wooden tongue depressor. Place the acrylic on the desired area, slightly overestimating the amount of acrylic needed. Wait for the acrylic to firm into a clay consistency before placing the appliance into the patient's mouth. The acrylic may slump or flow while you are waiting, and it is important to ensure the acrylic does not flow into the internal portion of the appliance. Therefore, the appliance is generally held so that the added acrylic is toward the floor, and the acrylic generally has to be remolded once or twice during this wait.

Once the acrylic is the consistency of clay (Figure 12-55), place the appliance in the patient's mouth, manipulate the mandible to the position that will be used to adjust the appliance, and ask the patient to close slowly into the soft acrylic. As the patient initially closes into the acrylic, observe whether it needs to be repositioned and, if needed, mold it into the proper position. Again manipulate the mandible and ask the patient to close slowly into the soft acrylic and stop as soon as the teeth touch the hard acrylic substructure. If the patient closes further than this first contact, the mandible shifts and the

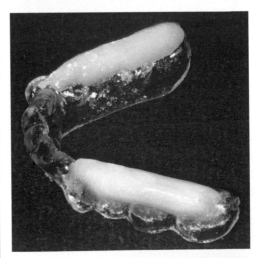

Figure 12-55. Hard thermoplastic stabilization appliance: acrylic of clay consistency added to the shell.

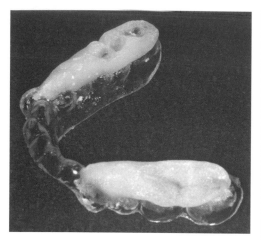

Figure 12-56. Hard thermoplastic stabilization appliance: hard acrylic, with cusp depths marked with pencil.

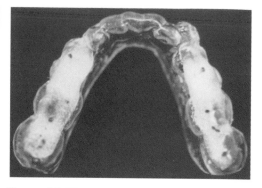

Figure 12-57. Hard thermoplastic stabilization appliance: centric contact Accufilm marks on an adjusted appliance.

cuspal indentations are not in the desired location.

The appliance is removed, placed in warm water to speed the curing process, and/or placed in a pressure-curing unit to decrease the added acrylic's porosity. Some patients wish to rinse their mouth with mouthwash at this time. Once the acrylic is hard, mark the cuspal depths with a pencil (Figure 12-56) and use the flat side of the acrylic bur to reduce the added acrylic until the pencil marks are almost erased. Repeatedly mark the appliance with black Accufilm and adjust the appliance so at least one centric mark is obtained from each posterior tooth, the patient feels that both sides hit evenly, and each side of the appliance has uniform centric marks independent of the other side (Figure 12-57).

Adjust the appliance so the patient can slide the mandible easily into excursive positions, disoccluding the posterior teeth with the closest posterior contact being 1/2 to 1 mm from the appliance. It is preferred that the maxillary canines provide the posterior disocclusion, but the canines generally do not touch the appliance, thereby preventing them from providing immediate disocclusion of the posterior teeth. Therefore, the occluding maxillary first bicuspid's lingual cusp

can be used to disocclude the posterior until the canine contacts the appliance and can disocclude the posterior teeth.

Use red Accufilm to mark the appliance in excursive positions and ask the patient to grind the teeth side to side and forward and backward on red Accufilm. Then ask the patient to tap in the centric position on black Accufilm to provide the appliance with black centric contact marks on top of the red excursive marks. Adjust the posterior portion of the appliance so no red posterior excursive marks are produced except for the maxillary first bicuspid's lingual cusps and/or canines (Figure 12-58).

Since the patient will be wearing this appliance during the day, after adjusting the splint in the traditional manner, adjust the

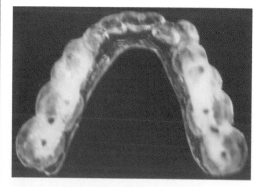

Figure 12-58. Hard thermoplastic stabilization appliance: red Accufilm marks of excursive contacts and black Accufilm marks of centric contacts on adjusted appliance.

appliance with the patient in an upright position. Reposition the dental chair into the sitting position and ask the patient to sit with feet to the side so they are on the floor. Mark and adjust the appliance with the same criteria.

Once the appliance's occlusion is adjusted, ensure the added acrylic is smooth and flowing. Sometimes, undesirable holes or concavities form when acrylic is added to the occlusal surface. These are easily filled by moistening the area with monomer and similarly mixing the acrylic, placing it in the concavity, and contouring it with a gloved finger. A smooth finish can be achieved by applying a little monomer over its surface and further smoothing it with a gloved finger.

Once the appliance is satisfactory, ask the patient to insert it. Inform the patient that the appliance will be smoothed later, but that you want to ensure that the posterior teeth hit the appliance as evenly as possible and determine whether the patient knows of anything that would make the appliance more comfortable. Once the appliance meets with the patient's approval, smooth the sides of the added acrylic and ask the patient whether it feels smooth enough.

I use this appliance only when the patient needs to wear an appliance during the day and needs one that is very esthetic and has minimal effect on speech. There is a concern that this appliance does not provide support for the maxillary anterior and that the maxillary anterior teeth might supraerupt if the patient wore this appliance full time. It appears this is not often a problem, because many people have maxillary anterior teeth that are so far anterior that their mandibular teeth rarely occlude with them, and the lower lip provides the support for these teeth.[22] To preclude the possibility of the maxillary anterior teeth supraerupting, if the patient needs to wear an appliance at night, it is recommended one be fabricated that will maintain the position of these teeth, i.e., a maxillary appliance or mandibular appliance with an anterior guidance ramp.

Soft Thermoplastic Stabilization Appliance

Soft thermoplastic material is also available in a large variety of thicknesses and is commonly used for fabricating athletic mouthguards. Similar to the hard thermoplastic material, once warmed and stretched across a patient's cast, it thins to approximately half its original thickness.

The 0.15-inch (3.8 mm)-thick and the 4.0-mm-thick material are the maximum thicknesses commercially available and generally provide an occlusal surface approximately 2 mm thick. This limited thickness is sometimes a problem and, if the patient has a significant occlusal discrepancy, this thickness may not be adequate for obtaining all of the desired occlusal contacts. Therefore, I routinely use this material for soft thermoplastic stabilization appliances, even though the resulting flanges are bulkier than I desire.

The practitioner need only to make an impression of the teeth in the arch for which the appliance will be made and request the laboratory fabricate a clear soft thermoplastic stabilization appliance, as specified in Appendix 7, "Laboratory Occlusal Appliance Instructions." The appliance rarely needs internal adjustments, but, if it does not completely seat or causes an uncomfortable pressure, determine the seating interference or ask the patient to identify the pressure area. (Accufilm does not adequately mark this appliance.) Adjust the internal surface with an acrylic or number 8 round bur. If the appliance cannot be made to fully seat comfortably, have it refabricated.

Once the appliance completely seats and is comfortable, evaluate its retention, which varies with the depth the material penetrated into the undercuts. This fluctuates with the temperature at which the material was warmed and the amount of force used by the vacuum suction or pressurized air. If the appliance is too retentive, use an acrylic or number 8 round bur and reduce the material that fits into the most retentive undercuts. If there is inadequate retention due to insufficient material penetrating into the undercuts, have the appliance refabricated.

The appliance's occlusal surface can be rapidly modified to provide a close approximation of the final occlusal surface.[42] In order that the patient does not disrupt this procedure and can perform the necessary movements, first discuss the procedure with the patient, demonstrate the mandibular manipulation, and ask the patient to practice the excursive movements.

With the appliance on the cast, use an alcohol torch to warm all areas of the appliance that the opposing teeth may touch. Evenly warm the appliance by repeatedly sweeping the flame from one side of the appliance to the other. Clinical experience has demonstrated that, when the appliance feels slightly tacky, it is ready to place in the mouth.

Once the appliance is seated on the teeth, manipulate the mandible to the position where the appliance will be adjusted, and ask the patient to close into the softened appliance. Ask the patient to stop when the last tooth desired to occlude with the appliance is only lightly touching or just about to touch the appliance; this retains the maximal thickness for the appliance. Then, ask the patient to slide the mandible across the appliance into the previously practiced excursive positions.

This creates occlusal imprints of the opposing cusp tips into the appliance's occlusal surface. Place the appliance on the cast and mark the bottom of each cusp indentation with dark ink so they can easily be observed as an acrylic bur is used to modify the occlusal surface. Any nonsupporting cusp indentations present are removed well below the depth of their indentation, whereas the supporting cusp indentations are reduced so the ink marks are just barely removed.

The indentations from the anterior teeth provide guidance to disocclude the posterior teeth. These indentations are retained, but, if there is material that extruded around the teeth, remove it and contour the area to allow for smooth excursive movements. The occlusal surface is contoured to form a flat plane, and the sides are contoured to flow smoothly onto the occlusal surface.

An indentation from at least one supporting cusp of every posterior tooth is desired. If the initial attempt did not obtain or almost obtain these imprints, the aforementioned steps may be repeated.

For the final adjustments, use the acrylic bur to adjust the occlusion marked on the appliance with articulating paper (Bausch Articulating Paper, Nashua, NH, USA), because Accufilm does not adequately mark this material. The articulating paper marks are not the point contacts typically observed on acrylic appliances, but broad marks (Figure 12-59).

Clinical experience has demonstrated that, even though the articulating paper marks appear uniform, the patient may detect the opposing teeth are not occluding evenly on the appliance. If the patient identifies heavier contacts that appear as even ar-

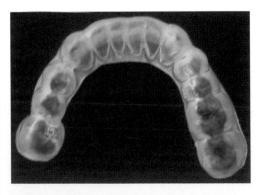

Figure 12-59. Soft thermoplastic stabilization appliance: centric articulating paper marks on an adjusted appliance.

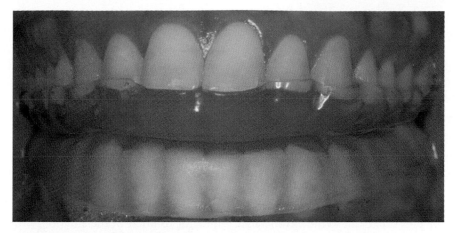

Figure 12-60. Soft thermoplastic stabilization appliance opposing an acrylic appliance.

ticulating paper marks, it is recommended that further adjustments of the appliance be made with the patient's guidance until it feels even to the patient.

The appliance is next adjusted so the anterior teeth disocclude the posterior teeth in excursive positions. The excursive movements are marked with articulating paper, and the new markings on the posterior portion of the appliance are adjusted.

The appliance may be polished with chloroform or halothane (a general inhalation anesthetic often used as a substitute for chloroform[54]). To obtain a smooth finish rapidly, seat the appliance on the cast and rub a dampened gauze firmly with either agent over any rough area of the appliance. Use water to rinse off any remaining polishing agent, ask the patient to insert the appliance, and ask whether there is anything that the patient would like done to improve the appliance.

Soft thermoplastic stabilization appliances can be fabricated for either the maxillary arch or the mandibular arch. Because of the bulkiness of its flanges, I generally fabricate this appliance for the mandibular arch. An appliance that is to be used as an athletic mouthpiece should be fabricated for the maxillary arch. I always adjust the occlusion of the athletic mouthpiece because it makes the mouthpiece more comfortable, less likely to cause occlusal changes, and less likely to cause the patient to develop TMD symptoms.

Occasionally a patient may have tooth or periodontal ligament pain, associated with heavy clenching, that does not fully resolve from the delivery of an acrylic stabilization appliance. It has been observed that providing a soft thermoplastic stabilization appliance opposed to the acrylic appliance (Figures 12-60 and 12-61) can provide additional benefit. This may be a result of the resilient material dissipating force when the patient clenches heavily.[55] It has also been observed that this appliance combination is beneficial for patients whose spouses complain that the noise created by the

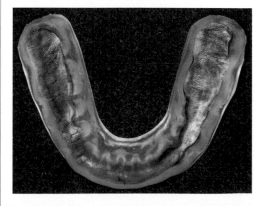

Figure 12-61. Articulating paper marks on an adjusted soft thermoplastic stabilization appliance opposing an acrylic appliance.

patient bruxing heavily on the acrylic appliance awakes them.

Dual Laminate Thermoplastic Stabilization Appliance

This material comes in sheets that have the soft thermoplastic material on one side and the hard thermoplastic material on the other thermally laminated together so they do not separate. The material is warmed and molded over the patient's cast by vacuum suction or pressurized air, so the soft material is against the teeth and the hard material is the external surface. This provides the appliance with most of the positive qualities of both the soft and hard thermoplastic appliances; i.e., the soft material feels comfortable to the supporting teeth, the soft material can compensate for minor errors so internal adjustments are rarely needed, the hard material bonds with self-curing acrylic giving it the versatility of an acrylic appliance, and the acrylic occlusal surface marks and adjusts with the precision of acrylic appliances.

In the construction of this appliance, I prefer the laboratory add the self-curing acrylic to the appliance's occlusal surface. Therefore, I send the laboratory a maxillary and mandibular cast and desired bite registration.

The laboratory technician mounts the models on the articulator, molds the dual laminate thermoplastic material over the cast, removes the excess material, and returns the cast to the articulator. At this stage, the laboratory technician is instructed to adjust the articulator's incisal pin so the closest opposing tooth is 1 mm from the dual laminate's occlusal surface. This provides a minimum acrylic thickness of 1 mm, which clinically appears appropriate for the needed intraoral adjustments.

The laboratory technician roughens the dual laminate's occlusal surface, moistens it with monomer, adds self-curing acrylic, and adjusts the acrylic occlusal surface (Figures 12-62 to 12-64). The added acrylic provides the same occlusal surface as would be established with the traditional acrylic appliance.

The laboratory technician is requested to carry the labial and buccal portions of this appliance to the gingival margin. The desired labial extent varies with the angulation of the anterior teeth, and the requested labial extent can be reduced as needed. If this appliance is difficult to insert or the anterior portion has too much retention, I generally correct this by reducing the labial extent, but leave at least 1 to 1½ mm of material labial to the incisal edge of the anterior teeth (the recommended labial extent used with acrylic appliances).

Similar to the soft thermoplastic appliances, the internal surface cannot be relined.

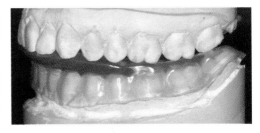

Figure 12-62. Dual laminate thermoplastic stabilization appliance: fabricated and adjusted on articulator.

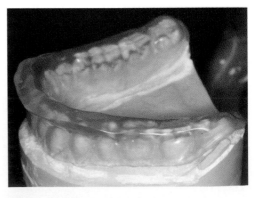

Figure 12-63. Dual laminate thermoplastic stabilization appliance: the occlusal surface of a fabricated appliance.

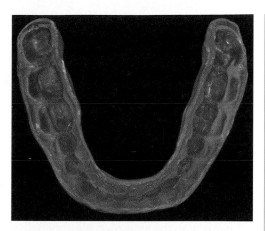

Figure 12-64. Dual laminate thermoplastic stabilization appliance: the internal surface of a fabricated appliance; note the thickness of buccal and lingual flanges, and the acrylic thickness lingual to the anterior teeth.

Adjust the internal surface with an acrylic or number 8 round bur and, if this does not make the appliance fully seat comfortably, have it refabricated.

External relines and adjustments are made in the same way as those for acrylic appliances. Since the soft internal layer occupies a portion of the interocclusal space, the vertical dimension of this appliance will be a little larger than that of comparable acrylic appliances.

APPLIANCE MANAGEMENT

Great variations in the protocols that practitioners use when delivering occlusal appliances have been observed. Some practitioners (as myself) attempt to refine the occlusion fully at the insertion appointment. Occasionally the lengthy appointment aggravates a patient's TMD symptoms to the degree that the patient wants to stop prior to completion of the adjustments.

Some practitioners make shorter insertion appointments, adjust the appliance so it is comfortable on the teeth that support it, and adjust the appliance's occlusion so one or two contacts are occluding on each side. At each follow-up appointment, its occlusion is further refined, and eventually the appliance becomes adjusted as described earlier.

Fully adjusting the appliance at its delivery has the advantage of the patient obtaining the maximal initial treatment effect from the appliance, but the long procedure may cause some temporary TMD aggravation. The stepwise adjustment protocol causes minimal TMD symptom aggravation during appliance delivery, but some patients have symptom aggravation from wearing an inadequately adjusted appliance; the uneven occlusal contacts may induce some shifting of the teeth, which may delay the practitioner from obtaining a stable occlusion on the appliance; and it takes the patient longer to obtain the appliance's maximal treatment effect.

Whenever patients are provided an appliance, it is recommended they also receive the "Occlusal Appliance Care Instructions" handout (Appendix 4) and it be reviewed with them. The instructions inform patients about common problems they may encounter, maintenance of the appliance, reasons the appliance will need additional adjustments and, if discomfort occurs, to stop wearing it and return to have the discomfort relieved.

The recommended wear pattern will vary with the symptoms that are being treated. Patients who awake with TMD symptoms that last up to several hours and/or who have minimal daytime symptoms are asked to wear the appliance only at night.

❂ FOCAL POINT

Patients who awake with TMD symptoms that last up to several hours and/or who have minimal daytime symptoms are asked to wear the appliance only at night.

If attempting to reduce significant daytime symptoms, I would like the patient to wear the appliance during the day (a) as a reminder to help him or her observe and break the daytime habits,[1,56] and (b) to maximize the effects from the stable occlusal environment. The patient is instructed to wear the appliance temporarily during the day and never eat with it. Nighttime appliance use often provides some prolonged benefits that carry over to help alleviate the daytime symptoms also. Therefore, I instruct these patients to wear the appliance temporarily 24 hours a day and, over several months, reduce its use slowly to primarily nighttime.

FOCAL POINT

If attempting to reduce significant daytime symptoms with an appliance, the patient is instructed to wear the appliance temporarily 24 hours a day (except when eating) and, over several months, reduce its use slowly to primarily nighttime.

Occasionally patients who wear an appliance 24 hours a day (including while eating), and never put their teeth into maximum intercuspation, over time lose the ability to occlude their teeth into maximum intercuspation. This situation may require orthognathic surgery to enable the patient to once again occlude into maximum intercuspation. One of the principal reasons patients are instructed to not eat with their appliance is that they generally put their teeth into maximum intercuspation while eating. Patients are allowed to wear their appliance 24 hours a day for only a relatively short period (a few months), during which they are closely observed to ensure they are not losing the ability to occlude into maximum intercuspation.

Some patients recognize that their TMD symptoms and parafunctional habits are related to certain activities, e.g., driving a car or using a computer. These patients are asked to wear their appliance during these activities (if they are willing) and at night. During the initial phase of daytime wear, patients observe the benefit they obtain from wearing the appliance during these activities and its cost (e.g., difficulty speaking and its visibility). From this, they decide how often

they will wear the appliance during the day. Alternative conservative therapies should be provided, as needed, so patients can stop their daytime appliance use and limit the wear to nighttime.[1]

Generally, as patients wear their new appliance, the masticatory muscles become less tense and the TMJ inflammation reduces. These changes within the masticatory system usually alter the occlusion on the appliance. It has been observed that these changes are often proportional to a patient's symptoms and, with repeated appliance adjustments, the occlusion stabilizes.[54,57] No matter how well the appliance was initially adjusted, the patient needs to return for follow-up to refine the occlusion for these adaptive changes, to ensure the appliance is not causing any correctable problems, to ensure the appliance is beneficial and, if needed, so that additional TMD therapies can be recommended.

The length of time between the insertion and follow-up appointment will vary with a patient's symptom severity and how well the appliance could be adjusted. If a patient's symptoms are severe and/or the appliance can not be adjusted adequately, the patient is given an appointment within a week. If a patient has minimal symptoms and a well-adjusted appliance was provided, the patient is generally given an appointment approximately 4 weeks later.

When the patient returns for follow-up, ask about any problems he or she may be having with the appliance. Occasionally a patient relates that he or she unintentionally removes the appliance while sleeping. It appears patients subconsciously remove their appliances at night because it aggravates them in some manner. Four different causes have been observed, and the patient generally stops removing it once the cause is corrected. The four problems I probe are whether the appliance is (a) too loose, (b) too tight, (c) not satisfactorily adjusted to the opposing dentition, or (d) too bulky.

The appropriate corrections typically stop this problem.

Generally patients report a significant reduction in the TMD symptoms upon awaking, and the daytime symptom reduction varies with how often a patient has worn the appliance during the day and/or learned to break the daytime habits.[1] If the appliance needs only minor adjustments, the occlusion should be perfected, but the patient often does not even notice the difference or have any additional symptom improvement.

Fortunately the percentage of patients who have no improvement from an appliance adjusted as previously described is relatively small. All patients who are provided an occlusal appliance should have received the "TMD Self-management Therapies" handout (Appendix 3) at the evaluation appointment. The end of this handout states, "A percentage of patients receiving TMD therapies report no symptom improvement (i.e., 10 to 20 percent of patients receiving occlusal appliances report no improvement)." Therefore, the patient has been warned about this possibility, but this does not decrease the disappointment felt by the practitioner as well as the patient if symptoms do not improve.

Typically our treatments in dentistry are successful, whereas, in medicine, practitioners are accustomed to having a percentage of patients not benefit from a therapy. The success of TMD therapies is similar to that of other medical procedures provided for patients with chronic pain. The percentage of patients reporting minimal improvement from the use of an occlusal appliance should be minimized by following the recommendations in "Integration of Conservative Therapies" in Chapter 19.

If a patient has not obtained the expected improvement from using an appropriately adjusted appliance for several weeks, consider reevaluating the patient to determine whether the chief complaint may be due to a non-TMD condition and/or whether non-TMD contributors (neck pain, fibromyalgia, etc.) were missed during the initial evaluation.[8] If a panoramic radiograph was not taken, the practitioner may desire to take one at this time.

◉ **QUICK CONSULT**
Failing to Relieve Symptoms

If a patient has not obtained the expected improvement from using an appropriately adjusted appliance for several weeks, consider reevaluating the patient to determine whether the chief complaint may be due to a non-TMD condition and/or whether non-TMD contributors (neck pain, fibromyalgia, etc.) were missed during the evaluation. If a panoramic radiograph was not taken, the practitioner may desire to take one at this time.

If a patient did not receive satisfactory improvement with use of the stabilization appliance, the practitioner may want to try a different mandibular position to determine whether it might make the appliance more effective. The most likely other position that would provide a beneficial effect is at the location where the masticatory system feels the most relaxed and comfortable for the patient.

Ask the patient to slide the mandible slowly anterior and determine whether there is a position at which the masticatory system feels more relaxed and comfortable. If the patient can locate such a position, the practitioner may find the appliance more effective with the mandible supported at this new position.

As the patient protruded the mandible to the new comfortable position, the condyle also translated. If the patient has a disc displacement with reduction, and a click or pop was detected within the TMJ as the condyle translated, clinically this suggests the condyle moved onto the disc's intermediate zone (called the *reduced position*). To confirm clinically that the disc-condyle is reduced, ask the patient to open from and close to this protruded position and, if the disc-condyle is reduced, the patient's typical TMJ click or pop will no longer be present. The bottom left diagram of the "TMJ Disc Displacements" handout (Appendix 2) may help readers to understand visually that, once the condyle is reduced, the patient can open and close from that position without creating the normal joint noise. Contrary to what one would expect, this clinical test is not accurately supported by magnetic resonance imaging (MRI) findings.[58,59]

If a patient has a disc displacement with reduction, and the clinical test suggests the new position is where the disc-condyle is reduced, the proposed new appliance would be an anterior positioning one. It is recommended the practitioner follow the guidance provided in Chapter 13, "Anterior Positioning Appliance," for this appliance. Acrylic can be added to the existing stabilization appliance to modify it into an anterior positioning appliance.

If the new comfortable position is only 1 or 2 mm anterior from the previously used position, and the patient can close repeatedly at this location, the practitioner may desire to adjust the appliance to provide a stabilization appliance with the centric contacts at the new position. If the patient cannot close repeatedly at this new location, the practitioner may want to add acrylic to provide occlusal indentations that will help the patient maintain the mandible at this comfortable position.

The indentations can be added to the occlusal surface of the appliance with self-curing acrylic (Figure 12-65). Follow the guidance provided in "External Reline" in this chapter, and ask the patient to close into the identified comfortable position. Trim and adjust the appliance as instructed in "Anterior Positioning Appliance" in Chapter 13. The wear schedule, warnings, and follow-up provided for the anterior positioning appliance would probably apply for this appliance.

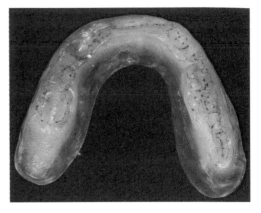

Figure 12-65. Appliance with occlusal indentations: Accufilm contact marks on an adjusted appliance.

If the patient could not find a comfortable position, but meets the criteria for an anterior positioning appliance, consider providing an anterior positioning appliance and follow the guidance provided in Chapter 13.

Patients provided a stabilization appliance generally have their conditions followed for several months to determine the amount of occlusal change that occurs between appointments and how sensitive the patient is to these changes. From these observations, the practitioner can determine the appropriate time for scheduling the next follow-up appointment. Typically patients are eventually placed on an annual recall.

Using the conservative TMD therapies discussed in "Integration of Conservative Therapies" in Chapter 19, I try to reduce the patient's symptoms satisfactorily so that the appliance needs to be worn only at night. I plan for the great majority of my patients to wear their appliance at night for many years. Periodically patients forget to wear their appliance at night, which provides an unintentional test of whether the appliance is still needed.

TMD tends to be a cyclic disorder that is often related to situations occurring in a patient's life, and there are many possible scenarios for how often the patient will need to wear the appliance. Some patients may need to wear it every night and others on a weekly basis, whereas some others may find at some point that they no longer need it. If patients do not wear their appliance, the teeth tend to shift and, over time, the appliance becomes more difficult and/or painful to insert and wear.

It is common to hear patients returning for a new appliance say that they no longer needed it and so stopped wearing it. Then, 1 or 2 years later, a situation in their life changes, and they once again need an appliance. Therefore, even though a patient no longer needs to wear the appliance, it is recommended that the appliance consistently be worn every night. When the appliance reaches the condition where it should be replaced and is no longer needed, this is an appropriate time to discontinue its use.

Appliance therapy should be viewed as one of many conservative TMD therapies. Used in conjunction with other conservative therapies, it augments the symptom improvement that patients can obtain. Appliance therapy should *not* be viewed as temporary treatment for which occlusal rehabilitation is the final treatment approach.[3,60]

REFERENCES

1. Pertes RA. Occlusal appliance therapy. In: Pertes RA, Gross SG (eds). Clinical Management of Temporomandibular Disorders and Orofacial Pain. Chicago: Quintessence, 1995:197–210.
2. Bush FM, Abbott FM, Butler JH, Harrington WG. Oral orthotics: design, indications, efficacy and care. In: Hardin JF (ed). Clark's Clinical Dentistry, volume 2, chapter 39. Philadelphia: JB Lippincott, 1998:1–33.
3. Widmalm SE. Use and abuse of bite splints. Compendium 1999;20(3):249–59.
4. Christensen GJ. Now is the time to observe and treat dental occlusion. J Am Dent Assoc 2000;132(1):100–2.
5. Lobbezoo F, Lavigne GJ. Do bruxism and temporomandibular disorders have a cause-and-effect relationship? J Orofac Pain 1997;11(1):15–23.
6. Clark GT, Beemsterboer PL, Solberg WK, Rugh JD. Nocturnal electromyographic evaluation of myofascial dysfunction in patients undergoing occlusal splint therapy. J Am Dent Assoc 1979;99:607–11.
7. Holmgren K, Sheikohleslam A, Riise C. Effect of full-arch maxillary occlusal splint on parafunctional activity during sleep in patients with nocturnal bruxism and signs and symptoms of craniomandibular disorders. J Prosthet Dent 1993;69:293–7.
8. American Academy of Orofacial Pain, with Okeson JP (ed). Orofacial Pain: Guidelines for Assessment, Diagnosis and Management. Chicago: Quintessence, 1996:150–3.
9. Messing SG. Splint therapy. In: Kaplan AS, Assael LA (eds). Temporomandibular Disorders: Diagnosis and Treatment. Philadelphia: WB Saunders, 1991:395–454.
10. Okeson JP. Management of Temporomandibular Disorders and Occlusion, 5th edition. St Louis: CV Mosby, 2003:112, 507–36.
11. Kreiner M, Betancor E, Clark GT. Occlusal stabilization appliances: evidence of their efficacy. J Am Dent Assoc 2001;132(6):770–7.
12. Rubinoff MS, Gross A, McCall WD Jr. Conventional and nonoccluding splint therapy compared for patients with myofascial pain dysfunction syndrome. Gen Dent 1987;35(6):502–6.
13. Wassell RW, Adams NR, Kelly PJ. Treatment of temporomandibular disorders by stabilization splints in general dental practice: 3 month results [abstract 3314]. J Dent Res (Special Issue) 1999;78:520.
14. Ekberg EC, Vallon D, Nilner M. The efficacy of appliance therapy in patients with temporomandibular disorders of mainly myogenous origin: a randomized, controlled, short-term trial. J Orofac Pain 2003;17(2):133–9.
15. Young PA. A cephalometric study of the effect of acrylic test palatal piece thickness on the physiologic rest position. J Philipp Dent Assoc 1966;19(1):5–15.
16. Nitzan DW. Arthrocentesis for management of severe close lock of the temporomandibular joint. Oral Maxillofac Surg Clin North Am 1994;6:245–57.
17. Nitzan DW. Temporomandibular joint "open lock" versus condylar dislocation: signs and symptoms, imaging, treatment, and pathogenesis. J Oral Maxillofac Surg 2002;60(5):506–11.

18. Dawson PE. New definition for relating occlusion to varying conditions of the temporomandibular joint. J Prosthet Dent 1995;74:619–27.

19. Academy of Prosthodontics. The glossary of prosthodontic terms, 7th edition. J Prosthet Dent 1990;81:39–110.

20. Obrez A, Turp JC. The effect of musculoskeletal facial pain on registration of maxillomandibular relationships and treatment planning: a synthesis of the literature. J Prosthet Dent 1998;79(4): 439–45.

21. Dylina TJ. A common-sense approach to splint therapy. J Prosthet Dent 2001;86:539–45.

22. Dawson PE. Evaluation, diagnosis and treatment of occlusal problems, 2nd edition. St Louis: CV Mosby, 1989:41–7, 72–84.

23. Makofsky H. The effect of head posture on muscle contact position: the sliding cranium theory. Cranio 1989;7(4):286–92.

24. Boero RP. The physiology of splint therapy: a literature review. Angle Orthod 1989;59(3): 165–80.

25. Clark GT. A critical evaluation of orthopedic interocclusal appliance therapy: design, theory, and overall effectiveness. J Am Dent Assoc 1984;108(3):359–64.

26. Douglass JB, Smith PJ. Loss of control of the vertical dimension of occlusion during interocclusal acrylic resin splint therapy: a clinical report. J Prosthet Dent 1992;67(1):1–4.

27. Dahlstrom L, Haraldson T, Janson ST. Comparative electromyographic study of bite plates and stabilization splints. Scand J Dent Res 1985;93(3):262–8.

28. Greene CS, Laskin DM. Splint therapy for the myofascial pain-dysfunction (MPD) syndrome: a comparative analysis. J Am Dent Assoc 1972;84:624–8.

29. Ito T, Gibbs CH, Marguelles-Bonnet R, Lupkiewicz SM, Young HM, Lundeen HC, Mahan PE. Loading on the temporomandibular joints with five occlusal conditions. J Prosthet Dent 1986;56(4):478–84.

30. Casey J, Dunn WJ, Wright E. In vitro wear of various orthotic device materials. J Prosthet Dent 2003;90(5):498–502.

31. Okeson JP. The effects of hard and soft occlusal splints on nocturnal bruxism. J Am Dent Assoc 1987;114:788–91.

32. Nevarro E, Barghi N, Rey R. Clinical evaluation of maxillary hard and resilient occlusal splints [abstract 1246]. J Dent Res (Special Issue) 1985;64:313.

33. Pettengill CA, Growney MR Jr, Schoff R, Kenworthy CR. A pilot study comparing the efficacy of hard and soft stabilizing appliances in treating patients with temporomandibular disorders. J Prosthet Dent 1998;79(2):165–8.

34. Huggins KH, Truelove EL, Dworkin SF, Mancl L, Sommers E, LeResche L. RTC of splints for TMD: clinical findings at 12 months [abstract 1490]. J Dent Res (Special Issue) 1999;78:292.

35. Williams WB. Pain release splint. Cranio Clin Int 1991;1:55–64.

36. Morgan DH, House LR, Hall WP, Vamvas SJ. Diseases of the Temporomandibular Apparatus: A Multidisciplinary Approach. St Louis: CV Mosby, 1982:266–74.

37. Ramfjord S, Ash MA. Occlusion, 3rd edition. Philadelphia: WB Saunders, 1983:362–5.

38. Singh BP, Berry DC. Occlusal changes following use of soft occlusal splints. J Prosthet Dent 1985;54:711–5.

39. Wright E, Anderson G, Schulte J. A randomized clinical trial of intraoral soft splints and palliative treatment for masticatory muscle pain. J Orofac Pain 1995;9:116–30.

40. Harkins S, Marteney JL, Cueva O, Cueva L. Application of soft occlusal splints in patients suffering from clicking temporomandibular joints. Cranio 1988;6:71–6.

41. Attanasio R. Intraoral orthotic therapy. Dent Clin North Am 1997;41(2):309–24.

42. Wright EF. Using soft splints in your dental office. Gen Dent 1999;47(5):506–12.

43. Giedrys-Leeper E. Night guards and occlusal splints. Dent Update 1990;17:325–9.

44. Boero RP. The physiology of splint therapy: a literature review. Angle Orthod 1989;59:165–80.

45. Mense S, Simons DG, Russell IJ. Muscle Pain: Understanding Its Nature, Diagnosis, and Treatment. Philadelphia: Lippincott Williams & Wilkins, 2001:21–3.

46. Manns A, Miralles R, Guerrero F. Changes in electrical activity of the postural muscles of the mandible upon varying the vertical dimension. J Prosthet Dent 1981;45:438–45.

47. Rugh JD, Drago CJ. Vertical dimension: a study of clinical rest position and jaw muscle activity. J Prosthet Dent 1981;45(6):670–5.

48. Manns A, Miralles R, Santander H, Valdivia J. Influence of the vertical dimension in the treat-

ment of myofascial pain-dysfunction syndrome. J Prosthet Dent 1983;50(5):700–9.

49. Dos Santos J Jr, Gurklis M. Chairside fabrication of occlusal biteplane splints using visible light cured material. Cranio 1995;13(2): 131–6.

50. Nelson SJ. Principles of stabilization bite splint therapy. Dent Clin North Am 1995;39(2): 403–21.

51. Swanberg DF, Henry MD. Avoiding implant overload. Implant Soc 1995;6(1):12–4.

52. Obrez A, Stohler CS. Jaw muscle pain and its effect on gothic arch tracings. J Prosthet Dent 1996;75:393–8.

53. Capp NJ, Clayton JA. A technique for evaluation of centric relation tooth contacts. Part II: Following use of an occlusal splint for treatment of temporomandibular joint dysfunction. J Prosthet Dent 1985;54(5):697–705.

54. Wilcox LR. Endodontic retreatment with halothane versus chloroform solvent. J Endod 1995;21(6):305–7.

55. Craig RG, Godwin WC. Properties of athletic mouth protectors and materials. J Oral Rehabil 2002;29(2):146–50.

56. Tuddey JJ. Problems and solutions. Cranio 1995;13(1):68.

57. Suvinen T, Reade P. Prognostic features of value in the management of temporomandibular joint pain-dysfunction syndrome by occlusal splint therapy. J Prosthet Dent 1989;61(3):355–61.

58. Kurita H, Kurashina K, Ohtsuka A, Kotani A. Change of position of the temporomandibular joint disk with insertion of a disk-repositioning appliance. Oral Surg Oral Med Oral Pathol Oral Radiol Endod 1998;85(2):142–5.

59. Kirk WS Jr. Magnetic resonance imaging and tomographic evaluation of occlusal appliance treatment for advanced internal derangement of the temporomandibular joint. J Oral Maxillofac Surg 1991;49(1):9–12.

60. Greene CS. The etiology of temporomandibular disorders: implications for treatment. J Orofac Pain 2001;15(2):93–105.

Chapter 13

Anterior Positioning Appliance

FAQ

Q: Why does eliminating the TMJ noise clinically suggest that the condyle is positioned into the disc's intermediate zone?

A: The bottom left diagram of the "TMJ Disc Displacements" handout (Appendix 2) may help readers to understand visually that, once the condyle is reduced, the patient can open from and close to that position without creating the normal joint noise.

This appliance, which is traditionally used for patients who have a disc displacement with reduction, temporarily holds the mandible in an anterior location, where the condyle is positioned onto the disc's intermediate zone, also referred to as the location where the condyle is reduced onto the disc (Figure 13-1). There appear to be two primary mechanisms by which the anterior positioning appliance reduces the TMD symptoms: (a) it removes the disc-condyle mechanical disturbance, and (b) it transfers the condylar loading forces from the retrodiscal tissue to the intermediate zone.

✖ FOCAL POINT

An anterior positioning appliance is traditionally used for patients who have a disc displacement with reduction. It temporarily holds the mandible in an anterior location where the condyle is reduced onto the disc (Figure 13-1).

When a patient occludes on this appliance, the condyle is maintained in the reduced position, causing the patient to be unable to make his or her normal TMJ clicking or popping noise. If the mechanical disturbance responsible for the joint noise irritates the TMJ, and the patient has parafunctional habits that continually stimulates this disturbance, wearing the appliance should minimize the consequent irritation.

If the patient were to clench while wearing this appliance, the force transmitted through the condyle would load the disc's intermediate zone rather than the retrodiscal tissue. Intuitively this should benefit patients with retrodiscal tissue inflammation.[1]

172

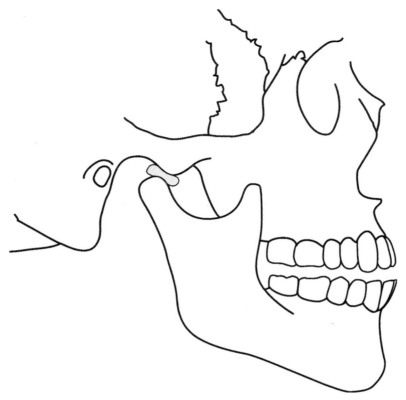

Figure 13-1. Condyle in the reduced position.

The retrodiscal tissue can also be protected from loading forces by a stabilization appliance. If a stabilization appliance is adjusted using the neutral position (described in "Mandibular Positions and Bite Registration" in Chapter 12), the condyle is not braced against the disc assembly. Therefore, when the patient clenches in maximum intercuspation (MI) on this stabilization appliance, there is minimal load transferred to the disc assembly or pressure created within the TMJ.[2] In this manner, the stabilization appliance can also unload the inflamed retrodiscal tissue.

Anterior positioning appliances have been shown to reduce TMJ pain, muscle pain, and TMJ noise for many patients.[3-5] Similarly stabilization appliances improve TMD symptoms for most patients, even if their pain is related to a disc-condyle mechanical disturbance or intermittent locking at the opening where the noise occurs.[6]

✪ FOCAL POINT

Anterior positioning appliances have been shown to reduce TMJ pain, muscle pain, and TMJ noise for many patients. Stabilization appliances similarly improve TMD symptoms for most patients, even if their pain is related to a disc-condyle mechanical disturbance or intermittent locking at the opening where the noise occurs.

It has been suggested that anterior positioning appliances may be more effective in reducing some TMD symptoms than are stabilization appliances.[7] Due to the probable efficacy of the stabilization appliance and the problems associated with the anterior positioning appliance, it is recommended that practitioners first use a stabilization appliance and other conservative TMD therapies. Only after these fail to provide adequate symptom relief is it recommended that an anterior positioning appliance be considered.[6,8-10]

Maintaining the mandible at the desired anterior location for an extended period may occasionally aggravate a patient's TMD symptoms. Clinically it has been observed that a patient who finds that this mandibular location aggravates his or her TMD symptoms will usually find that this appliance exacerbates the symptoms.

Intuitively it appears only patients who meet all of the following criteria have a high probability of gaining improvement from this appliance:

1. The patient's TMJ mechanical disturbance appears related to his or her pain.
2. The TMJ noise is eliminated by placing the mandible in the recommended anterior location.
3. The masticatory system feels more relaxed or comfortable with the mandible located in the recommended anterior location.

This principle of temporarily altering a joint so it functions in a more comfortable position is similarly used to treat other musculoskeletal disorders in the body.[11]

MANDIBULAR POSITION AND BITE REGISTRATION

For this appliance, the mandible should be located where the condyle is reduced onto the disc and the masticatory system feels more relaxed or comfortable. The mandible cannot be positioned excessively anterior, because generally the more anterior the mandible is placed, the more strained the masticatory system feels to the patient. I identify the desired mandible location and make the bite registration with the dental chair back about 10° to 20° from its maximum upright position.

If the patient has a normal maxillomandibular relationship, it is recommended to evaluate initially whether the mandibular location where the maxillary and mandibular anterior teeth touch end to end is feasible.

With the mandible at this location, ask the patient to open from and close to this position several times, and observe whether the click or pop has been eliminated.

If the noise is eliminated, this clinically suggests that this location positions the condyle so it is reduced onto the intermediate zone of the disc (Figure 13-1). The bottom left diagram of the "TMJ Disc Displacements" handout (Appendix 2) may help readers to understand visually that, once the condyle is reduced, the patient can open from and close to that position without creating the normal joint noise. Practitioners should bear in mind that this clinically identified mandibular location does not accurately identify the position for which all TMJs are fully reduced, but is the technique that is traditionally used and provides clinically acceptable results for this appliance.[12,13]

If the position does not eliminate the noise, ask the patient to protrude the mandible further and retest whether this position eliminates the TMJ noise. Once the noise is eliminated, ask the patient whether this is a more comfortable position than his or her normal mandibular posture.

If the chosen mandibular location eliminates the noise, but the position feels uncomfortable to the patient, ask the patient to retrude the mandible slightly and retest whether the noise continues to be eliminated but now feels comfortable. Experiment to find the mandibular location at which the TMJ noise is eliminated and the masticatory system feels more relaxed or comfortable. If such a mandibular location can be identified, this is the recommended location for the bite registration. If a mandibular location that meets these criteria cannot be identified, for this patient an anterior positioning appliance will probably not be more effective than the stabilization appliance.

If the anterior positioning appliance criteria are satisfied at the location where the anterior teeth meet end to end, this is a good location to use, for at this location the practitioner can visualize whether the mandible returns to the same position and it provides a stable position for the patient to hold the mandible.

If the identified mandibular location is different than where the anterior teeth meet end to end, patients can usually feel the desired mechanical disc-condyle relationship within their TMJ and can also easily maintain or return to this location. The practitioner may desire that the patient practice opening from and closing to this position several times, so the patient does not have difficulty finding this location while the bite registration is made.

The bite registration can be made by asking the patient to bite into softened wax or by syringing a bite registration material between the teeth, if the patient has a stable position to occlude while the material hardens. If the bite registration was made with the teeth occluding, ask the laboratory technician to open the articulator's vertical dimension approximately 1 mm.

DESIGN AND ADJUSTMENTS

Similar to the stabilization appliance, the anterior positioning appliance should cover all of the teeth in the arch, fit comfortably over them, and provide even occlusal contacts for all of the opposing posterior teeth, and its external surface should flow smoothly (Figure 13-2).

The maxillary anterior positioning appliance is constructed with a ramp immediately behind the mandibular anterior tooth contacts (Figure 13-3). When people sleep, their muscles relax and the mandible tends to drift posterior.[8] The ramp supports the mandible as it drops posterior, helps to maintain the desired disc-condyle relationship, and guides the mandible forward into the desired position when the patient attempts to occlude. A mandibular appliance can be constructed with a similar ramp, but there is a greater tendency for patients to

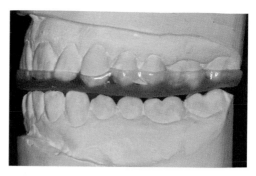

Figure 13-2. The maxillary anterior positioning appliance occluding with opposing teeth.

wear the mandibular appliance during the day, and mandibular appliances tend to be less effective.[6,9]

The appliance's internal adjustments are made as described for the stabilization appliance. Its external adjustments are made by marking the opposing tooth contacts with two sheets of black Accufilm by using the articulating forceps. Hold the forceps as described for the stabilization appliance, at a slight angle in the mouth so the patient can mark the third molar as well as the central incisor at the same time (see Figure 12-21).

Some practitioners fabricate the posterior occlusal surface of this appliance with cuspal indentations into which the opposing teeth fit,[14] whereas others recommend fabricating a flat posterior occlusal surface.[9] Both are

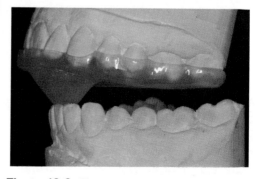

Figure 13-3. The maxillary anterior positioning appliance is constructed with a ramp. This ramp prevents the patient's mandible from retruding behind the appliance and guides the mandible forward into the desired position when the patient attempts to occlude.

acceptable, but I prefer the flat posterior occlusal surface because it is easier and faster for adjusting the appliance's occlusion.

Repeatedly mark and adjust the appliance, slowly developing even contacts from the opposing posterior teeth. Similar to the stabilization appliance, at least one contact from each posterior tooth should be obtained, and the anterior teeth should provide light or no marks in comparison with the posterior marks. Clinical experience has demonstrated that the appliance's occlusion should be well adjusted to provide its maximal effect.

◉ **QUICK CONSULT**
Adjusting Appliances
Clinical experience has demonstrated that the appliance's occlusion should be well adjusted to provide its maximal effect.

Once the desired centric contacts are obtained, adjust the protrusive guidance ramp. It should be long enough that the mandibular anterior teeth cannot retrude behind it. If the mandibular anterior teeth were to retrude behind the ramp while the patient is sleeping, he or she might clench in this unadjusted location and exacerbate the symptoms. Therefore, position the mandible into the neutral position to determine how far the patient can retrude the mandible. If the ramp is too short, add self-curing clear orthodontic acrylic to extend it. If the ramp is longer than necessary, remove the excess portion (Figure 13-3).

As the patient glides from the neutral position into the desired anterior position, use two sheets of black Accufilm in the articulating forceps to mark the opposing anterior tooth contacts on the ramp. Repeatedly mark and adjust the ramp so it provides the patient even gliding marks along the ramp for the teeth, canine to canine.

Similar to the stabilization appliance, smooth the appliance and ensure the appliance feels comfortable to the patient.

APPLIANCE MANAGEMENT

Originally anterior positioning appliances were used to hold the mandible in the described anterior location for 24 hours a day (including while eating). After a period of time, the patient's teeth were altered (through orthodontics and/or prosthodontic reconstruction) so MI coincided with this new mandibular location. Investigators following these cases observed that, despite the extensive treatment provided, patients could not maintain the desired disc-condyle relationship.[6,15,16]

The most comprehensive study I have read that followed the posttreatment changes observed 12 patients who were first provided anterior positioning appliance therapy and then orthodontics that established a stable occlusion at the predetermined anterior position. Comparing superimpositions of the patients' cephalometric radiographs, the investigator found that over time all of the patients had occlusal and TMJ changes, which included distal repositioning of the mandible, intrusion of the maxillary molars, and concomitant increase in overbite and overjet.[17]

Therefore, it is recommended that patients use the anterior positioning appliance only while they sleep and use their normal mandibular position during the day. In this manner, patients can maintain their normal MI and obtain TMD symptom relief by nighttime use.[9,10,18,19] One author indicates that nighttime wear appears to provide similar TMD symptom improvement as normally obtained from 24-hour wear.[10]

🗨 **FOCAL POINT**
It is recommended that patients use the anterior positioning appliance only while they sleep and use their normal mandibular position during the day.

When patients first wear the anterior positioning appliance at night, they commonly report that, once they have removed the appliance upon waking, it takes up to an hour for their teeth to occlude into MI. Over the next month, this time generally progressively shortens. A small percentage of the patients will find that it takes longer than several hours to close into MI, and this time may progressively lengthen. Out of fear that such patients may eventually not be able to occlude into MI, they should discontinue wearing this appliance, and the provider may choose to convert the appliance into a stabilization appliance.

Since the appliance was designed to hold the mandible at the location where the masticatory system feels more relaxed or comfortable, some patients have a tendency to wear their appliance 24 hours a day. If worn 24 hours a day, it may cause the patient to not be able to close into MI.[8,9,20] The inability to close into MI may be due to remodeling of condyles, proliferation of soft tissue posterior to the condyles, and/or myofibrotic contracture of the lateral pterygoid muscles.[8,9,18] This problem is usually reversible if caught early, but is usually permanent if it is a long-standing condition.[18,21] Therefore, instruct patients to wear this appliance only while they sleep and closely follow the cases to ensure they do not start to lose their ability to close into MI.[10,22]

An easy technique for observing whether a patient is beginning to lose the ability to close into MI is to follow whether there is a change among the opposing teeth that can hold shim stock when the patient closes into MI (Figure 13-4). It is recommended that these cases be followed every month, and it should be observed which opposing teeth can hold shim stock. Some variations are normal,[23] but if a patient begins to lose the ability to close into MI, the most posterior opposing teeth will start to lose their ability to hold shim stock. If this occurs, the patient should immediately discontinue wearing this appliance, and the provider may choose to convert the anterior positioning appliance into a stabilization appliance. If only minimal changes have occurred, these teeth should regain the ability to hold shim stock.

⊙ **QUICK CONSULT**

Observing for Maximum Intercuspation Changes

An easy technique for observing whether a patient is beginning to lose the ability to close into MI is to follow whether there is a change among the opposing teeth that can hold shim stock when the patient closes into MI (Figure 13-4).

Since significant complications are associated with the anterior positioning appliance, I do not view it as a potential long-term therapy. Once the pain and dysfunction have

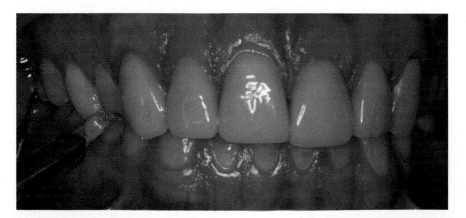

Figure 13-4. Monitoring occlusion; identifying which opposing teeth hold shim stock.

adequately decreased, the appliance should gradually be discontinued or replaced with a stabilization appliance.[6] I ask patients who have been wearing an anterior positioning appliance for a year to stop wearing it so we can test what occurs when they do not wear it. I expect to observe one of three situations: (a) Their pain does not reappear, suggesting they no longer need an appliance. (b) They have only morning pain without the appliance, so the appliance is converted into a stabilization appliance to treat this pain. (c) Their mechanical symptoms and pain return, so they continue to wear their anterior positioning appliance and their cases are followed monthly.

◉ QUICK CONSULT

Using Anterior Positioning Appliances

Since there are significant complications associated with the anterior positioning appliance, I do not view it as a potential long-term therapy.

Practitioners should bear the following in mind: (a) Anterior positioning appliance therapy is not intended to correct the disc-condyle relationship, but to facilitate the reduction in TMD symptoms, similar to other conservative TMD treatments.[24,25] (b) Even though a patient meets the anterior positioning appliance criteria, a stabilization appliance is generally similarly effective in reducing a patient's symptoms. Since the anterior positioning appliance needs to be carefully followed for complications whereas the stabilization appliance has minimal complications, it is recommended that the stabilization appliance be used first. If the patient meets the anterior positioning appliance criteria and continues to have significant pain or TMJ locking after receiving a stabilization appliance and other conservative therapies, then it would be appropriate to consider an anterior positioning appliance.

✺ FOCAL POINT

It is recommended practitioners use the stabilization appliance prior to using the anterior positioning appliance, because the stabilization appliance has minimal associated complications and patients who meet the anterior positioning appliance criteria typically do well with a stabilization appliance.

Counsel patients who are to receive an anterior positioning appliance about potential complications associated with it and the importance of returning for their follow-up appointments. I have had considerable difficulty with some patients returning for their required follow-up appointments, especially those who have responded quite well with the appliance. Therefore, prior to delivering this appliance, it is recommended that a statement be typed in the patient's record that the patient was advised that, if he or she does not return for follow-up appointments, the patient should discontinue wearing this appliance, and have the patient sign this entry.

REFERENCES

1. Dylina TJ. A common-sense approach to splint therapy. J Prosthet Dent 2001;86:539–45.
2. Nitzan DW. Arthrocentesis for management of severe close lock of the temporomandibular joint. Oral Maxillofac Surg Clin North Am 1994;6: 245–57.
3. Kurita H, Kurashina K, Baba H, Ohtsuka A, Kotani A, Kopp S. Evaluation of disk capture with a splint repositioning appliance: clinical and critical assessment with MR imaging. Oral Surg Oral Med Oral Pathol Oral Radiol Endod 1998;85(4):377–80.
4. Williamson EH, Rosenzweig BJ. The treatment of temporomandibular disorders through repositioning splint therapy: a follow-up study. Cranio 1998;16(4):222–5.
5. Hersek N, Uzun G, Cindas A, Canay S, Kutsal YG. Effect of anterior repositioning splints on the electromyographic activities of masseter and anterior temporalis muscles. Cranio 1998;16(1):11–6.

6. American Academy of Orofacial Pain, with Okeson JP (ed). Orofacial Pain: Guidelines for Assessment, Diagnosis and Management. Chicago: Quintessence, 1996:150–3.

7. Brown DT, Gaudet EL Jr. Temporomandibular disorder treatment outcomes: second report of a large-scale prospective clinical study. Cranio 2002;20(4):244–53.

8. Pertes RA. Occlusal appliance therapy. In: Pertes RA, Gross SG (eds). Clinical Management of Temporomandibular Disorders and Orofacial Pain. Chicago: Quintessence, 1995:197–210.

9. Okeson JP. Management of Temporomandibular Disorders and Occlusion, 5th edition. St Louis: CV Mosby Co, 2003:445–7, 507–36.

10. Schiffman EL. Recent advances: diagnosis and management of TMJ disorders. In: Hardin JF (ed). Clark's Clinical Dentistry, volume 2. Philadelphia: JB Lippincott, 1998:1–5.

11. McPoil TG, Hunt GC. Evaluation and management of foot and ankle disorders: present problems and future directions. J Orthop Sports Phys Ther 1995;21(6)381–8.

12. Kurita H, Kurashina K, Ohtsuka A, Kotani A. Change of position of the temporomandibular joint disk with insertion of a disk-repositioning appliance. Oral Surg Oral Med Oral Pathol Oral Radiol Endod 1998;85(2):142–5.

13. Kirk WS Jr. Magnetic resonance imaging and tomographic evaluation of occlusal appliance treatment for advanced internal derangement of the temporomandibular joint. J Oral Maxillofac Surg 1991;49(1):9–12.

14. Anderson GC, Schulte JK, Goodkind RJ. Comparative study of two treatment methods for internal derangement of the temporomandibular joint. J Prosthet Dent 1985;53(3):392–7.

15. Summer JD, Westesson P-L. Mandibular repositioning can be effective in treatment of reducing TMJ disk displacement: a long-term clinical and MRI imaging follow-up. Cranio 1997;15(2):107–20.

16. Moloney F, Howard JA. Internal derangements of the temporomandibular joint. III: Anterior repositioning splint therapy. Aust Dent J 1986;31(1):30–9.

17. Joondeph DR. Long-term stability of orthopedic repositioning. Angle Orthod 1999;69:201–9.

18. Bush FM, Abbott FM, Butler JH, Harrington WG. Oral orthotics: design, indications, efficacy and care. In: Hardin JF (ed). Clark's Clinical Dentistry, volume 2, chapter 39. Philadelphia: JB Lippincott, 1998:1–33.

19. Clark GT, Lanham F, Flack VF. Treatment outcome results for consecutive TMJ clinic patients. J Craniomandib Disord 1988;2(2):87–95.

20. Okeson JP. Long-term treatment of disk-interference disorders of the temporomandibular joint with anterior repositioning occlusal splints. J Prosthet Dent 1988;60(5):611–6.

21. Kai S, Kai H, Tabata O, Tashiro H. The significance of posterior open bite after anterior repositioning splint therapy for anteriorly displaced disk of the temporomandibular joint. Cranio 1993;11(2):146–52.

22. Messing SG. Splint therapy. In: Kaplan AS, Assael LA (eds). Temporomandibular Disorders: Diagnosis and Treatment. Philadelphia: WB Saunders, 1991:395–454.

23. Anderson GC, Schulte JK, Aeppli DM. Reliability of the evaluation of occlusal contacts in the intercuspal position. J Prosthet Dent 1993;70(4):320–3.

24. Attanasio R. Intraoral orthotic therapy. Dent Clin North Am 1997;41(2):309–24.

25. Orenstein ES. Anterior repositioning appliances when used for anterior disk displacement with reduction: a critical review. Cranio 1993;11(2):141–5.

Part IV

Multidisciplinary Treatment Approach

Occlusal appliance therapy is only one of a multitude of therapies available to treat TMD. Since TMD is a multifactorial disorder (having many etiologic factors), many therapies have been shown to have a positive impact on an individual patient's TMD symptoms.[1-3]

☯ FOCAL POINT

Occlusal appliance therapy is only one of a multitude of therapies available to treat TMD.

Physicians, physical therapists, chiropractors, massage therapists, and others treating the muscles and/or cervical region report positive responses to treatment of TMD symptoms.[4-8] Psychologists working with relaxation, stress management, cognitive-behavioral therapy, and other psychological aspects report reducing TMD symptoms with their therapies.[2,4,5] Orthodontists, prosthodontists, and general dentists observe a positive impact on TMD symptoms by improving the occlusal stability.[1,4,5] Surgeons report TMD symptom reduction from different TMJ surgical approaches.[9-11] Medications as well as self-management strategies used for other muscles and joints in the body have also been shown to reduce TMD symptoms.[2,4,5,12]

The literature advocates a large number of potentially reversible conservative therapies to treat TMD patients. Not all TMD therapies are equally effective, and no one treatment has been shown to be best for all TMD patients.[5,13] By using the information obtained from the patient interview and clinical exam, practitioners can select the most cost-effective evidence-based therapies that have the greatest potential for providing long-term symptom relief for a particular patient.[14]

Many of the therapies act through different mechanisms, enabling a practitioner to use multiple therapies simultaneously, which provides a synergistic effect. The most successful treatments often focus on therapies that decrease a patient's perpetuating contributing factors, which have kept the body from resolving the symptoms on its own.[15-17] These TMD management concepts are consistent with treatment of other orthopedic and rheumatologic disorders.[2,18]

☻ FOCAL POINT

Many of the therapies act through different mechanisms, enabling a practitioner to simultaneously use multiple therapies, which provides a synergistic effect.

The most successful treatments often focus on therapies that decrease a patient's perpetuating contributing factors, which have kept the body from resolving the symptoms on its own.

Most TMD patients can be successfully managed by general practitioners,[19] and TMD patients who receive TMD therapy obtain significant symptom relief, whereas patients who do not receive treatment have minimal symptom change.[3,20] A practitioner's experience and expertise, and the availability of modalities, may impact the treatment plan.[21]

While practitioners evaluate their patients, they must be cognizant that many disorders outside of the dentist's realm of treatment can contribute to the perpetuation of TMD symptoms, e.g., widespread pain, neck pain, rheumatic disorders, poor sleep, or depression.[22-24] Identifying (as delineated in Chapter 2, "Review of Initial Patient Questionnaire") and obtaining appropriate therapy for these disorders should greatly enhance the TMD symptom relief practitioners can obtain.[14]

A patient's prognosis is often related to the duration the problem has been present, the frequency and severity of the pain, the presence of other pains, the patient's previous response to therapy, and patient's cooperation.[22,24-26] In medical care, noncompliance is reported to be 15 to 93 percent, and poor compliance is remarkably similar across drugs, diseases, prognosis, and symptoms.[27,28] Educating the patient and a good patient-practitioner relationship are important factors in improving patient compliance.[28-30]

The time spent educating a patient is a significant factor in developing a high level of rapport and treatment compliance.[28-30] The time should be appropriate to educate the patient on clinical findings, diagnostic data, treatment options, and prognosis. This may require the practitioner or a trained staff member to show drawings to the patient, such as the "TMJ Disc Displacements" diagram in Appendix 2.

REFERENCES

1. Dawson PE. Evaluation, diagnosis and treatment of occlusal problems, 2nd edition. St Louis: CV Mosby, 1989.

2. American Academy of Orofacial Pain, with Okeson JP (ed). Orofacial Pain: Guidelines for Assessment, Diagnosis and Management. Chicago: Quintessence, 1996:141–58.

3. Gaudet EL, Brown DT. Temporomandibular disorder treatment outcomes: first report of a large scale prospective clinical study. Cranio 2000;18(1):9–22.

4. McNeill C. History and evolution of TMD concepts. Oral Surg Oral Med Oral Pathol Oral Radiol Endod 1997;83:51–60.

5. Greene CS. The etiology of temporomandibular disorders: implications for treatment. J Orofac Pain 2001;15(2):93–105.

6. Knutson GA, Jacob M. Possible manifestation of temporomandibular joint dysfunction on chiropractic cervical x-ray studies. J Manipulative Physiol Ther 1999;22:32–7.

7. Stiesch-Scholz M, Fink M, Tschernitschek H, Rossbach A. Medical and physical therapy of temporomandibular joint disk displacement without reduction. Cranio 2002;20(2):85–90.

8. Wright EF, Domenech MA, Fischer JR Jr. Usefulness of posture training for TMD patients. J Am Dent Assoc 2000;131(2):202–10.

9. Montgomery MT, Gordon SM, Van Sickels JE, Harms SE. Changes in signs and symptoms following temporomandibular joint disc repositioning surgery. J Oral Maxillofac Surg 1992;50(4):320–8.

10. Montgomery MT, Van Sickels JE, Harms SE. Success of temporomandibular joint arthroscopy in disk displacement with and without reduction. Oral Surg Oral Med Oral Pathol 1991;71(6):651–9.

11. McKenna SJ, Cornella F, Gibbs SJ. Long-term follow-up of modified condylotomy for internal derangement of the temporomandibular joint.

Oral Surg Oral Med Oral Pathol Oral Radiol Endod 1996;81(5):509–15.

12. Wright E, Anderson G, Schulte J. A randomized clinical trial of intraoral soft splints and palliative treatment for masticatory muscle pain. J Orofac Pain 1995;9(2):116–30.

13. Kaplan AS, Goldman JR. General concepts of treatment. In: Kaplan AS, Assael LA (eds). Temporomandibular Disorders: Diagnosis and Treatment. Philadelphia: WB Saunders, 1991: 388–94.

14. Wright EF. How daily TMD symptom patterns may affect treatment approach. Am Acad Orofac Pain Newsl 2000;5(3)15–6.

15. McNeill C. Management of temporomandibular disorders: concepts and controversies. J Prosthet Dent 1997;77:510–22.

16. Fricton JR, Chung SC. Contributing factors: A key to chronic pain. In: Fricton JR, Kroening RJ, Hathaway KM (eds). TMJ and Craniofacial Pain: Diagnosis and Management. St Louis: Ishiyaku EuroAmerica, 1988:27–37.

17. Fricton JR. Establishing the problem list: an inclusive conceptual model for chronic illness. In: Fricton JR, Kroening RJ, Hathaway KM (eds). TMJ and Craniofacial Pain: Diagnosis and Management. St Louis: Ishiyaku EuroAmerica, 1988:21–6.

18. McNeill C, Mohl ND, Rugh JD, Tanaka TT. Temporomandibular disorders: diagnosis, management, education, and research. J Am Dent Assoc 1990;120(3):253–63.

19. Egermark I, Carlsson GE, Magnusson T. A 20-year longitudinal study of subjective symptoms of temporomandibular disorders from childhood to adulthood. Acta Odontol Scand 2001;59(1):40–8.

20. Brown DT, Gaudet EL Jr. Temporomandibular disorder treatment outcomes: second report of a large-scale prospective clinical study. Cranio 2002;20(4):244–53.

21. Check RK, Carlson GL, Fricton JR, Gibilisco JA, Keller EA, Omlie MR, Speidel TM. Report of the ad hoc committee on craniomandibular and tem-

poromandibular joint disorders. Current concepts of diagnosis and treatment. Nov 14, 1988. Minnesota Dental Association.

22. Raphael KG, Marbach JJ, Klausner J. Myofascial face pain: clinical characteristics of those with regional vs. widespread pain. J Am Dent Assoc 2000;131(2):161–71.

23. Wright EF, Schiffman EL. Treatment alternatives for patients with masticatory myofascial pain. J Am Dent Assoc 1995;126(7):1030–9.

24. Garofalo JP, Gatchel RJ, Wesley AL, Ellis E. III Predicting chronicity in acute temporomandibular joint disorders using the Research Diagnostic Criteria. J Am Dent Assoc 1998;129(4):438–47.

25. Pertes RA, Bailey DR. General concepts of diagnosis and treatment. In: Pertes RA, Gross SG (eds). Clinical management of temporomandibular disorders and orofacial pain. Chicago: Quintessence, 1995:63.

26. Rammelsberg P, LeResche L, Dworkin S, Mancl L. Longitudinal outcome of temporomandibular disorders: a 5-year epidemiologic study of muscle disorders defined by research diagnostic criteria for temporomandibular disorders. J Orofac Pain 2003;17(1):9–20.

27. Miller NH, Hill M, Kottke T, Ockene IS. The multilevel compliance challenge: recommendations for a call to action. Circulation 1997; 95(4)1085–90.

28. Kaplan RM, Simon NJ. Compliance in medical care: reconsideration of self-predictions. Ann Behav Med 1990;12(2):66–71.

29. Blanpied P. Why won't patients do their home exercise programs? J Orthop Sports Phys Ther 1997;25(2):101–2.

30. Cameron C. Patient compliance: recognition of factors involved and suggestions for promoting compliance and therapeutic regimens. J Adv Nurs 1996;24(2):244–50.

Chapter 14

Self-management Therapy

FAQ

Q: What do you do when a patient cannot control his or her daytime habits or muscle tension adequately to reduce the daytime symptoms satisfactorily?

A: Some patients cannot adequately control their daytime habits or muscle tension to reduce their daytime symptoms satisfactorily. Most of these patients are referred to a psychologist for additional help with changing these, especially if other psychosocial needs are observed.

Self-management therapies are procedures a patient is instructed to perform on his or her own. They are convenient and inexpensive, compared with the patient going to a practitioner's office to receive the therapy.

⊚ QUICK CONSULT

Using Self-management Therapies

Self-management therapies are convenient and inexpensive, compared with a patient going to a practitioner's office to receive the therapy.

The most common of these therapies is a wide-ranging set of self-management instructions (e.g., Appendix 3, "TMD Self-management Therapies") that is generally given to all patients diagnosed with TMD.[1] These instructions

1. Encourage patients to rest the masticatory muscles by voluntarily limiting the activities for which they are used, i.e., avoiding hard or chewy foods and abstaining from activities that may aggravate the masticatory system (oral habits and overextending the jaw by yawning or prolonged dental appointments).

2. Encourage awareness and elimination of parafunctional habits, e.g., changing a clenching habit to lightly resting the tongue behind the maxillary anterior teeth and keeping the teeth apart and masticatory muscles relaxed.

3. Recommend instituting a home physiotherapeutic program, e.g., applying heat or cold to the most painful masticatory areas.

4. Recommend over-the-counter medications on an as-needed basis.

Additional self-management therapies that may be provided to TMD patients include instructing them in an exercise to stretch the closure muscles, an exercise to stretch the lateral pterygoid muscles, exercises to improve the posture, techniques to massage and/or compress the muscle *trigger points* (knots with the muscles), and techniques to break the daytime parafunctional habits.

The practitioner or a trained staff member needs to initially instruct and often motivate the patient to perform the self-management therapies. Once the patient discovers the benefit that is obtained by using them, he or she tends to be more self-motivated.

◉ **QUICK CONSULT**
Implementing Self-management Therapies
The practitioner or a trained staff member needs to initially instruct and often motivate the patient to perform the self-management therapies.

Here are a few techniques that may instill greater patient compliance: (a) give patients follow-up appointments at which they know they will be asked about performing the therapies; (b) obtain a promise that they will perform the therapy as requested; and (c) have them determine another routinely performed activity that will trigger them to do these therapies. For example, if a patient decides to use the heating pad while watching a nightly television program, hopefully when the show is broadcast it will remind the patient to apply the heating pad.

SELF-MANAGEMENT INSTRUCTIONS

A recommended self-management instructions handout is provided in Appendix 3, "TMD Self-management Therapies." It begins with a short background about TMD, providing information that patients used to often ask me. After the self-management instructions, the handout informs patients that TMD cannot be "cured" but has to be managed, the treatments are not fully predictable, and the treatment plan may need to be altered based on a patient's treatment response.

Home physiotherapeutics can involve using heat, cold, or alternating between heat and cold. Many practitioners prefer patients use heat,[2] whereas others prefer cold. No study has compared which is better for TMD patients, for specific TMD diagnoses, or for specific situations (other than the use of cold following trauma). Empirically most TMD patients appear to prefer heat,[3] but those with severe pain (9/10 or above) seem to find heat aggravates their pain, and so prefer cold. Other patients find their symptoms respond best by alternating between heat and cold.

One study that compared a moist heating pad to moist towels found that almost twice the percentage of patients using the moist heating pad did not require any additional treatment.[4] It is speculated the response difference is due to the heating pad maintaining the tissue at a consistently high temperature, whereas the towels cool down with time. Based on this study, I recommend patients use a heating pad rather than a device that cools over time.

Another study compared the intraoral buccal mucosa temperatures obtained by using moist and dry heating pads over the cheek.[5] The authors found there was no difference between the two methods, but a few patients did prefer the moist to the dry heat. Understanding that compliance is related to the complexity of the requested procedure[6] and that dry heat is simpler to use, I inform patients that a dry heating pad works just as well as a moist heating pad, but it is fine to use moist heat if the patient prefers.

Patients use many methods for applying cold. Some desire to apply an ice cube directly to their skin, others prefer to wrap it in a wash cloth, etc. Patients who routinely use cold seem to prefer to take a bag of frozen peas, loosen the peas by hitting the bag with the heel of their hand, and apply the bag to their skin. These patients generally mark the bag in some manner so they do not later accidentally cook these peas for a meal.

Many TMD patients find that eating tough or chewy foods aggravates their TMD symptoms. Some patients observe that simultaneously chewing on both sides of the mouth reduces their normal symptom aggravation. Therefore, patients are advised to eat a moderately soft diet, cut other foods into small pieces, and try evenly dividing the food on both sides of their mouth and chewing on both sides.

Caffeine tends to cause the muscles to tighten and contribute to poor sleep. Many individuals can relate to these effects because they have experienced consuming too much caffeine, which caused them to shake from uncontrollable muscle contractions and/or have difficulty sleeping. Clinically one well-known muscle researcher concluded that two or more cups of coffee or cans of soda a day aggravate muscle trigger points (the most common source of TMD pain).[3]

The amount of caffeine in beverages varies greatly.[7] As a general guide, I tell patients that a cup of coffee, a can of soda, and two cups of ice tea or hot tea are equivalent. It is recommended that TMD patients reduce their caffeine consumption to no more than one cup of coffee, one can of soda, or two cups of tea a day.

Many caffeine consumers have developed a chemical dependency to their caffeine intake and know that they will develop a severe headache if they do not drink sufficient caffeine. These patients can reduce their caffeine consumption slowly without developing headaches or tiredness. It has been observed that patients consuming more than a pot of coffee a day can usually reduce consumption to one pot a day without developing these problems. These patients are asked to maintain that level for 1 week. It has been observed also that these patients and those on lower amounts of caffeine can usually reduce consumption by one cup of coffee or can of soda a week without developing caffeine withdrawal symptoms.

The TMD symptom response from decreasing caffeine consumption is quite variable. Some patients report no change, whereas others have a dramatic reduction or even elimination of their TMD symptoms. Empirically, patients who consume higher doses of caffeine appear to be more likely to have a more favorable response to restriction of their caffeine consumption. I ask all patients to attempt to reduce their consumption to no more than one cup of coffee, one can of soda, or two cups of tea a day, and hold this consumption level during treatment. They are informed that, once treatment is complete, they are welcome to resume consuming caffeine at whatever level they prefer but should observe for any increase in their TMD symptoms related to this. With this knowledge, they can make an educated decision about the amount of caffeine they want to consume.

◉ **QUICK CONSULT**

Restricting Caffeine Consumption

Empirically, patients who consume higher doses of caffeine appear to be more likely to have a more favorable response to restriction of their caffeine consumption.

Some individuals tend to clench their teeth when they are irritated, driving a car, using a computer, or concentrating. Clenching or grinding the teeth requires the masticatory muscles to contract and often loads the TMJs. An excessive amount of this activity tends to overuse the masticatory muscles and/or excessively load the TMJs. This may be a primary contributor to masticatory muscle pain and/or TMJ inflammation.[8]

⊙ **QUICK CONSULT**

Informing Patients of Tendencies

Some individuals tend to clench their teeth when they are irritated, driving a car, using a computer, or concentrating. This may be a primary contributor to masticatory muscle pain and/or TMJ inflammation.

Similarly, chronically holding tension within these muscles can also overuse the masticatory muscles and/or excessively load the TMJs. Patients who have neck or shoulder pain often know they tend to hold excessive tension in the locations of their pain. For these patients, it is often helpful to use the comparison that holding tension in the neck or shoulders similarly contributes to their pain as holding tension in the masticatory system.

In an attempt to try to break these habits, patients are instructed to monitor themselves closely for clenching or grinding habits, especially while they are irritated, driving a car, using a computer, or otherwise concentrating. Some TMD patients relate they rest their teeth together only lightly, but frequently unconsciously squeeze their teeth together during these activities. Therefore, patients are asked to learn to keep their jaw muscles relaxed, teeth separated, and tongue lightly resting on the roof of the mouth just behind their upper front teeth.

⊙ **QUICK CONSULT**

Asking Patients to Observe for Habits

Some TMD patients relate they rest their teeth together only lightly, but frequently unconsciously squeeze their teeth together when they are irritated, driving a car, using a computer, or otherwise concentrating.

Additionally patients are instructed to observe for, and avoid, habits that put unnecessary strain on the masticatory muscles and TMJs, e.g., resting the mandible on the hand or biting their cheeks, lips, fingernails, cuticles, or any other objects they may put in their mouth.

Posture appears to play a role in TMD symptoms, so patients are asked to maintain good head, neck, and shoulder posture. They are requested to be especially vigilant of their posture while using a computer and to avoid poor postural habits, such as cradling a telephone against their shoulder. Posture-improving exercises are provided in Appendix 6, "Posture Improvement Exercises," and discussed further in "Posture Exercises" in this chapter.

Patients are informed that their sleep posture is also important. They are requested to avoid positions that strain their neck or jaw, such as stomach sleeping. If they sleep on their side, they are asked to ensure they keep their cervical spinal column in alignment and in a neutral position.

Studies show that relaxation is beneficial for reducing TMD symptoms.[9,10] Patients are requested to set aside time once or twice a day to relax and drain the tension from their jaw and neck. Patients often benefit from simple relaxation techniques such as sitting in a quiet room while listening to soothing music, taking a warm shower or bath, and slow deep breathing. Relaxing in this manner generally not only reduces the pain, but also enables patients to become aware of what tense and relaxed muscles feel like and to develop the capability to reduce their muscle tension immediately whenever they notice the muscles are tight.

Many TMD patients find that opening their mouth wide, such as in yawning, yelling, or prolonged dental procedures, aggravates their TMD symptoms. Therefore, patients are requested to avoid these activities.

Over-the-counter medications usually provide only minor TMD symptom relief. Patients who find these beneficial are instructed to take them as needed, but to avoid those that have caffeine (e.g., Anacin, Excedrin, and Vanquish).

To emphasize its importance, motivate the patient, and explain any confusion with performing these procedures, it is strongly recommended that the handout be reviewed with the patient. Based on the assumption that this handout will be reviewed with the patient, a few potential contributing factors (e.g., caffeine consumption or sleeping posture) were not asked about in the initial patient questionnaire, and it was assumed they would be identified at this time. This review may be performed by any staff member trained to provide this education.[11]

▼ **TECHNICAL TIP**

Motivating Patients to Perform Self-management Instructions

To emphasize its importance, motivate the patient, and explain any confusion with performing these procedures, it is strongly recommended that the handout be reviewed with the patient.

☻ **FOCAL POINT**

Based on the assumption that this handout will be reviewed with the patient, a few potential contributing factors (e.g., caffeine consumption or sleeping posture) were not asked about in the initial patient questionnaire, and it was assumed they would be identified at this time.

Clinical experience with this self-management instruction handout has shown that the amount of improvement patients obtain from it varies greatly. It is speculated this variation is primarily due to the compliance of the patients. Most report some TMD symptom improvement from applying these instructions, but most do not report a dramatic change. If a patient has minimal TMD symptoms, these instructions may be adequate. In one study using these instructions, it was observed that the average TMD symptom reduction was only 8 percent.[12]

CLOSURE MUSCLE-STRETCHING EXERCISE

Studies suggest that providing a TMD patient whose pain is primarily of muscle origin with stretching exercises will decrease the TMD pain and increase the range of motion.[13-15] One study demonstrated that the amount of improvement derived from stretching exercises was comparable to that obtained from an occlusal appliance.[14] The masseter, temporalis, and medial pterygoid muscles, which are responsible for closing the mandible, are often major contributors to TMD pain. Appendix 5, "Jaw Muscle-stretching Exercise," is a recommended stretching-exercise handout for these closure muscles. As with the self-management instructions, a trained staff member can effectively educate a patient and follow the patient's use of the jaw exercises.[14]

☻ **FOCAL POINT**

Studies suggest that providing a TMD patient whose pain is primarily of muscle origin with stretching exercises will decrease the TMD pain and increase the range of motion.

If a patient is reluctant to try stretching, it can be helpful to introduce the concept by explaining that the pain in these muscles is most probably due to their overuse, secondary to excessive parafunctional activity or excessive tension. As with an individual with leg muscle pain secondary to excessive leg exercises, an initial therapy for the muscle would be to stretch it prior to and after exercising. Since the patient may be performing the parafunctional activity or maintaining excessive muscle tension throughout the day and night, the patient may have the best results from stretching the closure muscles periodically throughout the day.

This exercise is exclusively for patients who have painful closure muscles (masseter, temporalis, and/or medial pterygoid). This exercise uses the opening muscles (lateral pterygoid, anterior digastric, and posterior digastric) to stretch the closure muscles; if a patient's pain is primarily in an opening muscle, this exercise may aggravate the symptoms. Additionally, if a patient has significant TMJ inflammation, the exercise may aggravate the TMJ, so it is recommended that this exercise not be provided to patients who have significant opening muscle or TMJ pain. A lateral pterygoid muscle-stretching exercise is provided in the next section.

▼ **TECHNICAL TIP**
Prescribing Stretching Exercise
If a patient has significant TMJ inflammation, the stretching exercise may aggravate the TMJ, so it is recommended that this exercise not be provided to patients who have significant TMJ pain.

The benefits derived from stretching exercises appear to be increased by patients applying heat to the area prior to stretching. A study compared the increase in range of motion of the shoulder when heat was applied to the area before stretching, when stretching was followed by an ice pack, when heat was applied before stretching followed by an ice pack, when stretching only, and when there was no stretching (control) (see Figure 14-1). The results suggest applying heat prior to stretching exercises provides the greatest improvement.[16] Therefore, if a patient performs this exercise and is using heat on the painful closure muscles, encourage performing this exercise after sufficiently warming the muscle. Some TMD patients warm their painful closure muscles with hot shower water. For patients who do this, similarly encourage performing the exercise after warming the muscle in this manner.

LATERAL PTERYGOID MUSCLE-STRETCHING EXERCISE

The lateral pterygoid muscle can be stretched to reduce pain and/or tightness within it.[17] To stretch the lateral pterygoid muscle, the practitioner should place his or her thumb on the most posterior ipsilateral mandibular teeth and wrap the fingers around the mandible, as depicted in Figure 14-2. Use of either the dominant or the nondominant hand may be preferred. Some

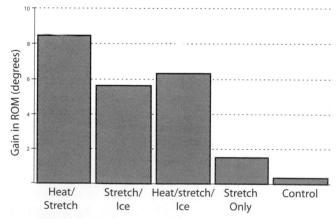

Heat and Ice with Stretching

Figure 14-1. Heat followed by a stretching exercise is more effective than stretching followed by ice; heat stretching, then ice; stretching only; or not using any of these.[16]

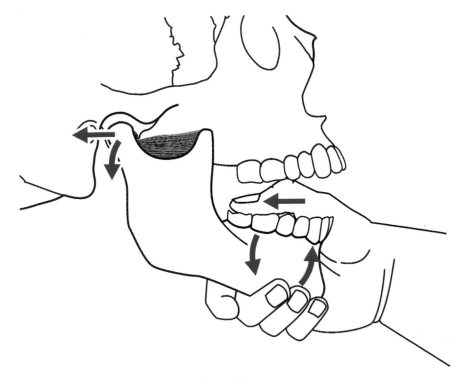

Figure 14-2. Stretching the lateral pterygoid muscle.

practitioners like to place gauze between the teeth and their thumb to prevent discomfort from pressing on the cusp tips.

▼ **TECHNICAL TIP**

Stretching the Lateral Pterygoid Muscle

To stretch the lateral pterygoid muscle, the practitioner should place his or her thumb on the most posterior ipsilateral mandibular teeth and wrap the fingers around the mandible, as depicted in Figure 14-2.

The practitioner should push down with the thumb and pull up on the chin. This rotates the mandible, distracts the condyle, and provides more room to mobilize the condyle. While distracting the condyle, slowly push the mandible posteriorly up to approximately 4 pounds of force and hold for about 30 seconds. Release the force, but maintain the hand position on the mandible. After about 10 seconds, repeat the 30-second

stretch of the lateral pterygoid muscle and perform the stretch six times. Ask the patient to practice this stretch on himself or herself and provide advice on performing the maneuver as needed.

Patients who have TMJ inflammation may aggravate their pain when pushing the mandible posteriorly and thus may need to modulate the force of the stretch so the TMJ inflammation is not aggravated. Patients are asked to perform a series of six stretches, six times a day, holding each stretch for approximately 30 seconds.

Anatomically it would appear the lateral pterygoid muscle is too deep for superficial heat to be beneficial, but patients with a lateral pterygoid muscle disorder continually report its use is beneficial. As described for the closure muscles (Appendix 5, "Jaw Muscle-stretching Exercise"), patients who use heat over this area should have better results with this exercise by performing it after the area has been warmed sufficiently.

POSTURE EXERCISES

Poor posture is extremely common among the general population and appears to be an adaptive, self-perpetuating trait for which individuals lack the cognitive ability or desire to self-correct. Forward head posture, the most common form of poor posture, is very prevalent among TMD patients[18] and might contribute to cervical dysfunction (pain and/or restricted movement).[19,20] With this posture, the head's center of gravity is forward of the spine's weight-bearing axis, increasing the strain within the posterior cervical muscles, ligaments, and apophyseal joints.[12]

Posture training usually entails exercises that are repetitively preformed within the pain-free range to stretch structures that poor posture tends to shorten, strengthen structures that poor posture tends to weaken, and create a cognitive awareness of the new desired posture.[21,22] Patients are asked to try to maintain this new posture, which is thought to prevent them from being in positions that cause undue stress, microtrauma, and overuse on structures of the head and neck.

In a randomized clinical trial, the exercises provided in Appendix 6, "Posture Improvement Exercises," were found to improve TMD and neck symptoms significantly. The treatment group received these posture exercises and the self-management instructions in Appendix 3, whereas the control group received only the self-management instructions. The treatment group reported a mean reduction in their TMD and neck symptoms of 42 and 38 percent, whereas the control group reported a mean reduction of 8 and 9 percent, respectively (Table 14-1). TMD patients who held their head further forward relative to the shoulders (having greater forward head posture) were significantly more likely to derive TMD symptom improvement from posture training and self-management instructions.[12]

Table 14-1. Benefits of posture exercises

	Average pain reduction[12]	
	Posture exercises and self-management	Self-management only
TMD	42%	8%
Neck	38%	9%

TMD symptom improvement correlated with pretreatment head and shoulder postural difference (p < 0.05) and neck symptom improvement (p < 0.005).

◉ QUICK CONSULT

Recommending Posture Exercises

The treatment group, using the exercises provided in Appendix 6, reported a mean reduction in TMD and neck symptoms of 42 and 38 percent, whereas the control group reported a mean reduction of 8 and 9 percent, respectively (Table 14-1).

Practitioners may wish to use the posture exercises in Appendix 6 to help their TMD patients obtain these benefits. Follow-up appointments are necessary to ensure the exercises are being performed properly and tend to motivate patients to comply better with the exercise schedule, especially if patients know they will be asked about their compliance and to demonstrate the exercises. Performing these exercises improperly may exacerbate the TMD or neck symptoms.

In addition to performing these exercises, patients must continually monitor their posture and maintain the desired new posture. Clinically this new cognizance can be combined easily with other self-monitoring that should improve TMD symptoms, e.g., continually monitor tongue posture, jaw posture, and jaw muscle tension. This self-monitoring enables patients to modify their posture or behavior as soon as they begin to revert to their old undesirable postures or behaviors.

Knowing that TMD patients with a greater forward head posture have a higher probability of deriving TMD symptom improvement from these exercises, observe the degree of the patient's forward head posture during the initial evaluation. The greater the forward head posture is, the more likely I am to recommend these exercises.

MUSCLE MASSAGE

This is an ancient practice that is used to treat myofascial pain (the most common source of TMD pain).[23,24] There are many massage techniques, modifications, and theories to account for their effectiveness, but all provide their beneficial effect by inactivating trigger points.[17] Trigger points are the hypersensitive knots that may be found in muscles, and inactivating them decreases the muscle's pain and increases its range of motion.

A massage generally begins by lightly stroking the skin and gradually increasing the stroking pressure. As the stroking pressure increases, trigger points begin to stand out and are felt as nodular obstructions to the smooth flow of the movement. With each pressure stroke, the trigger points are compressed and eventually inactivated. Some massage therapists will apply considerable pressure directly over the identified trigger points (*trigger-point compression*) to help inactivate them.

There are currently no clinical trials in which massage therapy alone was used to treat TMD symptoms.[9] The most applicable study available is one in which patients with chronic tension headache derived significant pain relief and greater neck range of motion from 10 aggressive massage sessions.[25]

The symptom improvement obtained from a massage is only temporary, just as one would not expect permanent benefits from taking a medication or performing an exercise.[26] Since the benefits are temporary, patients who only passively receive a massage must continually return for repeated massages to maintain the benefits.[1] On the other

hand, patients who are instructed to perform their own muscle massage may derive benefits similar to those achieved by a therapist, but without the expense and loss of time.

TMD patients whose pain is primarily of muscle origin are more likely to benefit from massage therapy, and a practitioner may desire to teach and encourage patients to massage the painful areas of their masseter, temporalis, and/or neck muscles multiple times throughout the day.[1,27] Massage of the symptomatic muscles is not part of the "TMD Self-management Therapies" handout (Appendix 3), but patients can easily be instructed in self-massage when provided the self-management handouts.

▼ TECHNICAL TIP
Massaging Muscles

TMD patients whose pain is primarily of muscle origin are more likely to benefit from massage therapy, and a practitioner may desire to teach and encourage patients to massage the painful areas of their masseter, temporalis, and/or neck muscles multiple times throughout the day.

Patients instructed to use self-massage achieve additional benefit if it is combined with trigger-point compression. It has also been proposed that the massage is more effective when it is performed with the muscle in a comfortably stretched position.[17] Some patients find additional benefit by massaging their muscles with one of the over-the-counter topical muscle creams, e.g., Icy Hot (which should not be used in combination with capsaicin). Typically I discuss massage only when a patient expresses an interest, because the other self-management therapies provided in the handout are already overwhelming for most patients.

TRIGGER-POINT COMPRESSION

One of the elements of muscle massage that inactivates trigger points, this therapy has also been termed myotherapy,[28] ischemic compression,[29] and trigger-point pressure release.[17] Moderately active trigger points can usually be inactivated through one compressive treatment, whereas chronic trigger points may take several treatments.[28] Muscles that can be compressed against bone or held between the fingers (as the anterior portion of the masseter muscle) may be the best candidates for this therapy.

The technique is generally performed with the muscle in a comfortably stretched position; a thumb or knuckle applies pressure on the trigger point for approximately 1 minute. Over the minute, as the discomfort decreases, the applied pressure is increased to tolerance. Heat and active muscle stretching should follow the trigger-point compression.[29]

Many TMD patients have additional trigger points in the neck and shoulders. A common technique to compress the cervical trigger points is to take two tennis balls and tie them together (using duct tape or placing them in a sock with a knot tied at the end to keep them together). The patient lies on the floor and positions the tennis balls so the neck is balanced between the two balls and the cervical trigger points are compressed. Trigger points in the shoulder can be similarly compressed by the patient lying on a single tennis ball.

▼ **TECHNICAL TIP**

Compressing Cervical Trigger Points

A common technique to compress the cervical trigger points is for the patient to take two tennis balls, tie them together (i.e., using duct tape), lie on the floor, position the tennis balls so the neck is balanced between the two balls, and apply pressure onto the cervical trigger points.

As with muscle massage, trigger-point compression is only a temporary therapy that needs to be continually repeated. To keep the inactivated trigger points from reactivating, the contributing factors perpetuating the disorder have to be identified and adequately controlled.[3,30] The most common perpetuating factors for the development of trigger points are the cumulative effect of long-standing repetitive overuse of the muscle, chronic muscle tension, and emotional stress. For the masticatory system, repetitive overuse would most likely be from parafunctional habits, whereas, for the cervical region, it would most likely be from poor posture.[30]

Trigger-point compression can be incorporated with muscle massage and is not part of the "TMD Self-management Therapies" handout (Appendix 3). Patients can easily be instructed in this when provided the self-management handouts, but I typically do not discuss trigger-point compression with patients. One exception may be when a patient who is performing the posture exercises has persistent cervical trigger points, but for some reason cannot escalate care to have the cervical region treated by someone with greater expertise in cervical dysfunction. In this situation, I may recommend the patient use the tennis ball technique to compress the persistent cervical trigger points.

BREAKING DAYTIME HABITS

TMD symptoms related to nocturnal contributing factors are present when patients wake up and usually last a few minutes to an hour or so. If the TMD symptoms last longer, worsen as the day progresses, or occur later in the day, daytime habits (parafunctional, emotionally induced muscle tension, etc.) generally are contributing to them.[27,31]

✪ **FOCAL POINT**

If TMD symptoms last longer than an hour upon awaking, worsen as the day progresses, or occur later in the day, daytime habits (parafunctional, emotionally induced muscle tension, etc.) generally are contributing to them.

To help patients understand the relationship between their habits and TMD symptoms, the following analogy can be helpful. A man went to the physician because the man's right biceps and elbow were hurting and the elbow was popping and locking (I use the same muscle and joint complaints as the patient's masticatory muscle and joint complaints).

The doctor pressed on the man's right biceps and elbow, and observed their tenderness. He then pressed on the patient's right shoulder, left shoulder, and left arm (as I say these locations, I look at them), and found they were not tender. The doctor said (using an inquisitive facial expression), "This is odd; I wonder what could be causing this localized tenderness in the right arm". As I say this, I put my right hand on my knee, push down on the knee so my arm muscles flex, and make my right arm quiver. The doctor looked over at his right arm and said (using an astonished facial expression), "What are you doing with your right arm?" The man replied, "You should ignore this, because it is just a nervous habit I have when I get a little anxious or frustrated; it helps me get rid of my nervous energy." The doctor said, "No wonder you have pain in your right arm; anyone continually doing that would have your type of localized pain. You have to stop your crazy habit if you want to get rid of your pain." I take my hand off of the knee, continue to flex the muscles in the arm, and make them quiver. The patient said he could stop that habit, do this instead, and could still get rid of his nervous energy in this manner. The doctor said, "No, you have to learn to let your arm relax and hang loose" (demonstrating this with my arms at the same time). "Once you learn to keep your arm relaxed, your biceps and elbow pain will disappear."

I tell the patient (demonstrating it with the arm) that pressing against the knee is similar to putting the teeth together and squeezing, whereas holding the arm out with the muscles flexed is similar to holding tension in the jaw muscles. You have to learn to let your jaw muscles relax and allow your jaw to hang loose (at the same time, I drop my arms and just let them hang). When you do this, your lips will lightly touch and you will find your teeth are separated by an eighth to a quarter of an inch.

In Questions 26 through 28 of the "Initial Patient Questionnaire" (Appendix 1), patients identify the percent of the day they are aware of touching their teeth together and the daytime oral habits they are aware of performing. Patients should be strongly encouraged (a) to always keep the tongue lightly resting on the roof of the mouth and the teeth apart, (b) to stop any clenching or grinding of the teeth (the nighttime activity is beyond their control), (c) to stop performing any other oral habits they may have (e.g., chewing on cheeks, chewing objects, or biting nails or cuticles), and (d) to observe for any additional oral habits that may be contributing to their TMD symptoms.

These habits usually occur when patients are focused on other things, especially when they are busy, stressed, or concentrating (e.g., using the computer). Therefore, they generally need cues to alert themselves to check for whether they are performing these harmful habits. The cues may be external, such as a timer that alerts them every 5 minutes. Based on the pain intensity's fluctuations, patients can normally tell when their major contributing habits occur, which is the most beneficial time to use the cues. Clinically it has been observed that it is best to work with the patients and have them determine what they will use for their **external cues**, in addition to when and how they will use them.

◉ QUICK CONSULT

Using External Cues

Daytime habits usually occur when patients are focused on other things, especially when they are busy, stressed, or concentrating (e.g., using the computer). Therefore, they generally need cues to alert themselves to check for whether they are performing these harmful habits.

If the habits are prominent while driving, some patients choose to place a portion of a yellow Post-it note over the car's speedometer, so that, every time they check their speed, they are reminded to also check for oral habits. In one situation in which the habits were prominent during computer use, one patient decided to place a rolled piece of tape (sticky side out) over the keyboard's "Z" key. This patient felt she would hit this key about every five minutes and, when the sticky side of the tape was touched, it would alert her to check for oral habits.

Over time, external cues tend to lose their startling effect, blend into the background, and stop alerting patients to check for oral habits. As this occurs, patients may desire to change the external cues or change to internal cues. **Internal cues** are aspects within the body that patients can also use to alert themselves about their oral habits. The most common internal cues that TMD patients use are the teeth touching the opposing teeth or an occlusal appliance, their pain intensity, and muscle tension. Clinically patients appear to have the best long-term success if they have learned to use internal cues to maintain their new behaviors or postures. Some patients prefer to first work with external cues and later progress to internal cues.

Some patients find using a diary that hourly records their activity and pain intensity helps them to better identify the activities related to their major contributing habits and reinforces the need to break these habits. Some patients choose to become very cognizant about their major contributing habits, constantly monitor for them, and use them as internal cues to alert themselves to change the activity. For example, an individual who tends to hold tension in the masseter muscle uses masseter muscle tension as the internal

cue and relaxes the masseter muscle whenever tension is noticed. If patients notice themselves reverting to their old harmful behaviors or postures, they need to institute the desired behavior or posture.

⊙ QUICK CONSULT
Recommending Diary
Some patients find using a diary that hourly records their activity and pain intensity helps them to better identify the activities related to their major contributing habits and reinforces the need to break these habits.

Some patients desire to use their pain intensity as their internal cue. As patients notice an increase in pain, they alert themselves, ask what they are doing to cause this, and change it. Once they satisfactorily control their habits so the pain decreases to a low level or becomes intermittent, ask patients to change their internal cue, *from* pain intensity *to* muscle tightness or tension. In this manner, they alert themselves whenever they begin to tighten their muscles and subsequently intentionally relax them. Patients usually find this enables them to keep their muscle tension from progressing and thereby prevents the pain from developing. Clinically it has been observed that patients who can master using muscle tightness or tension as their internal cue seem to have the greatest long-term success in eliminating their daytime TMD symptoms and maintaining this benefit.

Some patients find breaking these habits and using the "TMD Self-management Therapies" handout (Appendix 3) decrease their TMD symptoms satisfactorily. This is primarily observed among patients who are motivated to get better on their own and predominately have diurnal (daytime) pain.

Some other patients find wearing an occlusal appliance during the day helps them to continually be more attuned to parafunctional habits and what they are doing with their oral cavity, thereby enabling them to catch and alter their daytime habits.[32-34] If a daytime appliance is desired, some practitioners use the 2-mm hard thermoplastic appliance discussed in "Hard Thermoplastic Stabilization Appliance" in Chapter 12. If a patient also awakes with TMD symptoms, some practitioners will provide a maxillary stabilization appliance to wear at night.

For various reasons, some practitioners provide a maxillary or mandibular stabilization appliance for their patients to wear temporarily during the day. A patient who also awakes with TMD symptoms is instructed to wear the appliance at night, too. If patients use an appliance during the day, I refer to it as a habit-breaking appliance and instruct them that its purpose is to help alert them whenever their opposing teeth touch the appliance. I try to have patients break their daytime habits within several months and then request they limit the use of the appliance to nighttime and only a few hours during the day, if at all. Some patients find they still prefer to continue wearing their appliance for certain activities, e.g., driving a car.

◉ QUICK CONSULT
Using a Habit-breaking Appliance

If patients use an appliance during the day, I refer to it as a habit-breaking appliance and instruct them that its purpose is to help alert them whenever their opposing teeth touch the appliance.

Some patients cannot adequately control their daytime habits or muscle tension to reduce their daytime symptoms satisfactorily. Most of these patients are referred to a psychologist for additional help with changing these, especially if other psychosocial needs are observed. These therapies and the referral process are discussed in Chapter 16, "Cognitive-Behavioral Intervention."

REFERENCES

1. Wright EF, Schiffman EL. Treatment alternatives for patients with masticatory myofascial pain. J Am Dent Assoc 1995;126(7):1030–39.
2. Nelson SJ, Ash MM Jr. An evaluation of a moist heating pad for the treatment of TMJ/muscle pain dysfunction. Cranio 1988;6(4):355–9.
3. Simons DG, Travell JG, Simons LS. Travell & Simons' Myofascial Pain and Dysfunction: The Trigger Point Manual, volume 1, 2nd edition. Baltimore: Williams & Wilkins, 1999:140–1, 145, 149.
4. Nelson SJ, Santos J, Barghi N, Narendran S. Using moist heat to treat acute temporomandibular muscle pain dysfunction. Compendium 1991;12(11):808–16.
5. Poindexter RH, Wright EF, Murchison DF. Comparison of moist and dry heat penetration through orofacial tissues. Cranio 2002;20(1): 28–33.
6. Miller NH, Hill M, Kottke T, Ockene IS. The multilevel compliance challenge: recommendations for a call to action. Circulation 1997;95(4)1085–90.
7. What caffeine can do for you—and to you. Consumer Rep Health 1997;9(9):97–101.
8. American Society of Temporomandibular Joint Surgeons. Guidelines for diagnosis and management of disorders involving the temporomandibular joint and related musculoskeletal structures [White paper]. Cranio 2003;21(1):68–76.
9. Myers CD, White BA, Heft MW. A review of complementary and alternative medicine use for treating chronic facial pain. J Am Dent Assoc 2002;133(9):1189–96.
10. Winocur E, Gavish A, Emodi-Perlman A, Halachmi M, Eli I. Hypnorelaxation as treatment for myofascial pain disorder: a comparative study. Oral Surg Oral Med Oral Pathol Oral Radiol Endod 2002;93(4):429–34.
11. Dworkin SF, Huggins KH, Wilson L, Mancl L, Turner J, Massoth D, LeResche L, Truelove E. A randomized clinical trial using research diagnostic criteria for temporomandibular disorders-axis II to target clinic cases for a tailored self-care TMD treatment program. J Orofac Pain 2002;16(1): 48–63.
12. Wright EF, Domenech MA, Fischer JR Jr. Usefulness of posture training for TMD patients. J Am Dent Assoc 2000;131(2):202–10.

13. Maloney GE, Mehta N, Forgione AG, Zawawi KH, Al-Badawi EA, Driscoll SE. Effect of a passive jaw motion device on pain and range of motion in TMD patients not responding to flat plane intraoral appliances. Cranio 2002;20(1): 55–66.

14. Magnusson T, Syren M. Therapeutic jaw exercises and interocclusal therapy: a comparison between two common treatments of temporomandibular disorders. J Swed Dent 1999;22:23–37.

15. Dall Arancio D, Fricton J. Randomized controlled study of exercises for masticatory myofascial pain [abstract 76]. J Orofac Pain 1993;7(1): 117.

16. Lentell G, Hetherington T, Eagan J, Morgan M. The use of thermal agents to influence the effectiveness of a low-load prolong stretch. J Orthop Sports Phys Ther 1992;16(5):200–7.

17. Mense S, Simons DG, Russell IJ. Muscle Pain: Understanding Its Nature, Diagnosis, and Treatment. Philadelphia: Lippincott Williams & Wilkins, 2001:153.

18. Fricton JR, Kroening R, Haley D, Siegert R. Myofascial pain syndrome of the head and neck: a review of clinical characteristics of 164 patients. Oral Surg Oral Med Oral Pathol 1985;60:615–23.

19. Mannheimer JS, Rosenthal RM. Acute and chronic postural abnormalities as related to craniofacial pain and temporomandibular disorders. Dental Clin North Am 1991;35(1):185–209.

20. Griegel-Morris P, Larson K, Nueller-Klaus K, Oatis CA. Incidence of common postural abnormalities in the cervical, shoulder and thoracic regions and their association with pain in two age groups of healthy subjects. Phys Ther 1992;72: 425–31.

21. Decker KL, Bromaghim CA. Utilizing physical therapy in the treatment of temporomandibular disorders. In: Clark JW, Curtis JW (eds). Clark's Clinical Dentistry, volume 2, chapter 41. Philadelphia: JB Lippincott, 1994:1–14.

22. Liddle EJ. A comparison of round shoulder posture with thoraco-cervical-shoulder pain and an asymptomatic control group [MS thesis]. Oklahoma City: University of Oklahoma Health Sciences Center, 1994:1–6.

23. Sundqvist B, Magnusson T. Individual prediction of treatment outcome in patients with temporomandibular disorders. Swed Dent J 2001;25(1): 1–11.

24. Yap AUJ, Dworkin SF, Chua EK, List T, Tan KBC, Tan HH. Prevalence of temporomandibular disorder subtypes, psychologic distress, and psychosocial dysfunction in Asian patients. J Orofac Pain 2003;17(1):21–8.

25. Puustjarvi K, Airaksinen O, Pontinen PJ. The effects of massage in patients with chronic tension headache. Acupunct Electrother Res 1990;15(2): 159–62.

26. Field TM. Massage therapy effects. Am Psychol 1998;53(12):1270–81.

27. Okeson JP. Management of Temporomandibular Disorders and Occlusion, 5th edition. St Louis: CV Mosby, 2003:371, 384, 393.

28. Prudden, B. Myotherapy: Bonnie Prudden's Complete Guide to Pain Free Living. New York: Dial, 1984:35–40.

29. Travell JG, Simons DG. Myofascial Pain and Dysfunction: The Trigger Point Manual—The Upper Extremities, volume 1. Baltimore: Williams & Wilkins; 1983:86–7.

30. Hong CZ. Considerations and recommendations regarding myofascial trigger point injection. J Musculoske Pain 1994;2(1):29–59.

31. Wright EF. How daily TMD symptom patterns may affect treatment approach. Am Acad Orofac Pain Newsl 2000;5(3)15–6.

32. Taddey JJ. Problems and solutions. Cranio 1995;13(1):68.

33. Kreiner M, Betancor E, Clark GT. Occlusal stabilization appliances: evidence of their efficacy. J Am Dent Assoc 2001;132(6):770–7.

34. Pertes RA. Occlusal appliance therapy. In: Pertes RA, Gross SG (eds). Clinical Management of Temporomandibular Disorders and Orofacial Pain. Chicago: Quintessence, 1995:197–210.

Chapter 15

Physical Medicine

In the field of TMD, physical medicine procedures are referred to as *adjunctive TMD therapies* and generally provide additional improvement in TMD symptoms. If patients have not changed their perpetuating contributing factors, many of the improvements obtained through physical medicine procedures are only temporary, unless patients are taught to perform these procedures and continually use them on their own.

◉ QUICK CONSULT

Using Physical Medicine Procedures

In the field of TMD, physical medicine procedures are referred to as *adjunctive TMD therapies* and generally provide additional improvement in TMD symptoms.

◑ FOCAL POINT

If patients have not changed their perpetuating contributing factors, many of the improvements obtained through physical medicine procedures are only temporary, unless patients are taught to perform these procedures and continually use them on their own.

Myofascial pain, which is the most common source of TMD pain,[1,2] is characterized by localized tender nodules, know as *trigger points*, within the muscles. *TMJ inflammation* is another common source of TMD

pain, which is characterized by TMJ tenderness. *Cervical dysfunction* (pain and/or restricted movement) is a third prevalent disorder among TMD patients, causing them to not obtain the usual TMD symptom improvement.[3-5] Most physical medicine procedures used to improve TMD symptoms are directed at one or more of these three disorders.

Many of the physical medicine therapies used to inactivate trigger points provide only temporary improvement. To keep the trigger points inactivated, the therapy typically needs to be continually repeated or the contributing factors perpetuating the trigger-point activation must be adequately controlled.[6,7] Trigger-point activation is generally a cumulative effect from various perpetuating factors, with the most common being repetitive overuse of the muscle, chronic muscle tension, and emotional stress.[7] Parafunctional habits are the most frequent cause of repetitive overuse of the masticatory system, whereas poor posture is the most frequent cause of repetitive overuse of the cervical region.[7]

A university chronic facial pain center found that 15 percent of their new patients had received treatment for their pain by chiropractors, 4 percent by acupuncturists, 2 percent by massage therapists, and 0.5 percent by homeopaths. For patients whose pain was due to TMD, massage (54 percent) and chiropractics (50 percent) were most frequently rated as very helpful.[8] A substantial number of physicians believe massage therapy, chiropractics, acupuncture, and magnetic therapy are legitimate physical medical therapies to treat pain, and these are discussed in this chapter.[9]

In addition to physical medicine therapies, cognitive-behavioral intervention provides other commonly used adjunctive TMD therapies that have also been shown to reduce TMD symptoms (see Chapter 16, "Cognitive-Behavioral Intervention"). Some of the adjunctive TMD therapies are directed primarily at peripheral structures, whereas others provide primarily a central effect. Those primarily acting on the peripheral tissues are heat or cold applications, masticatory muscle exercises, physical therapy modalities, massage, trigger-point compression, trigger-point injections, chiropractics, and magnetic therapy, whereas treatments primarily having a central effect include acupuncture, relaxation therapy, biofeedback, and stress management.

Adjunctive TMD therapies are discussed separately, but are generally used in combination with other therapies.[10-12] Not all of the physical medicine procedures discussed are recommended for TMD patients, but are presented in order that practitioners may make informed treatment decisions.

In the literature, comparisons are made between adjunctive TMD therapies and occlusal appliances. When these are discussed in Chapters 15 and 16, the appliances are acrylic stabilization appliances unless specified differently.

MUSCLE MASSAGE

Massage therapists can treat myofascial pain by compressing and inactivating trigger points during the massage. Muscle massage, which generally decreases the pain and increases the mobility of the region, is discussed in Chapter 14, "Self-management Therapies."

Most massage therapists want to treat myofascial pain by repeating the massage weekly, which is time consuming and costly for patients. Muscle massage can decrease myofascial pain and increase a muscle's mobility. If patients are taught to use self-massage and topical liniments (e.g., Icy Hot), they may have an effective adjunctive treatment to use whenever they desire it. A survey of patients with TMD found that 24 percent reported using muscle massage for their TMD symptoms and rated it as one of the most beneficial of the alternative treatments surveyed.[13]

⊙ **QUICK CONSULT**

Recommending Self-massage and Topical Liniments

If patients are taught to use self-massage and topical liniments, they may have an effective adjunctive treatment to use whenever they desire it.

TRIGGER-POINT COMPRESSION

This is one component of massage therapy that inactivates trigger points, thereby decreasing the pain and increasing the mobility of the region. Some muscle therapists are specifically trained to use this technique in treating myofascial pain.[14] Trigger-point compression is discussed in Chapter 14, "Self-management Therapies," and patients instructed in this technique may have an effective tool for maintaining trigger-point inactivation.

TRIGGER-POINT INJECTION

This is another technique used to inactivate trigger points. Clinically it is often observed that patients relate the injection allowed them to relax and stretch their muscle, thereby decreasing the symptoms from the muscle.

Typically 1 percent procaine or 2 percent lidocaine without vasoconstrictor is injected into the active trigger point. This generally provides immediate relief, and it is recommended practitioners stretch the injected muscle and apply superficial heat after the injection.[7,15] The relief normally lasts days (much longer than the local anesthetic effect), and the pain never quite returns to the original level. Weekly sequential injections are generally provided, which enables the practitioner to obtain a stair-step reduction in the pain.[7,16,17]

Other agents that have been used in trigger-point injections are nonsteroid anti-inflammatory drugs, corticosteroid, and botulinum toxin type A. The time between injections varies with the agent used; e.g., botulinum injections generally provide 3 to 6 months of symptom relief.[15,18,19]

As with other adjunctive therapies, if the perpetuating factors have not been adequately reduced, the trigger points will tend to reactivate.[7] Generally trigger-point injections are provided only after traditional conservative management in addition to exercises and other physical therapy modalities have failed to have a lasting effect.[20]

◉ **QUICK CONSULT**

Recommending Trigger-point Injections

Generally trigger-point injections are provided only after traditional conservative management in addition to exercises and other physical therapy modalities have failed to have a lasting effect.

Trigger-point injections into the masticatory and neck muscles can be provided by dentists, and a recommended step-by-step detailed technique is presented by Hong.[7,21] Practitioners desiring to refer a patient for this therapy will find that some physicians provide these injections in their office, and most pain clinics have practitioners experienced in providing them.

PHYSICAL THERAPY

This encompasses a wide variety of evaluation techniques and treatments commonly used for musculoskeletal disorders. Physical therapy generally entails conservative noninvasive therapies that are typically used in combination with other treatments for TMD.[22,23] It is appropriate and common for dentists to refer TMD patients to physical therapists to reduce TMD pain or improve TMJ function, range of motion, and daytime or sleeping postures, or to evaluate and treat neck symptoms.[24,25]

The goal in physical therapy is to improve TMD symptoms and teach patients to maintain this improvement. Therefore, patients do not need to continually return for treatment, minimizing the cost and time spent in therapy.

◐ **FOCAL POINT**

The goal in physical therapy is to improve TMD symptoms and teach patients to maintain this improvement. Therefore, patients do not need to continually return for treatment, minimizing the cost and time spent in therapy.

Physical therapists often provide TMD patients with education and a combination of therapies. Patients most frequently receive exercises rather than passively receiving treatments that do not require them to participate actively in their own improvement.[26] Most of the passive treatments are referred to as *physical therapy modalities*, which may include superficial heat, superficial cold, combination of heat and cold, ultrasound (deep heat), phonophoresis (deep heat with an anti-inflammatory or anesthetic medication driven by the ultrasound waves), electrical stimulation, microcurrent electrical nerve stimulation (MENS), transcutaneous electrical nerve stimulator (TENS), and iontophoresis (a charged anti-inflammatory or anesthetic medication driven by an electrical gradient).

The literature suggests that *exercises* have the greatest potential for therapeutic benefit and enable patients to maintain this improvement. Therefore, physical therapists now tend to use more active therapies than in the past.[26,27]

A randomized clinical trial found that TMD patients given the posture improvement exercises (Appendix 6) and TMD self-management instructions (Appendix 3), on average, reported a 42 percent reduction in their TMD symptoms and 38 percent reduction in neck symptoms. Patients who held their head further forward relative to their shoulders had a higher probability of deriving TMD symptom improvement from the exercises and instructions.[28] Practitioners may desire to refer TMD patients who have more significant forward head posture to physical therapy for posture exercises or directly instruct and follow the cases of patients with the posture improvement exercises (Appendix 6).

The efficacy of physical therapy increases when performed in conjunction with occlusal appliance therapy.[22,23] I often consider referring TMD patients to physical therapy for any of the following:

1. *The patient has neck pain.* TMD patients with neck pain do not respond to TMD therapy as well as those without neck pain.[3] Some TMD symptoms primarily come from the neck, and some TMD patients who have their cervical trigger points inactivated report a substantial decrease in their TMD pain.[7,29]

2. *The patient has cervicogenic headaches.* Cervicogenic headaches are headaches that originate in the neck,[30] and clinically it appears TMD patients tend to hold more tension in their masticatory muscles when they have a headache. Therefore, TMD patients with cervicogenic headaches who have their neck treated should have fewer headaches and may also obtain substantial TMD symptom improvement.

3. *The patient has moderate to severe forward head posture.* These patients may obtain significant TMD symptom improvement from posture exercises in combination with TMD self-management instructions[28] and be most likely to derive substantial TMD symptom improvement from these.

4. *The patient's TMD symptoms increase with abnormal postural activities.* Instructing these patients in body mechanics (teaching patients how to perform tasks without straining the body) should help them maintain good posture, thereby reducing their TMD symptoms.[31,32]

5. *The patient desires help in changing poor sleep posture.* Stomach sleeping perpetuates TMD and neck symptoms. Physical therapists are trained to help change the sleep position of patients who cannot stop sleeping on their stomach.

6. *The patient did not obtain adequate TMD symptom relief from other therapies.* Physical therapists are trained to treat musculoskeletal disorders throughout the body and can apply their skills to the masticatory system.

7. *The patient is to have TMJ surgery.* Patients who receive physical therapy after TMJ surgery may have better results.[33,34] It is appropriate for these patients to be referred for physical therapy prior to surgery in order that they may learn about and possibly start the postsurgical exercises, and schedule the recommended postsurgical appointments.

Two examples of physical therapy referrals are provided in Appendix 9, "Examples of Physical Therapy Consultations." To refer a TMD patient to a physical therapist, the practitioner can write the following on the prescription pad or office stationery:

1. The patient's chief complaint.
2. The patient's TMD diagnosis, e.g., myofascial pain and TMJ inflammation.

3. What the practitioner prescribes the physical therapist to perform. I generally write "Please evaluate and treat;" this allows the physical therapist to perform whatever treatment that is believed necessary. Many third-party payers also require the requested frequency and duration of treatment be documented; two to three times a week for a month is a reasonable request.

4. Any precautions the physical therapist should be aware of (e.g., previous surgery, tumor, screws, or wires in the region) and medical disorders that could complicate therapy (e.g., angioedema).

As with dentistry, TMD is not a primary field of physical therapy education. Physical therapists' TMD knowledge greatly varies with the university attended, and much of it is generally obtained from continuing education courses. Very few physical therapists have specialized training or extensive experience treating TMD patients, and great variations are observed in their abilities to treat TMD patients.

For most TMD patients, satisfactory results are obtained in treating a masticatory disorder when the physical therapist adequately resolves the cervical symptoms. For this reason, it is generally observed that the greatest success is with physical therapists who have additional training in treating the spinal column or cervical region.

⊙ **QUICK CONSULT**
Selecting a Physical Therapist

For most TMD patients, satisfactory results are obtained in treating a masticatory disorder when the physical therapist adequately resolves the cervical symptoms. For this reason, it is generally observed that the greatest success is with physical therapists who have additional training in treating the spinal column or cervical region.

If a practitioner is not aware of an appropriate physical therapist to whom to refer a patient, many physical therapists with skills or interest in such special areas as TMD, the neck, or the spinal column will list them in their telephone book's yellow pages ad. Practitioners can also talk with other dentists in the area who refer their TMD patients to physical therapists, to determine who they have found can obtain satisfactory results.

Physical therapy is a benefit of most medical insurance policies. Some third-party payers require their patients use in-house or contracted physical therapists, and some require the consults to go through a physician. Because of the complexities with the medical insurance or if the dentist is not knowledgeable about the physical therapists in the area, practitioners may desire to write the aforementioned items on their prescription pad and request that patients see their primary care providers for the referral. Some patients may desire to speak with their third-party payer concerning referral procedures and co-payment prior to making the physical therapy appointment.

ACUPUNCTURE

Many articles and studies tout acupuncture's ability to treat numerous ailments, and Americans visit acupuncturists up to 12 million times every year.[35] The key to acupuncture's pain relief is suspected to be the release of various endorphins [serotonin, norepinephrine, and possibly γ-aminobutyric acid (GABA)] within the central nervous system, and this effect is substantially reversed by naloxone.[35-38]

Acupuncturists generally need six to eight treatment sessions for TMD symptoms to respond adequately, and patients need to return periodically for additional sessions to maintain these benefits.[20,39] My clinical observations of TMD patients whose treatment is limited to acupuncture are that most need an acupuncture treatment every 2 or 3 weeks to maintain their symptom relief.

Two randomized clinical trials that com-

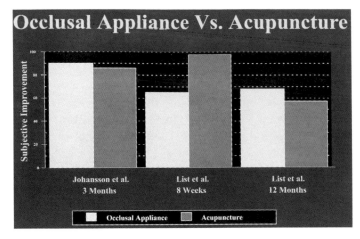

Figure 15-1. Initially, acupuncture was more effective than appliance therapy, but over time acupuncture lost its effectiveness and appliance therapy was superior.

pared the efficacy of acupuncture and orthopedic appliance therapy for TMD patients are summarized in Figure 15-1.[40-42] In one study, patients were allowed to cross over and receive the treatment provided to the other group at the 6-month follow-up. Among the patients who received the orthopedic appliance and chose to receive acupuncture, only 17 percent had any further subjective improvement from acupuncture.[40]

These studies suggest that, after six to eight acupuncture treatment sessions, patients initially obtain good symptom relief, but this decreases over time, and patients who do not derive satisfactory improvement from an orthopedic appliance tend not to receive additional improvement from acupuncture. Acupuncture can provide significant TMD symptom improvement, but there are simpler and less invasive therapies that provide sustained and comparable symptom relief.

✪ FOCAL POINT

Acupuncture can provide significant TMD symptom improvement, but there are simpler and less invasive therapies that provide sustained and comparable symptom relief.

CHIROPRACTICS

Chiropractic training varies considerably from school to school; therefore, chiropractors' treatment approaches and capabilities also vary greatly.[42] Some chiropractors attempt to relieve TMD-type symptoms through cervical spine manipulation, whereas other chiropractors will work directly with the masticatory system.[43-46]

There is no known clinical trial that has evaluated changes in TMD symptoms from chiropractic therapy, but TMD patients are referred to chiropractors for adjunctive TMD therapy.[47,48] These referrals are generally made when patients have coexisting neck pain, because it negatively impacts TMD, and cervical spine manipulation has been shown to reduce neck pain and cervicogenic headaches.[46,49]

Chiropractics is one of many avenues that can be used to treat cervical dysfunction (pain and/or restricted movement). After two or three chiropractic treatments, if cervical dysfunction is resolved and the improvement can be maintained, this would appear to have been an effective treatment approach. On the other hand, if adequate relief is not obtained or the improvement maintained without continued spinal manipulation, then it is recommended that the patient receive more traditional interventions rather than further chiropractic therapy. There are no studies to suggest when a chiropractic referral would be the preferred intervention for cervical pain or dysfunction.

⊙ **QUICK CONSULT**

Recommending Chiropractic Treatments

After two or three chiropractic treatments, if adequate neck pain relief is not obtained or the improvement is not maintained without continued spinal manipulation, then it is recommended that the patient receive more traditional interventions rather than further chiropractic therapy.

MAGNETIC THERAPY

Magnetic fields have been used to control pain for centuries, but scientific support has only recently become evident.[50,51] Studies demonstrate that magnetic exposure increases the peripheral blood flow, but the exact mechanism for this effect is not well understood, and there is no clear explanation for the significant and rapid pain relief observed by patients using magnets.[51]

No known clinical trial has evaluated the efficacy of magnetic therapy for TMD symptoms, but it has been shown to be beneficial for persistent neck pain, headache, and other muscle or arthritis-like pains.[52-54] No known adverse effects are related to magnetic field exposure.[51]

Support for magnetic therapy is growing, but magnets are expensive, with small ones costing about $25 and magnet-filled mattress pads selling for several hundred dollars. Therapeutic magnets vary in strength from 300 to 5000 Gauss, which is much stronger than refrigerator magnets (generally about 50 Gauss).[51,55]

A therapeutic magnet produces a magnetic field that extends only several millimeters beyond its surface; therefore, magnets are placed in direct contact with the painful area.[55] Consequently magnetic bracelets or necklaces that dangle from a patient's body should have minimal beneficial effect.

Clinically it has been observed that a number of patients have found magnetic therapy beneficial for their TMD pain, whereas a few others have found that the coldness of the magnet aggravates their pain. Esthetic considerations limit the use of magnets to primarily evening and nighttime.

REFERENCES

1. Sundqvist B, Magnusson T. Individual prediction of treatment outcome in patients with temporomandibular disorders. Swed Dent J 2001;25(1):1–11.
2. Yap AUJ, Dworkin SF, Chua EK, List T, Tan KBC, Tan HH. Prevalence of temporomandibular disorder subtypes, psychologic distress, and psychosocial dysfunction in Asian patients. J Orofac Pain 2003;17(1):21–8.
3. Raphael KG, Marbach JJ, Klausner J. Myofascial face pain: clinical characteristics of those with regional vs. widespread pain. J Am Dent Assoc 2000;131(2):161–71.
4. Clark GT, Green EM, Dornan MR, Flack VF. Craniocervical dysfunction levels in a patient sample from a temporomandibular joint clinic. J Am Dent Assoc 1987;115:251–6.
5. Clark GT, Green EM, Dornan MR, Flack VF. Craniocervical dysfunction levels in a patient sample from a temporomandibular joint clinic. J Am Dent Assoc 1987;115(2):251–6.
6. Simons DG, Travell JG, Simons LS. Travell & Simons' Myofascial Pain and Dysfunction: The Trigger Point Manual, volume 1, 2nd edition. Baltimore: Williams & Wilkins, 1999:140–1.
7. Hong CZ. Considerations and recommendations regarding myofascial trigger point injection. J Musculoske Pain 1994;2(1):29–59.
8. Myers CD, White BA, Heft MW. A review of complementary and alternative medicine use for treating chronic facial pain. J Am Dent Assoc 2002;133(9):1189–96.
9. Berman BM, Singh BK, Lao L, Singh BB, Ferentz KS, Hartnoll SM. Physicians' attitudes toward

complementary or alternative medicine: a regional survey. J Am Board Fam Pract 1995;8(5):361–6.

10. Gam AN, Warming S, Larsen LH, Jensen B, Hoydalsmo O, Allon I, Andersen B, Gotzsche NE, Petersen M, Mathiesen B. Treatment of myofascial trigger-points with ultrasound combined with massage and exercise: a randomized controlled trial. Pain 1998;77(1):73–9.

11. Hawk C, Byrd L, Jansen RD, Long CR. Use of complementary healthcare practices among chiropractors in the United States: a survey. Altern Ther Health Med 1999;5(1):56–62.

12. Crockett DJ, Foreman ME, Alden L, Blasberg B. A comparison of treatment modes in the management of myofascial pain dysfunction syndrome. Biofeedback Self Regul 1986;11(4):279–91.

13. DeBar LL, Vuckovic N, Schneider J, Ritenbaugh C. Use of complementary and alternative medicine for temporomandibular disorders. J Orofac Pain 2003;17(3):224–36.

14. Prudden B. Myotherapy: Bonnie Prudden's Complete Guide to Pain Free Living. New York: Dial, 1984:35–40.

15. Mense S, Simons DG, Russell IJ. Muscle Pain: Understanding Its Nature, Diagnosis, and Treatment. Philadelphia: Lippincott Williams & Wilkins, 2001:267–71.

16. Hong C. Considerations and recommendations regarding myofascial trigger point injection. J Musculoske Pain 1994;2(1):29–59.

17. Hameroff SR, Crago BR, Blitt CD, Womble J, Kanel J. Comparison of bupivacaine, etidocaine, and saline for trigger-point therapy. Anesth Analg 1981;60:752–5.

18. Tan EK. Treating severe bruxism with botulinum toxin. J Am Dent Assoc 2000;131(2):211–6.

19. Freund B, Schwartz M. The use of botulinum toxin for the treatment of temporomandibular disorder. Oral Health 1998;88(2):32–7.

20. Wright EF, Schiffman EL. Treatment alternatives for patients with masticatory myofascial pain. J Am Dent Assoc 1995;126(7):1030–9.

21. Rosenbaum RS, Gross SG, Pertes RA, Ashman LM, Kreisberg MK. The scope of TMD/orofacial pain (head and neck pain management in contemporary dental practice). J Orofac Pain 1997;11(1):78–83.

22. Colt J, Winber S. Relative efficacy of orthotic therapy, physical therapy and a combination of the two in the treatment of non-derangement temporomandibular disorders [abstract P27]. J Orofac Pain 1994;8(1):109.

23. Grieder A, Vinton PW, Cinotti WR, Kangur TT. An evaluation of ultrasonic therapy for temporomandibular joint dysfunction. Oral Surg Oral Med Oral Pathol 1971;31(1):25–30.

24. Riley III JL, Robinson ME, Wise EA, Campbell LC, Kashikar-Zuck S, Gremillion HA. Predicting treatment compliance following facial pain evaluation. Cranio 1999;17(1):9–15.

25. Dental Practice Parameters Committee. American Dental Association's dental practice parameters: temporomandibular (craniomandibular) disorders. J Am Dent Assoc Suppl 1997;128(Feb):29–32–S.

26. Di Fabio RP. Physical therapy for patients with TMD: a descriptive study of treatment, disability and health status. J Orofac Pain 1998;12(2):124–35.

27. Magnusson T, Syren M. Therapeutic jaw exercises and interocclusal therapy: a comparison between two common treatments of temporomandibular disorders. J Swed Dent 1999;22:23–37.

28. Wright EF, Domenech MA, Fischer JR Jr. Usefulness of posture training for TMD patients. J Am Dent Assoc 2000;131(2):202–10.

29. Carlson CR, Okeson JP, Falace DA, Nitz AJ, Lindroth JE. Reduction of pain and EMG activity in the masseter region by trapezius trigger point injection. Pain 1993;55(3):397–400.

30. Jaeger B. Are "cervicogenic" headaches due to myofascial pain and cervical spine dysfunction? Cephalalgia 1989;9(3):157–64.

31. Palazzi C, Miralles R, Soto MA, Santander H, Zuniga C, Moya H. Body position effects on EMG activity of sternocleidomastoid and masseter muscles in patients with myogenic cranio-cervical-mandibular dysfunction. Cranio 1996;14(3):200–9.

32. Mannheimer JS, Rosenthal RM. Acute and chronic postural abnormalities as related to craniofacial pain and temporomandibular disorders. Dental Clin North Am 1991;35(1)185–209.

33. Kuwahara T, Bessette RW, Maruyama T. The influence of postoperative treatment on the results of TMJ meniscectomy. Part II: Comparison of chewing movement. Cranio 1996;14(2):121–31.

34. Austin BD, Shupe SM. The role of physical therapy in recovery after temporomandibular joint surgery. J Oral Maxillofac Surg 1993;51:495–8.

35. Loitman JE. Pain management: beyond pharmacology to acupuncture and hypnosis. J Am Med Assoc 2000;283(1):118–9.

36. Pert A, Dionne R, Ng L, Bragin E, Moody TW, Pert CB. Alterations in rat central nervous system endorphins following transauricular electroacupuncture. Brain Res 1981;224(1):83–93.

37. Cheng RS, Pomeranz B. A combined treatment with D-amino acids and electroacupuncture produces a greater analgesia than either treatment alone; naloxone reverses these effects. Pain 1980;8(2):231–6.

38. Okeson JP. Bell's Orofacial Pains, 5th edition. Carol Stream, IL: Quintessence, 1995:83.

39. List T, Helkimo M, Andersson S, Carlsson GE. Acupuncture and occlusal splint therapy in the treatment of craniomandibular disorders. Part I: A comparative study. Swed Dent J 1992;16:125–41.

40. List T, Helkimo M. Acupuncture and occlusal splint therapy in the treatment of craniomandibular disorders. II: A 1-year follow-up study. Acta Odontol Scand 1992;50(6):375–85.

41. Johansson A, Wenneberg B, Wagersten C, Haraldson T. Acupuncture in treatment of facial muscular pain. Acta Odontol Scand 1991;49(3):153–8.

42. Kaptchuk TJ, Eisenberg DM. Chiropractic: origins, controversies, and contributions. Arch Intern Med 1998;158:2215–22.

43. Curl DD. Acute closed lock of the temporomandibular joint: manipulation paradigm and protocol. Chiropractic Technique 1991;3(1): 13–18.

44. Curl DD. Chiropractic management of capsulitis and synovitis of the temporomandibular joint. J Orofac Pain 1993;7(3):283–94.

45. Boline PD, Kassak K, Bronfort G, Nelson C, Anderson AV. Spinal manipulation vs amitriptyline for the treatment of chronic tension-type headaches: a randomized clinical trial. J Manipulative Physiol Ther 1995;18(3):148–54.

46. Nilsson N, Christensen HW, Hartvigsen J. The effect of spinal manipulation in the treatment of cervicogenic headache. J Manipulative Physiol Ther 1997;20:326–30.

47. Kaplan AS, Goldman JR. General concepts of treatment. In: Kaplan AS, Assael LA (eds). Temporomandibular Disorders: Diagnosis and Treatment. Philadelphia: WB Saunders, 1991:388–94.

48. Raphael KG, Klausner JJ, Nayak S, Marbach JJ. Complementary and alternative therapy use by patients with myofascial temporomandibular disorders. J Orofac Pain 2003;17(1):36–41.

49. Raphael KG, Marbach JJ. Widespread pain and the effectiveness of oral splints in myofascial face pain. J Am Dent Assoc 2001;132(3):305–16.

50. Takeshige C, Sato M. Comparisons of pain relief mechanisms between needling to the muscle, static magnetic field, external qigong and needling to the acupuncture point. Acupunct Electro Ther Res 1996;21(2):119–31.

51. Vallbona C, Richards T. Evolution of magnetic therapy from alternative to traditional medicine. Phys Med Rehabil Clin North Am 1999;10(3):729–54.

52. Foley-Nolan D, Barry C, Coughlan RJ, O'Connor P, Roden D. Pulsed high frequency (27 MHz) electromagnetic therapy for persistent neck pain: a double blind, placebo-controlled study of 20 patients. Orthopedics 1990;13(4):445–51.

53. Sherman RA, Robson L, Marden LA. Initial exploration of pulsing electromagnetic fields for treatment of migraine. Headache 1998;38(3): 208–13.

54. Vallbona C, Hazlewood CF, Jurida G. Response of pain to static magnetic fields in postpolio patients: a double-blind pilot study. Arch Phys Med Rehabil 1997;78(11):1200–3.

55. Schindler M. Boost your pain-fighting power with magnets. Prevention 1999;51(3):112–7, 171.

Chapter 16

Cognitive-Behavioral Intervention

FAQs

Q: Are all psychologists able to help TMD patients satisfactorily control their daytime oral parafunctional and muscle tension habits?

A: Few psychologists have specialized training or extensive experience in using cognitive-behavioral intervention to treat TMD symptoms, and those not experienced in treating TMD patients would initially appreciate suggestions of specific behaviors that need to be changed.

Q: Since relaxation has been shown to be beneficial for TMD symptoms, wouldn't it be helpful if I provide my TMD patients with a relaxation audiotape program?

A: Clinically it has been observed that, when TMD patients are handed an audiotape program, few have the motivation to listen to the tape and practice the therapy consistently.

Q: How could a biofeedback machine help patients learn to relax their muscles?

A: Biofeedback enables patients to observe how different relaxation techniques can change their muscle tension and, with the feedback system, they usually can learn to relax their masticatory muscles and reduce their TMD symptoms.

It is well recognized that daytime parafunctional habits, tension, stress, anxiety, anger, depression, catastrophizing (thinking the worst of situations), pain-related beliefs, not coping well with "life's stuff," etc., negatively impact patients' TMD symptoms and their ability to improve from conservative TMD therapy.[1-4] Cognitive-behavioral interventions are adjunctive TMD therapies that attempt to help patients reduce their daytime parafunctional habits and psychosocial contributing factors.

☯ **FOCAL POINTS**

It is well recognized that daytime parafunctional habits, tension, stress, anxiety, anger, depression, catastrophizing (thinking the worst of situations), pain-related beliefs, not coping well with "life's stuff," etc., negatively impact patients' TMD symptoms and their ability to improve from conservative TMD therapy.

Cognitive-behavioral interventions are adjunctive TMD therapies that attempt to help patients reduce their daytime parafunctional habits and psychosocial contributing factors.

The "TMD Self-management Therapies" handout (Appendix 3) provides patients with some techniques they can use to reduce these contributors. Patients with minor daytime habits and minor psychosocial contributors can often satisfactorily reduce their habits when they realize how these contribute to their pain. Patients with significant persistent daytime habits and/or psychosocial contributors often need additional help from a practitioner trained in cognitive-behavioral interventions.[5]

◉ **QUICK CONSULT**

Differentiating Patients' Needs

Patients with minor daytime habits and minor psychosocial contributors can often satisfactorily reduce their habits when they realize how these contribute to their pain, whereas those with significant persistent daytime habits and/or psychosocial contributors often need additional help from a practitioner trained in cognitive-behavioral interventions.

Clinical trials demonstrate that the "average" patient who receives cognitive-behavioral therapy gains comparable TMD symptom improvement as that acquired

from occlusal appliance therapy (see Figures 16-1 and 16-2).[6-8] If used in conjunction with an occlusal appliance, patients generally obtain additional symptom improvement (Figure 16-2).[6] It has also been demonstrated that TMD patients with poor psychosocial adaptation have significantly greater symptom improvement when the dentist's TMD therapy is combined with cognitive-behavioral intervention.[9]

☯ **FOCAL POINTS**

Clinical trials demonstrate that the "average" patient who receives cognitive-behavioral therapy gains comparable TMD symptom improvement as acquired from occlusal appliance therapy (see Figures 16-1 and 16-2).

If cognitive-behavioral therapy is used in conjunction with an occlusal appliance, patients' symptoms generally improve more than from either single therapy (Figure 16-2).

During the initial TMD evaluation, patients commonly deny having daytime parafunctional habits and psychosocial contributors. Many questions in the "Initial Patient Questionnaire" (Appendix 1) are designed to help identify these contributing factors. While contemplating the answers they will mark on the questionnaire, many patients reason what treatment may be recommended if they disclose psychosocial contributors, so some modify their answers. On occasion, patients did not respond to therapy as anticipated and, on further questioning, were found to have not been honest with these "Initial Patient Questionnaire" answers, primarily because they were not open to receiving the needed cognitive-behavioral therapy.

◉ **QUICK CONSULT**

Identifying Daytime Habits and Psychosocial Contributors

During the initial TMD evaluation, patients commonly deny having daytime parafunctional

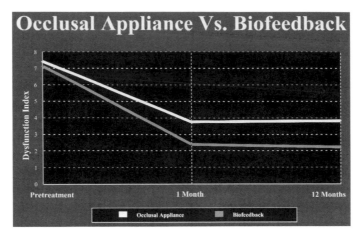

Figure 16-1. Appliance therapy and biofeedback can provide significant TMD improvement.[7]

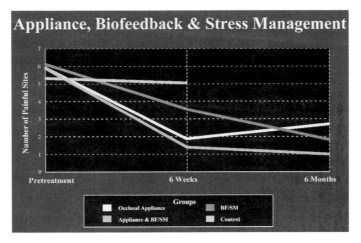

Figure 16-2. Appliance therapy (*Appliance*) and biofeedback with relaxation and stress management (**BF/SM**) can provide significant TMD improvement.[6]

habits and psychosocial contributors, but the "Initial Patient Questionnaire" (Appendix 1) is designed to help identify these contributing factors.

Cognitive-behavioral interventions primarily encompass habit reversal, relaxation, hypnosis, biofeedback, stress management, and cognitive therapy (focuses on changing patients' distorted thoughts). These therapies are generally provided by psychologists in a combined comprehensive strategy thought most effective for the patient and/or disor-

der. Their long-term efficacy for TMD symptoms has been demonstrated,[10] and they are more effective for patients with daytime symptoms.[11]

⊙ **QUICK CONSULT**

Comprehending Cognitive-Behavioral Interventions
Cognitive-behavioral interventions primarily encompass habit reversal, relaxation, hypnosis, biofeedback, stress management, and cognitive therapy (focuses on changing patients' distorted thoughts).

Relaxation is often used with most of these cognitive intervention therapies, and patients are often requested to practice relaxing at least once a day. Practitioners should keep in mind that these therapies are time consuming, and the patient must be motivated to practice them so maximum benefit is obtained and maintained over time.

◉ **QUICK CONSULT**
Understanding Patient's Role
Practitioners should keep in mind these therapies are time consuming, and the patient must be motivated to practice them so maximum benefit is obtained and maintained over time.

It has been observed that, to identify which therapies may be most beneficial for a patient, some psychologists prefer to perform psychological testing prior to the cognitive-behavioral intervention. Other psychologists may provide a standard brief cognitive-behavioral intervention and test only those patients who do not improve sufficiently. A standard brief cognitive-behavioral intervention has been shown to be beneficial for most TMD patients, but is not sufficient for some, such as those with dysfunctional chronic pain.[3,12,13]

▼ **TECHNICAL TIP**
Treating with a Standard Brief Cognitive-Behavioral Intervention
A standard brief cognitive-behavioral intervention has been shown to be beneficial for most TMD patients, but is not sufficient for some, such as those with dysfunctional chronic pain.

For many years, my patients who needed cognitive-behavioral intervention were primarily referred to a minimal intervention program, which entailed three sessions that were 2 hours long and 1 week apart. This intervention was sufficient for most of my TMD patients and, if satisfactory improvement was not obtained, psychological testing

was performed to identify which additional therapies may be most beneficial.[12]

Minimal intervention programs for patients with TMD will often have them use diaries and implement interventions (e.g., habit reversal, progressive muscle relaxation, and cognitive coping skills) that are thought to be most useful for the majority of them.[14] If a sufficient number of patients are referred for this therapy, the psychologist may be able to provide it in a classroom setting. This would minimize the cost of the therapy, and most of my patients related they preferred the group setting rather than individual instruction.[12]

Clinically it is observed that patients generally need to implement three phases to obtain substantial daytime symptom improvement. The degree of TMD symptom improvement and required assistance will vary with the severity of the patient's habits and psychosocial factors. These phases are as follows:

1. Patients must learn how to make their masticatory muscles relax (or drain the tension from these muscles) and learn what relaxed masticatory muscles feel like. For some patients, relaxation training is insufficient, and they will need biofeedback to help them learn to relax their muscles.
2. Patients must learn to identify when they are performing parafunctional habits and/or their masticatory muscles are tense. This is usually done through internal and/or external cues (explained in "Breaking Daytime Habits" in Chapter 14).
3. When patients are performing parafunctional habits, they must learn to stop them and relax their muscles; when their masticatory muscles are tense, they must learn to drain the tension from these muscles. These activities generally occur when patients are frustrated, busy, etc. Some patients do not want to release their tension or anger and may need stress

management or cognitive therapy to help them with this.

Few psychologists have specialized training or extensive experience in using cognitive-behavioral intervention to treat TMD symptoms. There are many alternatives for selecting a psychologist who can provide this therapy.

Behavioral psychology is a specialty, and psychologists with this training should be able to apply their training easily to TMD patients. Some psychologists have specialized training in pain management and should be experienced in using relaxation and biofeedback in addition to treating psychological conditions common among patients with chronic pain. Numerous psychologists use relaxation, biofeedback, and techniques for breaking other behaviors, e.g., smoking cessation and weight loss.[15,16] These psychologists should be able to apply these techniques readily in treating TMD patients. Psychologists not experienced in treating TMD patients would initially appreciate suggestions of specific behaviors that need to be changed.

The Biofeedback Certification Institute of America (BCIA) is an organization that requires practitioners meet specific biofeedback education and training requirements, plus pass a written examination. Their web site (www.bcia.org) enables individuals to search for certified practitioners in a selected city and state. Biofeedback is used for many disorders other than TMD, so psychologists found through this source will probably also appreciate suggestions of specific behaviors that need to be changed.

Many dentists have worked with a psychologist for problems such as dental anxiety and needle phobia. Practitioners can telephone one of the psychologists with whom they worked and ask whether someone in the community has expertise in treating TMD symptoms. Referring patients to a psychologist can be as easy as giving them the psychologist's name and asking them to make an appointment. The patient would tell the psychologist the problem during the initial visit, and the psychologist would assess the patient and generally telephone the dentist to discuss the problem and the treatment approach.

Practitioners may prefer to write a note or summary on their prescription pad or office stationery. I give the psychologist a summary of my thoughts, such as examples provided in Appendix 10.

Some medical organizations or third-party payers may require the practitioner to write a consult as in the appendix. Some require their patients to use in-house or contracted psychologists, and some require the consults to go through their physicians. Patients may need to speak with their third-party payer regarding referral procedures and copayments prior to the practitioner making the referral.

Cognitive-behavioral intervention is a benefit of most medical insurance policies. Because of the complexities of the medical insurance, or if the practitioner is not knowledgeable about the psychologists in the area, the practitioner may write a summary on a prescription pad and request the patient see his or her primary care provider for the referral.

BREAKING DAYTIME HABITS

Typically TMD symptoms that occur when patients first awake are primarily due to nighttime parafunctional habits, whereas symptoms that occur or worsen during the day or evening are primarily due to daytime parafunctional habits or patients holding an excessive amount of tension in their masticatory muscles. Theoretically patients with significant daytime pain can become aware of their muscle tightness or parafunctional habits, break them, and thus dramatically reduce or eliminate their daytime pain.

Understanding the Cause of the Daily Symptom Pattern

Typically TMD symptoms that occur when patients first awake are primarily due to night-time parafunctional habits, whereas symptoms that occur or worsen during the day or evening are primarily due to daytime parafunctional habits or patients holding an excessive amount of tension in their masticatory muscles.

These daytime parafunctional or muscle-tightening habits are often subconscious, and the patient may be totally unaware of performing them. Patients will often unconsciously cross their ankles while they are sitting in the dental chair, and correlating this with their oral habits has often been found helpful. It is explained to them that, if they had knee pain that was aggravated by crossing their ankles, they would need to change this unconscious ankle-crossing habit. Since their pain is in the jaw, they need to identify and break their oral habits.

Question 26 ("What percent of the day are your teeth touching?") of the "Initial Patient Questionnaire" will give the practitioner a sense of the patient's awareness of possible clenching activity. Many TMD patients lightly rest their teeth together and unconsciously squeeze them together when they become busy, concentrate, are irritated, drive a car, or use a computer. A pain diary will often help a patient correlate the activities that are most associated with the parafunctional or muscle-tightening activities. Often, treating these habits entails having the patient break the behaviors and reduce the intensity level of the associated activities.

If a patient appears sufficiently motivated and has minimal daytime symptoms and/or minimal psychosocial contributors, it is recommended that the patient attempt to break the daytime parafunctional habits as part of the self-management therapies. The occlusal appliance can also be temporarily used as a reminder to help patients observe and break their daytime habits (for specific recommendations, see "Appliance Management" in Chapter 12).

▼ TECHNICAL TIP

Breaking Daytime Habits

If a patient appears sufficiently motivated and has minimal daytime symptoms and/or minimal psychosocial contributors, it is recommended that the patient attempt to break the daytime parafunctional habits as part of the self-management therapies.

Habit-reversal therapy has been effectively used by psychologists for over 25 years to treat nervous repetitive motion habits such as lip biting, cheek biting, tongue biting, nail biting, and tooth clenching.[17-20] Habit reversal in conjunction with relaxation can significantly decrease daytime parafunctional habits and TMD symptoms.[13,21] As patients identify their nervous habits, they generally discover they have many,[17] so patients must be instructed to observe for and avoid all habits that put unnecessary strain on the masticatory muscles and TMJs, e.g., biting their cheeks, lips, fingernails, cuticles, and any other objects they may put in their mouth.

Habit-reversal therapy entails (a) patients becoming aware of their habits, (b) patients developing a competing response (i.e., tongue up and teeth apart), and (c) motivating patients to use the competing response when the habits are most prevalent (often identified through their pain diary).[17] Psychologists will generally ask patients to use external and internal cues to identify their habits, help them to learn to use the competing response, and teach them how to relax their tight muscles (or drain the tension held in these muscles). This enables patients to stop their parafunctional habits and keep their masticatory muscles relaxed.

RELAXATION

A similar physiological relaxation response can be produced by progressive muscle relaxation, imagery, hypnosis, yoga, prayer, or meditation.[22,23] This response counters the hyperarousal state individuals may have from overstimulation of their fight-or-flight mechanism.

▼ **TECHNICAL TIP**

Reducing Hyperarousal State

Relaxation counters the hyperarousal state individuals may have from overstimulation of their fight-or-flight mechanism.

Relaxation has been shown to reduce TMD symptoms[3,8,12] and is traditionally provided in conjunction with habit-reversal and biofeedback therapies.[7,13,21] Generally patients find relaxation not only temporarily reduces their pain, but also helps them become aware of what tense and relaxed masticatory muscles feel like and develop the capability to relax these muscles rapidly whenever they notice their muscles are tight.

Unfortunately practitioners cannot simply hand a relaxation audiotape or compact-disk program to patients and expect them to listen to it and receive the benefits. When TMD patients are handed an audiotape program, few have the motivation to listen to the tape and practice the therapy consistently.[24] Most TMD patients appear to need a trained relaxation instructor to motivate them to practice and assist them with problems they may encounter.

Occasionally patients prefer to practice this therapy on their own. They can be given the options of using a relaxation tape or compact disk purchased from a bookstore; quietly listening to soothing music; taking a warm, relaxing shower or bath; quietly sitting and taking slow deep breaths; etc. Some patients may prefer to do this while using a heating pad. They should be encouraged to use the therapy form that provides them the greatest degree of relaxation and enjoyment. The more pleasurable the experience is, the greater is the probability of long-term compliance.

Each of these techniques should help patients obtain the physiological relaxation response and teach them what relaxed muscles feel like. Hopefully patients will thus develop the ability to reestablish this relaxed state whenever they choose. The next step is for them to identify when they are tensing their masticatory muscles or performing parafunctional habits, and consciously stop these habits and induce the relaxed state they have learned.

HYPNOTHERAPY

Hypnotherapy or hypnosis, which has been used for pain management since the mid-1980s, assists patients to reach a deep level of relaxation. Some patients and/or psychologists may prefer hypnosis for treating TMD symptoms and it has been shown to be beneficial for treating those symptoms (Figure 16-3).[25,26]

Hypnotic sessions generally last between 20 and 60 minutes.[25] Throughout the hypnotic session, patients maintain control of their thoughts and can come out of the relaxed state whenever they desire.[25] Explaining this to patients generally reduces any fear of adverse reactions.

During hypnotherapy for TMD, patients are usually given hypnotic suggestions to release all physical and emotional stress and anxiety. They are generally given an audiocassette or compact disk of one of the hypnotic sessions, which they listen to repeatedly at home, enabling them to practice reaching this relaxed state and to deal with any residual or future stress or anxiety.[25,27] Often, listening to the tape just prior to sleep enables patients to sleep more peacefully and decreases nocturnal parafunctional habits.[28]

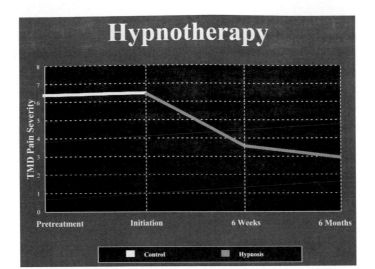

Figure 16-3. The TMD treatment effect from hypnotherapy.[26]

BIOFEEDBACK

This was developed in the 1960s to provide patients a manner for observing changes in certain physiological measures (e.g., muscle activity, blood pressure, and skin temperature).[29] Feedback of muscle activity [electromyelography (EMG)] is routinely used with TMD patients, who are taught how to lower their masticatory muscle EMG activity to relax these muscles.[30] The feedback enables patients to observe how different relaxation techniques can change their muscle tension and, with the feedback system, they usually can learn to relax their masticatory muscles and reduce their symptoms. This is similar to how someone wanting to lower their weight would find feedback from a scale beneficial.

Biofeedback is routinely supplemented with relaxation to increase the treatment effect. A study that compared TMD patients who were restricted to only one of these two therapies found the average decrease in pain was 35 percent for the biofeedback group and 56 percent for the relaxation group.[31] This suggests relaxation is actually the more beneficial component when these therapies are combined. Studies demonstrate that biofeedback with relaxation has a similar efficacy as occlusal appliance therapy, and biofeedback with relaxation provides long-term TMD symptom relief.[32,33]

⊙ **QUICK CONSULT**

Understanding Biofeedback with Relaxation Therapy Efficacy

The study suggests relaxation is actually the more beneficial component of the biofeedback with relaxation therapy.

In general, TMD patients with significant daytime parafunctional habits complain about daytime or evening symptoms, whereas patients with significant nighttime parafunctional habits complain of symptoms when they first awake. Studies suggest that biofeedback with relaxation is more effective for patients with daytime parafunctional habits, whereas an occlusal appliance worn at night is more effective for patients with nighttime parafunctional habits.[34-36] It is important for patients receiving biofeedback to be taught to transfer the learned techniques from the therapist's office into their everyday life. It is occasionally found that some biofeedback therapists do not help their patients incorporate this relaxed state into the stressful, hectic portion of the patient's day, and thus these patients often derive minimal benefit from the therapy.

Comparing Biofeedback with Relaxation and an Occlusal Appliance

Studies suggest that biofeedback with relaxation is more effective for patients with daytime parafunctional habits, whereas an occlusal appliance worn at night is more effective for patients with nighttime parafunctional habits.

At one facility where I practiced, patients with significant daytime symptoms were routinely taught habit-reversal and relaxation techniques. Patients who related they could relax their entire body except for their masticatory muscles found biofeedback often exceptionally beneficial in reducing their remaining daytime symptoms.

Generally patients with daytime muscle-tightening or parafunctional habits will have significant TMD symptom improvement from breaking these habits, biofeedback with relaxation (relaxation being the more important component), and/or an occlusal appliance temporarily worn during the day to increase their awareness of these habits.

STRESS MANAGEMENT

Stress management is a cognitive approach to deal with the stresses, irritations, or frustrations that patients encounter. Some studies suggest the average TMD patient does not cope as well with stress as patients without TMD.[37] TMD patients tend to tighten their masticatory muscles in these situations,[38] and stress management teaches coping skills to help them better manage these situations and their thoughts about them.

TMD patients tend to tighten their masticatory muscles in stressful, irritating, or frustrating situations, and stress management teaches coping skills to help them better manage these situations and their thoughts about them.

Many muscle-contracture headaches are caused by minor stresses (compared with major stresses) in an individual's life.[39] Clinically TMD similarly appears often to be related to the minor stresses, and TMD patients commonly discount the contribution of stress. Many say their life is not stressful, but acknowledge they often hold tension in their jaw, neck, and/or shoulders and are frustrated or irritated a considerable amount of the time [see Question 22 of the "Initial Patient Questionnaire" (Appendix 1)]. TMD symptoms tend to become aggravated when patients are busier, more frustrated, or irritated, and sometimes it takes a daily pain/busyness diary for them to see these associations.

It is observed that TMD patients generally agree with these tendencies when the terms "busy," "frustrated," "irritated," and "hold tension in your muscles" are used rather than the word "stress." It is then explained that they need to learn to release the tension held in their masticatory muscles and learn coping skills to minimize the amount of time they feel busy, frustrated, or irritated. With this discussion, patients are usually open to work with someone to learn relaxation and/or stress management.

Avoiding the Word "Stress"

It is observed that TMD patients tend to deny they are stressed, but agree they are busy, frustrated, irritated, and hold tension in their muscles. Therefore, I avoid using the word "stress," and use the terms "busy," "frustrated," "irritated," and "hold tension in your muscles."

TMD patients often receive stress management in combination with biofeedback and relaxation therapies, and this combination generally provides a significant reduction in TMD symptoms that is maintained over time.[6]

REFERENCES

1. Turner JA, Dworkin SF, Mancl L, Huggins KH, Truelove EL. The roles of beliefs, catastrophizing, and coping in the functioning of patients with temporomandibular disorders. Pain 2001; 92(1–2):41–51.

2. Turner JA, Whitney C, Dworkin SF, Massoth D, Wilson L. Do changes in patient beliefs and coping strategies predict temporomandibular disorder treatment outcomes? Clin J Pain 1995;11(3): 177–88.

3. Dworkin SF, Turner JA, Wilson L, Massoth D, Whitney C, Huggins KH, Burgess J, Sommers E, Truelove E. Brief group cognitive-behavioral intervention for temporomandibular disorders. Pain 1994;59(2):175–87.

4. Gremillion HA. Multidisciplinary diagnosis and management of orofacial pain. Gen Dent 2002;50(2):178–86.

5. Gremillion HA. The prevalence and etiology of temporomandibular disorders and orofacial pain. Tex Dent J 2000;117(7):30–9.

6. Turk DC, Zaki HS, Rudy TE. Effects of intraoral appliance and biofeedback/stress management alone and in combination in treating pain and depression in patients with temporomandibular disorders. J Prosthet Dent 1993;70(2):158–64.

7. Dahlstrom L. Conservative treatment of mandibular dysfunction: clinical, experimental and electromyographic studies of biofeedback and occlusal appliances. Swed Dent J Suppl 1984;24:1–45.

8. Carlson CR, Bertrand PM, Ehrlich AD, Maxwell AW, Burton RG. Physical self-regulation training for the management of temporomandibular disorders. J Orofac Pain 2001;15(1):47–55.

9. Dworkin SF, Turner JA, Mancl L, Wilson L, Massoth D, Huggins KH, LeResche L, Truelove E. A randomized clinical trial of a tailored comprehensive care treatment program for temporomandibular disorders. J Orofac Pain 2002;16(4): 259–76.

10. Gardea MA, Gatchel RJ, Mishra KD. Long-term efficacy of biobehavioral treatment of temporo-

mandibular disorders. J Behav Med 2001; 24(4):341–59.

11. Wright EF. How daily TMD symptom patterns may affect treatment approach. Am Acad Orofac Pain Newslett 2000;5(3):15–6.

12. Bogart RK, Wright E, Dunn WJ, McDaniel R, Hunter C, Peterson AL. Efficacy of group cognitive behavioral intervention for temporomandibular disorders (TMD) patients [abstract 3907]. J Dent Res (Special Issue A) 2002;81:478.

13. Townsen D, Nicholson RA, Buenaver L, Bush F, Gramling S. Use of a habit reversal treatment for temporomandibular pain in a minimal therapist contact format. J Behav Ther Exp Psychiatry 2001;32(4):221–39.

14. Auerbach SM, Laskin DM, Frantsve LM, Orr T. Depression, pain, exposure to stressful life events, and long-term outcomes in temporomandibular disorder patients. J Oral Maxillofac Surg 2001;59(6):628–33.

15. El-Zayadi AR, Selim O, Hamdy H, El-Tawil A, Moustafa H. Heavy cigarette smoking induces hypoxic polycythemia (erythrocytosis) and hyperuricemia in chronic hepatitis C patients with reversal of clinical symptoms and laboratory parameters with therapeutic phlebotomy. Am J Gastroenterol 2002;97(5):1264–5.

16. Jeffery RW, McGuire MT, French SA. Prevalence and correlates of large weight gains and losses. Int J Obes Relat Metab Disord 2002;26(7): 969–72.

17. Miltenberger RG, Fuqua RW, Woods DW. Applying behavior analysis to clinical problems: review and analysis of habit reversal. J Appl Behav Anal 1998;31(3):447–69.

18. Twohig MP, Woods DW. Evaluating the duration of the competing response in habit reversal: a parametric analysis. J Appl Behav Anal 2001;34(4):517–20.

19. Woods DW, Murray LK, Fuqua RW, Seif TA, Boyer LJ, Siah A. Comparing the effectiveness of similar and dissimilar competing responses in evaluating the habit reversal treatment for oraldigital habits in children. J Behav Ther Exp Psychiatry 1999;30(4):289–300.

20. Jones KM, Swearer SM, Friman PC. Relax and try this instead: abbreviated habit reversal for maladaptive self-biting. J Appl Behav Anal 1997;30(4):697–9.

21. Gramling SE, Neblett J, Grayson R, Townsend D. Temporomandibular disorder: efficacy of an oral

habit reversal treatment program. J Behav Ther Exp Psychiatry 1996;27(3):245–55.

22. Benson H. Hypnosis and the relaxation response. Gastroenterology 1989;96(6):1609–11.

23. Benson H. The relaxation response: history, physiological basis and clinical usefulness. Acta Med Scand Suppl 1982;660:231–7.

24. Okeson JP, Moody PM, Kemper JT, Haley JV. Evaluation of occlusal splint therapy and relaxation procedures in patients with temporomandibular disorders. J Am Dent Assoc 1983;107(3):420–4.

25. Loitman JE. Pain management: beyond pharmacology to acupuncture and hypnosis. J Am Med Assoc 2000;283(1):118–9.

26. Simon EP, Lewis DM. Medical hypnosis for temporomandibular disorders: treatment efficacy and medical utilization outcome. Oral Surg Oral Med Oral Pathol Oral Radiol Endod 2000;90(1):54–63.

27. Dubin LL. The use of hypnosis for temporomandibular joint (TMJ). Psychiatr Med 1992;10(4):99–103.

28. Somer E. Hypnotherapy in the treatment of chronic nocturnal use of a dental splint prescribed for bruxism. Int J Clin Exp Hypn 1991;39(3):145–54.

29. Schutt NL, Bernstein DA. Relaxation skills for the patient, dentist, and auxiliaries. Dent Clin North Am 1986;30(Suppl 4):S93–S105.

30. Cott A, Parkinson W, Fabich M, Bedard M, Marlin R. Long-term efficacy of combined relaxation: biofeedback treatments for chronic headache. Pain 1992;51:49–56.

31. Funch DP, Gale EN. Biofeedback and relaxation therapy for chronic temporomandibular joint pain: predicting successful outcome. J Consult Clin Psychol 1984;52(6):928–35.

32. Myers CD, White BA, Heft MW. A review of complementary and alternative medicine use for treating chronic facial pain. J Am Dent Assoc 2002;133(9):1189–96.

33. Gardea MA, Gatchel RJ, Mishra KD. Long-term efficacy of biobehavioral treatment of temporomandibular disorders. J Behav Med 2001;24(4):341–59.

34. Pierce CJ, Gale EN. A comparison of different treatments for nocturnal bruxism. J Dent Res 1988;67:597–601.

35. Hijzen TH, Slangen JL, Van Houweligen HC. Subjective, clinical and EMG effects of biofeedback and splint treatment. J Oral Rehabil 1986;13:529–39.

36. Dahlstrom L, Carlsson SG. Treatment of mandibular dysfunction: the clinical usefulness of biofeedback in relation to splint therapy. J Oral Rehabil 1984;11:277–84.

37. De Leeuw JRJ, Steenks MH, Ros WJG, Bosman F, Winnubst JAM, Scholte AM. Psychosocial aspects of craniomandibular dysfunction: an assessment of clinical and community findings. J Oral Rehabil 1994;21:127–43.

38. Gremillion HA, Waxenberg LB, Myers CD, Benson MB. Psychological considerations in the diagnosis and management of temporomandibular disorders and orofacial pain. Gen Dent 2003;51(2):168–72.

39. Brantley PJ, Jones GN. Daily stress and stress-related disorders. Ann Behav Med 1993;15(1):17–25.

Chapter 17

Pharmacological Management

FAQs

Q: Don't muscle relaxants also help reduce the anxiety related to stress?
A: It has been speculated that muscle relaxants may be particularly effective for patients with an acute condition related to a short-term stressful situation, because they can generally help alter a patient's perception of the situation or its emotional impact.

Q: Will dentists be accused of treating psychological disorders if we prescribe tricyclic antidepressants for our patients with TMD?
A: At the low doses tricyclic antidepressants are used in treating TMD, they do not provide an antidepressant effect, euphoria, or mood elevation, and have low abuse potential.

Q: Are glucosamine and chondroitin beneficial in treating any of the TMJ disorders?
A: Studies evaluating patients with TMD found glucosamine and chondroitin beneficial in treating TMJ inflammation, TMJ noise, and TMJ osteoarthritis.

Clinical experience and controlled studies demonstrate that pharmacological management can generally reduce a patient's pain and sometimes speed recovery. Practitioners tend to have a favorite medication to prescribe to their TMD patients, even though no one drug has been shown best for the wide spectrum of TMD conditions. Many of the pharmacological principles used for musculoskeletal disorders of other areas of the body apply for the pharmacological management of TMD, because medications generally affect the rest of the musculoskeletal system as they do the masticatory musculoskeletal system.[1] TMD is often comparable to repetitive motion disorders in other parts of the body.[2]

Practitioners tend to have a favorite medication to prescribe to their TMD patients, even though no one drug has been shown best for the wide spectrum of TMD conditions.

Patients with chronic TMD symptoms typically need to change their perpetuating factors to obtain long-term control of their symptoms. Clinically it is observed that some patients with chronic symptoms who are initially prescribed medication(s) that provide adequate symptom relief prefer to stay on these medication(s) long term rather than change their perpetuating factors. Therefore, prescribing muscle relaxants to patients who have chronic TMD symptoms is avoided, unless they have an acute exacerbation. Patients with chronic symptoms who desire a prescription are typically prescribed medications that can be used long term, i.e., nonsteroid anti-inflammatory drugs (NSAIDs) on an as-needed basis and/or tricyclic antidepressants. If possible, chronic TMD symptoms are preferably controlled through nonpharmaceutical management, e.g., self-management therapies, occlusal appliance therapy, or habit-breaking techniques.

Understanding Some Patients' Treatment Desires
Clinically it is observed that some patients with chronic symptoms who are initially prescribed medication(s) that provide adequate symptom relief prefer to stay on these medication(s) long term rather than change their perpetuating factors.

Using Pharmaceutical Management
If possible, chronic TMD symptoms are preferably controlled through nonpharmaceutical management, e.g., self-management therapies, occlusal appliance therapy, or habit-breaking techniques.

TMD pharmacological management most commonly involves over-the-counter analgesics (including NSAIDs) and prescription anti-inflammatory drugs, muscle relaxants, low-dose tricyclic antidepressants, nutritional supplements, and topical analgesic cream. The "TMD Self-management Therapies" handout (Appendix 3) recommends over-the-counter medications for patients who prefer to try one. Practitioners must weigh the medication's potential benefits against its side-effect risks, along with their competence in managing patients taking the medication.[1]

There are reports that the selective serotonin reuptake inhibitor (SSRI) antidepressants, in addition to many other medications, may contribute to TMD symptoms.[3,4] The knowledge regarding which medications are more prone to cause this side effect is currently insufficient to recommend a patient's physician change the medication. Therefore, if it is believed a medication is contributing to a patient's TMD symptoms, this possibility is discussed with the patient, this medication is considered a possible contributing factor, and the patient is treated in the usual protocol, presented in this book.

Psychoactive medications prescribed for psychiatric disorders should be provided by psychiatrists or physicians as part of comprehensive mental health therapy.[5]

ANALGESICS

The salicylates, acetaminophen, ibuprofen, naproxen sodium, ketoprofen, and capsaicin are the major analgesics available without a prescription in the United States. Acetaminophen produces few gastric problems and does not interfere with the clotting mechanism, but chronic use (more than 5,000 pills in a lifetime) has been associated with approximately a 2.5-fold increase in kidney failure.[6]

NSAIDs are the most common analgesics used for management of TMD, and patients whose pain is primarily caused by an inflammatory condition may obtain significant improvement from a NSAID.[7,8] Although NSAIDs are generally well tolerated, they have a dose-related association with a wide spectrum of adverse effects.[9] A meta-analysis study suggests that NSAID users have a threefold greater risk of developing serious adverse gastrointestinal events than do nonusers.[10] Also, a retrospective analysis of patients with end-stage kidney disease requiring hemodialysis demonstrated an association between chronic NSAID use (more than 5,000 pills in a lifetime) and a ninefold increase risk of end-stage kidney disease[6] (see the discussion of NSAIDs in "Anti-inflammatory Medications" in this chapter).

Capsaicin (Zostrix), another analgesic agent that has been advocated for treatment of TMD, is specifically designed for topical application[11] (see "Topical Analgesic Cream" in this chapter).

ANTI-INFLAMMATORY MEDICATIONS

TMD therapy uses anti-inflammatory medications primarily to reduce inflammation within the TMJ. As the medication reduces TMJ inflammation, the associated pain and dysfunction corresponding decrease.[7,12] Practitioners should remember that chronic TMJ inflammation is generally secondary to excessive parafunctional activity overloading the TMJ.[13,14] Therefore, clinically it is common to observe anti-inflammatory medications reducing TMJ inflammation and associated symptoms while the patient is taking the medication; but, if a patient with chronic symptoms has not adequately reduced his or her parafunctional habits, the TMJ inflammation and associated symptoms return after the medication is stopped.

◉ **QUICK CONSULTS**

Observing the Effects of Anti-inflammatory Medications

Clinically it is common to observe anti-inflammatory medications reducing TMJ inflammation and associated symptoms while the patient is taking the medication; but, if a patient with chronic symptoms has not adequately reduced his or her parafunctional habits, the TMJ inflammation and associated symptoms return after the medication is stopped.

Anti-inflammatory medication is generally beneficial for patients with acute TMJ inflammation caused by conditions such as acute disc displacement without reduction or secondary to acute trauma. Patients with acute TMJ disc displacement without reduction typically find that anti-inflammatory medication reduces the inflammation associated with the pain, enabling them to stretch the retrodiscal tissue and move their disc further anterior. With the disc more anterior, patients regain their opening, thereby decreasing the disc's interference, and the inflammation is less likely to return.

For mild or moderate pain related to TMJ inflammation in which I would like a patient to take an anti-inflammatory medication, naproxen or naproxen sodium is generally recommended. For more severe pain (6 of 10 or greater) related to TMJ inflammation, a short course of oral corticosteroids followed by a NSAID is generally prescribed. These regimens are discussed further in their corresponding following sections.

The nutritional supplements glucosamine and chondroitin have also been shown to be beneficial for patients with TMJ inflammation and to have minimal side effects.[15,16] If it is preferred that a patient use an anti-inflammatory medication long term, the nutritional supplements or a NSAID taken on an as-needed basis would be reasonable choices (see "Nutritional Supplements" in this chapter).

Nonsteroidal Anti-inflammatory Drugs

NSAIDs usually provide some relief for mild to moderate TMJ inflammation and/or muscle pain. No individual NSAID has been found to be superior in analgesic effect, and individual patient response is highly variable. Therefore, if a patient does not obtain satisfactory improvement with one NSAID, this does not indicate that a different NSAID would not be of benefit.[7,17]

The typical NSAIDs and dosages I use are *ibuprofen* (Motrin), 800 mg t.i.d. or q.i.d.; *naproxen* (Naprosyn), 500 mg b.i.d.; and *naproxen sodium* (Anaprox), 550 mg b.i.d. A 550-mg tablet of naproxen sodium (Anaprox), which is sold over the counter as Aleve (220 mg naproxen sodium), is equivalent to a 500-mg Naprosyn tablet. Clinically it appears to me that patients who have primarily muscle pain find ibuprofen more effective, whereas those whose pain is primarily from TMJ inflammation find naproxen or naproxen sodium more effective. If a NSAID is used to treat a patient with acute TMJ inflammation, I generally prescribe naproxen, 500 mg b.i.d., for 2 or 3 weeks. Clinically it is observed that naproxen appears to lose its effectiveness if a patient uses this dose long term. Therefore, I ask patients to take 500 mg naproxen twice a day for 2 to 3 weeks and then only as needed (no more than a couple of times a week), if they desire to continue using it.

▼ TECHNICAL TIP
Observing Ibuprofen and Naproxen Differences
Clinically it appears to me that patients who have primarily muscle pain find ibuprofen more effective, whereas those whose pain is primarily from TMJ inflammation find naproxen or naproxen sodium more effective.

Clinically it is observed that most TMD patients do not obtain sufficient symptom relief to merit taking a NSAID on a continuous basis, but some patients prefer to take one on an as-needed basis. Some NSAIDs are encapsulated to produce sustained release, whereas others are enteric coated to decrease gastric irritation.[9]

◉ QUICK CONSULTS
Observing the Effects of NSAID Treatment
Clinically it is observed that most TMD patients do not obtain sufficient symptom relief to merit taking a NSAID on a continuous basis, but some patients prefer to take one on an as-needed basis.

For patients who cannot tolerate the NSAID side effects, selective COX_2 *inhibitors* have an efficacy comparable to other NSAIDs and cause minimal COX_1 adverse effects.[18-20] The COX_2 inhibitors celecoxib (Celebrex), rofecoxib (Vioxx), meloxicam (Mobic), and valdecoxib (Bextra) are available in the United States. Keep in mind that these medications are expensive, and NSAIDs generally do not provide TMD patients with much relief.

Due to the potential adverse effects from long-term NSAID use (discussed in "Analgesics" in this chapter), patients are generally not maintained on a NSAID long term, except on an as-needed basis. If a patient needs to be on a NSAID long term, the preferred NSAID and dose are determined, and the patient is referred to a physician for long-term monitoring and management. NSAIDs are primarily ingested, but they have also been given through trigger-point injections,[21] TMJ phonophoresis,[22] and topical applications.[23]

◉ QUICK CONSULTS
Prescribing a NSAID Long Term
Due to the potential adverse effects from long-term NSAID use, patients are generally not maintained on a NSAID long term, except on an as-needed basis.

▼ TECHNICAL TIP
Maintaining Patients on NSAIDs
If a patient needs to be on a NSAID long term, the preferred NSAID and dose are determined, and the patient is referred to a physician for long-term monitoring and management.

Steroidal Anti-inflammatory Drugs

Corticosteroids are potent anti-inflammatory medications that can be used to treat moderate to severe pain (6 of 10 or greater) from inflammation. Due to their potential adverse effects from extended use, a short course is typically prescribed for TMD patients, followed by a NSAID. An expedient method of providing a 6-day declining dose of corticosteroid is by prescribing a *Medrol Dosepak*, which is 21 methylprednisolone tablets conveniently packaged with easy-to-follow directions.[7]

If an oral corticosteroid is the preferred treatment, both Medrol Dosepak and 2 to 3 weeks of naproxen can be prescribed. Patients are routinely requested to start the naproxen on day 4 of Medrol Dosepak use; this decreases the likelihood of gastric upset in the beginning when the corticosteroid dose is high, and extends the anti-inflammatory response.

▼ **TECHNICAL TIP**

Prescribing an Oral Corticosteroid

If an oral corticosteroid is the preferred treatment, both Medrol Dosepak and 2 to 3 weeks of naproxen can be prescribed, in which the patient starts the naproxen on day 4 of Medrol Dosepak use.

The prescriptions are written as follows: Medrol Dosepak, 1 package, take as directed on package (m. dict. on package), and naproxen, 500 mg b.i.d., start on the 4th day of the Dosepak. Practitioners who are limited to a formulary that does not carry Medrol Dosepak can prescribe it in the same manner, but would have to write the dose schedule on a separate sheet of paper for the patient. Prescribe methylprednisolone (Medrol) 4 mg × 21, take as directed (m. dict.), and write these instructions:

Day 1: 2 tablets before breakfast, 1 after lunch, 1 after dinner & 2 at bedtime
Day 2: 2 tablets before breakfast, 1 after lunch, 1 after dinner & 1 at bedtime
Day 3: 1 tablet before breakfast, 1 after lunch, 1 after dinner & 1 at bedtime
Day 4: 1 tablet before breakfast, 1 after lunch & 1 at bedtime
Day 5: 1 tablet before breakfast & 1 at bedtime
Day 6: 1 tablet before breakfast

Corticosteroids are most often taken orally, but can be provided for TMD patients through topical application, phonophoresis, iontophoresis, and injection into the TMJ or another source of the inflammation.[7,12,24,25] TMJ corticosteroid injections are beneficial for reducing TMJ inflammation, but chronic injections can cause condylar degeneration; therefore, they are usually limited to two injections during any 1-year period.[7,26,27] Surgeons generally also use a corticosteroid at the end of arthrocentesis and arthroscopic procedures to obtain its potent anti-inflammatory response postoperatively.[7]

MUSCLE RELAXANTS

These decrease skeletal muscle tone and are generally prescribed for TMD patients with acute muscle pain or to decrease muscle activity temporarily.[3,12,19] Most muscle relaxants are primarily *central acting* agents, and their mechanism of action is not clearly understood. The oral doses are well below the levels needed to induce muscle relaxation locally, leading some investigators to believe the observed muscular relaxation is primarily accomplished through sedation and reduction of psychoemotional stress.[7,28,29] It has been speculated that muscle relaxants may be particularly effective for patients with an acute condition related to a short-term stressful situation, because they can generally help alter a patient's perception of the situation or its emotional impact.[7,29] The more common central-acting muscle relaxants include diazepam (Valium), carisoprodol (Soma), methocarbamol (Robaxin), chlorzoxazone (Paraflex), and cyclobenzaprine (Flexeril).

Occasionally I would like to decrease a patient's nocturnal muscle activity temporarily and can generally accomplish this pharmaceutically by prescribing a central-acting muscle relaxant.[3] For instance, at the initial examination, a patient may relate that, for the past month, he or she routinely awakes with an acute TMJ disc displacement without reduction that lasts half an hour and has been worsening over the past few days. A concern is that, before a stabilization appliance can be provided, the disorder may worsen and the TMJ may not unlock one morning. Therefore, the patient is prescribed a central-acting muscle relaxant to take at bedtime (e.g., 5 mg diazepam, 1 to 2 tablets h.s.) to decrease the nocturnal muscle activity and thereby decrease the probability of the disorder worsening.

▼ TECHNICAL TIP
Decreasing Nocturnal Muscle Activity

Occasionally I would like to decrease a patient's nocturnal muscle activity temporarily and can generally accomplish this pharmaceutically by prescribing a central-acting muscle relaxant.

Another situation in which I would consider prescribing patients a central-acting muscle relaxant to decrease their nocturnal muscle activity would be one in which the patient relates at the initial examination that he or she awakes with significant pain and would like some relief prior to my being able to provide a stabilization appliance. A central-acting muscle relaxant taken prior to bed should decrease a patient's nocturnal muscle activity temporarily, thereby decreasing the morning pain. This should reduce

pain caused by either the muscle or TMJ inflammation. If the pain is primarily due to TMJ inflammation, naproxen or naproxen sodium may also provide adequate benefit.

The primary muscle relaxants and dosages often prescribed for TMD are *diazepam* (Valium), 2 to 10 mg h.s. (low doses may be able to be taken during the day), *methocarbamol* (Robaxin); 500 mg h.s. or t.i.d.; and *cyclobenzaprine* (Flexeril), 10 mg h.s. (half a tablet may be taken in the morning and afternoon). Robaxin and Flexeril are expensive compared with diazepam, all are sedating, and all are preferably taken only at bedtime.

Diazepam has been shown beneficial in treating muscle pain.[30,31] I prefer to prescribe diazepam, because it is very inexpensive and patients seem to have heard of Valium and know that it is not to be taken long term, so I have not had problems with patients wanting to do so.

◉ QUICK CONSULTS
Prescribing Muscle Relaxants

I prefer to prescribe diazepam, because it is very inexpensive and patients seem to have heard of Valium and know that it is not to be taken long term.

Patients are generally prescribed 5-mg tablets of diazepam and asked to take 1 to 2 tablets at bedtime. On occasion, patients would like to take a muscle relaxant during the day. I discuss starting with one-fourth to one-half of the 5-mg diazepam tablet in the morning and afternoon. If a practitioner prefers, diazepam can be prescribed in 2-mg tablets. I add to the prescription "if does not cause drowsiness" and discuss with the patient trying the medication in such a manner that it will not be dangerous if it causes drowsiness. It is observed that patients are generally responsible when practitioners take the time to discuss these issues.

Rarely do I have a patient take a central-acting muscle relaxant for more than 3 weeks. Some patients have a combination of acute TMJ inflammation and muscle pain, for which they may be prescribed a central-acting muscle relaxant together with a NSAID, acetaminophen, or aspirin.[7,12]

Baclofen (Lioresal) is a *peripheral acting* muscle relaxant that works at the spinal chord level. Since the masticatory muscles are primarily innervated by the fifth cranial nerve (the posterior digastric muscle is innervated by the seventh cranial nerve), it is understandable that most of my TMD patients relate baclofen is not beneficial for their masticatory symptoms, but they generally find it valuable for their neck pain. Occasionally 1 tablet of 10 mg baclofen, q4h p.r.n., is prescribed for neck pain and, since it does not act centrally, it typically does not cause sedation. It is preferable that patients have their neck symptoms treated by nonpharmaceutical therapies, i.e., improving their posture and learning neck exercises (usually taught by a physical therapist). Sometimes baclofen is prescribed prior to the patient getting an appointment with the physical therapist and on an as-needed basis for residual symptoms.[7,32]

TRICYCLIC ANTIDEPRESSANTS

TCAs were originally prescribed to treat depression, but over the last 40 years have been used to treat chronic musculoskeletal disorders and neuropathic pain in doses well below those used for depression.[29,33] At these low doses, they do not induce euphoria or mood elevation, and have low abuse potential.[34]

A meta-analysis of 39 placebo-controlled studies that evaluated TCAs for patients with chronic pain indicates TCAs can provide statistically significant pain relief.[33] Their primary therapeutic effect is thought to be related to their ability to increase the neurotransmitters serotonin and norepinephrine at the synapses within the central nervous system.[35,36]

TCAs have been reported to decrease

TMD pain, decrease masticatory nocturnal electromyelographic (EMG) activity, and provide masticatory muscle relaxation for TMD patients.[7,37-39] Individual TMD patient response is highly variable, and some individuals will find no benefit from taking TCAs.[3,40,41]

Disturbed sleep is a common problem among TMD patients that tends to worsen the TMD symptoms, and TMD patients with disturbed sleep tend not to improve as much from conservative TMD therapy as do other patients.[42-44] Sedation is a side effect for most TCAs and, if the TCA is properly chosen and titrated, it might improve the quality of a patient's deep restorative sleep in addition to providing the traditional TCA benefits.[7,36]

⊙ **QUICK CONSULTS**

Prescribing TCAs

Sedation is a side effect for most TCAs and, if the TCA is properly chosen and titrated, it might improve the quality of the patient's deep restorative sleep in addition to providing the traditional TCA benefits.

Amitriptyline (Elavil), nortriptyline (Pamelor), and desipramine (Norpramin) are frequently used TCAs in the treatment of chronic pain,[36] and the degree of sedation the average patient receives from these varies from extensive to none. Clinically one of these TCAs is selected based on the degree of sleep disturbance the patient reports and whether the medication is needed while the patient is asleep or awake. Patients are asked to titrate the medication within the limits of the prescription so it provides the most desirable effect.

Amitriptyline (Elavil) has substantial sedation associated with it, and clinically it is observed that amitriptyline is most effective for patients who have a significant sleep problem and awake with pain. I recommend 10 to 50 mg 1 to 6 hours prior to bed. The patient is asked to start with 10 mg 3 to 4 hours prior to bed and increase the dose slowly, adjust the time the medication is taken prior to bed that is best for him or her, and balance the benefits and side effects of medications within the limits of the prescription.

Nortriptyline (Pamelor) has much less sedation associated with it, and clinically it is observed that nortriptyline is most effective for patients who have no or mild sleep disturbance and awake with pain. I recommend 10 to 50 mg 0 to 3 hours prior to bed. The patient is asked to start with 10 mg 1 hour prior to bed and increase the dose slowly, adjust the time the medication is taken prior to bed that is best for him or her, and balance the benefits and side effects of medications within the limits of the prescription. Some patients find a low dose in the morning and afternoon beneficial if the dose does not cause drowsiness.

Desipramine (Norpramin) essentially has no sedation associated with it, and I use it for patients with daytime pain. I recommend 25 mg in the morning and afternoon, as needed, balancing the benefits and side effects of medications within the limits of the prescription. Some patients have reported to me that taking it at bedtime keeps them from falling asleep.

Occasionally I will prescribe amitriptyline or nortriptyline to be taken prior to bed in combination with desipramine to be taken in the morning and afternoon. The beneficial effects from taking TCAs typically occur within 3 days.[7,36] When prescribing a TCA, it is strongly recommended that the side effects be reviewed with the patient. These medications are associated with many side effects (listed in most medication manuals) that can have a profound effect on patients.

TCAs can be used long term; they are nonhabituating and very rarely cause organ toxicity with long-term use.[36] If a patient needs to be on a TCA long term, the TCA and preferred dose range are determined and the patient referred to a physician for long-term monitoring and management.

Compared with TCAs, serotonin reuptake inhibitor (SSRI) antidepressants are not as effective for treating chronic pain.[7,12,35] The SSRIs are very good medications for treating depression with comparatively minimal side effects and have the potential to increase parafunctional activity.[3,4]

NUTRITIONAL SUPPLEMENTS

Studies on other joints of the body demonstrate *glucosamine* and *chondroitin* are beneficial (comparable to or better than ibuprofen) for joint pain and osteoarthritis, and cause minimal side effects.[45-47] Studies evaluating TMD patients found glucosamine and chondroitin beneficial for TMJ inflammation, TMJ noise, and TMJ osteoarthritis.[15,16]

Their most appropriate doses have never been evaluated, but studies typically use 500 mg glucosamine three times a day and/or 400 mg chondroitin three times a day. If a patient is interested in trying these agents, these doses are generally recommended. Glucosamine is inexpensive compared with chondroitin and may provide adequate benefits by itself. Therefore, patients are asked to start with glucosamine alone and, if it does not provide adequate relief, then add chondroitin. Symptom relief from these supplements is slower than with NSAIDs, and it is recommended patients use them for 30 days before deciding whether they are beneficial.[48]

These agents are available as nutritional supplements, they are not FDA evaluated or recommended, and the number of toxicity studies (particularly long term) is limited. Studies in the United States have revealed that a number of preparations have less agent in each tablet than the container's label states.[49] An independent laboratory evaluates the contents of over-the-counter supplements and reveals on their Web site (www.consumerlab.com) which brands contain the amount claimed on the label. Since these are over-the-counter items, patients with prescription insurance benefits may be reluctant to purchase them.

Another nutritional supplement that may benefit patients with TMD symptoms, although its efficacy has not been substantiated by clinical trials among TMD patients, is *magnesium*. Clinically it appears to act as a mild muscle relaxant, has been demonstrated to be beneficial in treating headaches and myofascial pain, and is often recommended to be taken in combination with calcium.[50-52] If a TMD patient would like to try magnesium, 250 mg twice a day, taken in combination with calcium, is recommended; some brands have the two combined into 1 tablet.

Practitioners who find that a patient takes other nutritional supplements to reduce TMD symptoms may desire these supplements be discontinued if medications are going to be prescribed. These supplements include *feverfew*, which appears to provide a mild anti-inflammatory effect; *valerian*, which appears to provide a muscle-relaxant effect; and *kava*, which also appears to provide a muscle-relaxant effect. Practitioners who discover a patient is taking kava should recommend he or she stop taking it, because of its association with liver toxicity.[53]

TOPICAL ANALGESIC CREAM

Capsaicin (Zostrix) is a topical analgesic cream that is reported also to have anti-inflammatory properties.[54,55] Its mechanism of action is not clearly understood. It has been advocated for treatment of arthritis and neuropathic pain in other parts of the body, and its value in TMD therapy may be promising.[56-58] A randomized clinical trial among TMD patients with pain in the TMJ area requested patients apply one of two creams four times a day. After 4 weeks, the group using capsaicin reported statistically significant symptom improvement, but this was not significantly better than the placebo-cream group's improvement.[56]

Capsaicin comes in two strengths (0.025 percent and 0.075 percent) that are available over the counter. Its active ingredient is the substance that makes chili peppers hot, so patients should be warned to wash their hands after applying the cream (because they may later rub their eyes), and a common side effect is skin redness or irritation for the first couple of days.

Capsaicin should be applied three to four times a day, and should not be used in conjunction with other local agents, e.g., Icy Hot or a heating pad. Because of the skin-irritation side effect, I generally prescribe the 0.025 percent formula to patients with light complexion and the 0.075 percent formula to patients with dark complexion. My clinical experience is that patients generally find it beneficial and often relate they believe the warm sensation it provides is the cause of its positive effect.

▼ **TECHNICAL TIP**
Prescribing Capsaicin
My clinical experience is that patients generally find it beneficial and often relate they believe the warm sensation it provides is the cause of its positive effect.

REFERENCES

1. No authors listed. Management of temporomandibular disorders. National Institutes of Health Technology Assessment Conference Statement. J Am Dent Assoc 1996;127(11): 1595–606.

2. Hong CZ. Considerations and recommendations regarding myofascial trigger point injection. J Musculoske Pain 1994;2(1):29–59.

3. Winocur E, Gavish A, Voikovitch M, Emodi-Perlman A, Eli I. Drugs and bruxism: a critical review. J Orofac Pain 2003;17(2):99–111.

4. Friedlander AH, Friedlander IK, Marder SR. Bipolar I disorder: psychopathology, medical management and dental implications. J Am Dent Assoc 2002;133(9):1209–17.

5. Magni G, Moreschi C, Rigatti-Luchini S, Merskey H. Prospective study on the relationship between depressive symptoms and chronic musculoskeletal pain. Pain 1994;56(3):289–97.

6. Perneger TV, Whelton PK, Klag MJ. Risk of kidney failure associated with the use of acetaminophen, aspirin, and nonsteroidal antiinflammatory drugs. N Engl J Med 1994;331(25):1675–9.

7. Ganzberg S, Quek SYP. Pharmacotherapy. In: Pertes RA, Gross SG (eds). Clinical management of temporomandibular disorders and orofacial pain. Chicago: Quintessence, 1995:211–26.

8. Jager RG, Absi EG. A comparison of naproxen and placebo in the treatment of temporomandibular joint dysfunction [abstract 31]. J Orofac Pain 1995;9(1):105.

9. Paulus HE, Bulpitt KJ. Nonsteroidal antiinflammatory drugs. In: Klippel JH, Weyand CM, Wortmann RL (eds). Primer on the Rheumatic Diseases, 11th edition. Atlanta: Arthritis Foundation, 1997:422–6.

10. Gabriel SE, Jaakkimainen L, Bombardier C. Risk for serious gastrointestinal complications related to use of nonsteroidal anti-inflammatory drugs: a meta-analysis. Ann Intern Med 1991;115(10): 787–96.

11. Winocur E, Gavish A, Halachmi M, Eli I, Gazit E. Topical application of capsaicin for the treatment of localized pain in the temporomandibular joint area. J Orofac Pain 2000;14(1):31–6.

12. Dionne RA. Pharmacologic treatments for temporomandibular disorders. Oral Surg Oral Med Oral Pathol Oral Radiol Endod 1997;83:134–42.

13. Stegenga B. Osteoarthritis of the temporomandibular joint organ and its relationship to disc displacement. J Orofac Pain 2001;15(3):193–205.

14. American Society of Temporomandibular Joint Surgeons. Guidelines for diagnosis and management of disorders involving the temporomandibular joint and related musculoskeletal structures [White paper]. Cranio 2003;21(1):68–76.

15. Thie NM, Prasad NG, Major PW. Evaluation of glucosamine sulfate compared to ibuprofen for the treatment of temporomandibular joint osteoarthritis: a randomized double blind controlled 3 month clinical trial. J Rheumatol 2001;28(6): 1347–55.

16. Shankland WE II. The effects of glucosamine and chondroitin sulfate on osteoarthritis of the TMJ: a preliminary report of 50 patients. Cranio 1998; 16(4):230–5.

17. Syrop SB. Initial management of temporomandibular disorders. Dent Today 2002;21(8): 52–7.

18. Jeske AH. Selecting new drugs for pain control: evidence-based decisions or clinical impressions? J Am Dent Assoc 2002;133(8):1052–6.

19. Mehlisch DR. The efficacy of combination analgesic therapy in relieving dental pain. J Am Dent Assoc 2002;133(7):861–71.

20. Wynn RL. The new COX-2 inhibitors: rofecoxib (Vioxx) and celecoxib (Celebrex). Gen Dent 2000;48(1):16–20.

21. Simons DG, Travell JG, Simons LS. Travell & Simons' Myofascial Pain and Dysfunction: The Trigger Point Manual, volume 1, 2nd edition. Baltimore: Williams & Wilkins, 1999:147.

22. Shin S-M, Choi J-K. Effect of indomethacin phonophoresis on the relief of temporomandibular joint pain. Cranio 1997;15(4):345–8.

23. Svensson P, Houe L, Arendt-Nielsen L. Effect of systemic versus topical nonsteroidal anti-inflammatory drugs on postexercise jaw-muscle soreness: a placebo-controlled study. J Orofac Pain 1997;11(4):353–62.

24. Padilla M, Clark GT, Merrill RL. Topical medications for orofacial neuropathic pain: a review. J Am Dent Assoc 2000;131(2):184–95.

25. Quek S. Treating masseter trigger points with a peripheral nerve block: a novel idea worth considering. AAOP News 1999;5(1):12–3.

26. Kopp S, Wenneberg B, Haraldson T, Carlsson GE. The short-term effect of intra-articular injections of sodium hyaluronate and corticosteroid on temporomandibular joint pain and dysfunction. J Oral Maxillofac Surg 1985;43(6): 429–35.

27. Kopp S, Wenneberg B, Haraldson T, Carlsson GE. The short-term effect of intra-articular injections of sodium hyaluronate and corticosteroid on temporomandibular joint pain and dysfunction. J Oral Maxillofac Surg 1985;43(6):429–35.

28. Stiesch-Scholz M, Fink M, Tschernitschek H, Rossbach A. Medical and physical therapy of temporomandibular joint disk displacement without reduction. Cranio 2002;20(2):85–90.

29. Okeson JP. Management of Temporomandibular Disorders and Occlusion, 5th edition St Louis: CV Mosby, 2003:371–2.

30. Singer E, Dionne R. A controlled evaluation of ibuprofen and diazepam for chronic orofacial muscle pain. J Orofac Pain 1997;11(2):139–46.

31. Montgomery MT, Nishioka GJ, Rugh JD, Thrash WJ. Effect of diazepam on nocturnal masticatory muscle activity [abstract 96]. J Dent Res 1986;65:180.

32. Waldman HJ. Centrally acting skeletal muscle relaxants and associated drugs. J Pain Symptom Manage 1994;9:434–41.

33. Onghena P, Van Houdenhove B. Antidepressant-induced analgesia in chronic non-malignant pain: a meta-analysis of 39 placebo-controlled studies. Pain 1992;49(2):205–19.

34. Brown RS, Bottomley WK. The utilization and mechanism of action of tricyclic antidepressants in the treatment of chronic facial pain: a review of the literature. Anesth Prog 1990;37(5):223–9.

35. Watson CPN. Antidepressant drugs as adjuvant analgesics. J Pain Symptom Manage 1994;9: 392–405.

36. Pettengill CA, Reisner-Keller L. The use of tricyclic antidepressants for the control of chronic orofacial pain. Cranio 1997;15(1):53–6.

37. Sharav Y, Singer E, Schmidt E, Dionne RA, Dubner R. The analgesic effect of amitriptyline on chronic facial pain. Pain 1987;31(2):199–209.

38. Kreisberg MK. Tricyclic antidepressants: analgesic effect and indications in orofacial pain. J Craniomandib Disord 1988;2(4):171–7.

39. Rizzatti-Barbosa CM, Nogueira MTP, de Andrade ED, Ambrosano GMB, de Albergaria Barbosa JR. Clinical evaluation of amitriptyline for the control of chronic pain caused by temporomandibular joint disorders. Cranio 2003;21(3):221–5.

40. Mohamed SE, Christensen LV, Penchas J. A randomized double-blind clinical trial of the effect of amitriptyline on nocturnal masseteric motor activity (sleep bruxism). Cranio 1997;15(4):326–32.

41. Raigrodski AJ, Christensen LV, Mohamed SE, Gardiner DM. The effect of four-week administration of amitriptyline on sleep bruxism: a double-blind crossover clinical study. Cranio 2001;19(1):21–5.

42. Fricton JR, Olsen T. Predictors of outcome for treatment of temporomandibular disorder. J Orofac Pain 1996;10(1):54–65.

43. Ursin R, Endresen IM, Vaeroy H, Hjelmen AM. Relations among muscle pain, sleep variables, and depression. J Musculoske Pain 1999;7(3): 59–72.

44. Bailey DR. Sleep disorders: overview and relationship to orofacial pain. Dent Clin North Am 1997;41(2):189–209.

45. Reginster JY, Deroisy R, Rovati LC, Lee RL, Lejeune E, Bruyere O, Giacovelli G, Henrotin Y, Dacre JE, Gossett C. Long-term effects of glucosamine sulphate on osteoarthritis progression: a randomized, placebo-controlled clinical trial. Lancet 2001;357(9252):251–6.

46. Leeb BF, Schweitzer H, Montag K, Smolen JS. A metaanalysis of chondroitin sulfate in the treatment of osteoarthritis. J Rheumatol 2000;27(1): 205–11.

47. McAlindon TE, Gulin J, Felson DT. Glucosamine and chondroitin treatment for osteoarthritis of the knee or hip: meta-analysis and quality assessment of clinical trials [abstract 994]. Arthritis Rheum 1998;41:S198.

48. Drovanti A, Bignamini AA, Rovati AL. Therapeutic activity of oral glucosamine sulfate in osteoarthrosis: a placebo-controlled double-blind investigation. Clin Ther 1980;3(4): 260–72.

49. Deal CL, Moskowitz RW. Nutraceuticals as therapeutic agents in osteoarthritis: the role of glucosamine, chondroitin sulfate, and collagen hydrolysate. Rheum Dis Clin North Am 1999;25(2):379–95.

50. Gremillion HA. Multidisciplinary diagnosis and management of orofacial pain. Gen Dent 2002;50(2):178–86.

51. Altura BM, Altura BT. Tension headaches and muscle tension: is there a role for magnesium? Med Hypotheses 2001;57(6):705–13.

52. Mauskop A, Altura BM. Role of magnesium in the pathogenesis and treatment of migraines. Clin Neurosci 1998;5(1):24–7.

53. Reisner L. Prescribing/drug interactions with alternative medications. In: American Academy of Orofacial Pain, 28th Annual Scientific Meeting, April 6, 2003.

54. Stiles A, Mitrirattanakul S. The use of topical medications in the management of peripheral neuropathic pain. AAOP News 1999;5(2):10–1.

55. Zhang WY, Li Wan Po A. The effectiveness of topically applied capsaicin: a meta-analysis. Eur J Clin Pharmacol 1994;46(6):517–22.

56. Winocur E, Gavish A, Halachmi M, Eli I, Gazit E. Topical application of capsaicin for the treatment of localized pain in the temporomandibular joint area. J Orofac Pain 2000;14(1):31–6.

57. Watson CPN. Topical capsaicin as an adjuvant analgesic. J Pain Symptom Manage 1994;9: 425–33.

58. Deal CL, Schnitzer TJ, Lipstein E, Seibold JR, Levey MD, Albert D, Renold F. Treatment of arthritis with topical capsaicin: a double-blind trial. Clin Ther 1991;13(3):383–95.

Chapter 18

Other Dental Procedures

FAQs

Q: In which situations would you recommend a dentist treat TMD by adjusting a patient's occlusion?

A: The only time I would recommend a patient's occlusion be adjusted at the initial visit is for patients whose TMD symptoms developed due to the placement of a restoration that was not in harmony with the rest of the dentition.

Q: Why do many dentists believe orthodontics is a sound TMD therapy?

A: During the active orthodontic phase, patients tend to have fewer TMD signs, and it has been proposed that teeth being orthodontically moved are so sensitive to percussion and opposing tooth contact that patients decrease their parafunctional habits. This may be the reason some practitioners and patients develop the illusion that orthodontics provides clinically significant long-term benefits in the treatment of TMD.

The more harmonious a person's occlusion is (degree of occlusal stability), the more orthopedically stable the masticatory system is when the individual clenches or bruxes the teeth.[1,2] Virtually no one is gifted with an "ideal" occlusion, and the improvement in an individual's occlusal stability should decrease the negative impact clenching or bruxing has on the masticatory system.[2-4] Stabilization appliances can generally improve a patient's occlusal stability, and it has been speculated this is one of the mechanisms by which stabilization appliances can reduce TMD symptoms.[5,6]

☻ FOCAL POINT

Virtually no one is gifted with an "ideal" occlusion, and the improvement of an individual's occlusal stability should decrease the negative impact clenching or bruxing has on the masticatory system.

TMD patients often have increased tone in their lateral pterygoid muscles and/or TMJ inflammation, making it difficult to position the mandible in centric relation and/or obtain a reproducible closure position.[7,8] Some TMD patients have a lateral pterygoid myospasm, which causes the condyle to be held in a partially translated position, and therefore these patients temporarily have a distorted occlusion. Some TMD patients initially hold their mandible in such an abnormal position from muscle and/or TMJ disorders that they cannot even close into maximum intercuspation.

For these reasons (among others), most practitioners recommend that TMD patients not be initially treated through occlusal therapy.[9-13] The only time I would recommend a patient's occlusion be adjusted at the initial visit is for patients whose TMD symptoms developed due to the placement of a restoration that was not in harmony with the rest of the dentition.[2,3,11] In this situation, it is generally much more cost effective to refine the restoration's occlusion than provide traditional TMD therapy. This typically resolves the TMD symptoms, but it must be kept in mind that TMD symptoms may develop for other reasons following the placement of a restoration (see Chapter 8, "TMD Secondary to Dental Treatment").

Since virtually no one has an "ideal" occlusion, practitioners can usually find dental procedures that could potentially improve the occlusal stability for nearly everyone. Before practitioners contemplate such procedures, they must compare the procedure's perceived benefits with its costs, e.g., price, time, and adverse sequelae.

There are many dental conditions for which improving a patient's occlusion may be warranted, e.g., inadequate teeth to chew food properly, adverse occlusal forces causing tooth mobility, fremitus, tooth or restoration fracture, tooth sensitivity, and damage to supporting structures.[9,14] If the purpose of therapy is to reduce TMD symptoms, many

different dental procedures have been advocated, but, as a whole, studies have found insufficient symptom improvement to justify these procedures.[15-17]

It is easy to get caught in this controversy, but practitioners must realize most TMD patients with constant chronic symptoms (a) will be given a stabilization appliance that is worn at night which should provide an "ideal" occlusion, and (b) will be taught not to touch their teeth together during the day, except momentarily for swallowing and the occasional bumping while eating. By using these two therapies, the teeth almost never touch. If the teeth rarely touch, the occlusion is not a significant factor in any residual TMD symptoms and any occlusal therapy probably would provide minimal to no benefit.

Patients with intermittent pain are generally provided the treatment that addresses the contributing factors related to their pain; i.e., patients who awake with pain are given a stabilization appliance that is worn at night, and those with daytime pain are taught not to touch their teeth together during the day. Therefore, any occlusal therapy probably would similarly have minimal impact on any residual TMD symptoms.

For patients having trouble breaking their daytime habits in order to reduce their daytime TMD pain satisfactorily, I typically ask them to wear their stabilization appliance when the habits are worse and/or escalate behavioral therapy rather than provide occlusal therapy. It is felt that this generally provides more cost-effective therapy and is likely to provide additional health benefits as coping strategies are learned for the situations that are causing the excessive muscle tension.

Some TMD patients have had their teeth equilibrated or received full-mouth reconstructions one or more times and continue to have significant TMD symptoms.[18,19] I have evaluated many TMD patients who had considerable pain despite having had multiple full-mouth equilibrations, and one patient who developed TMD symptoms as a result of being provided an ideal occlusion by a full-mouth reconstruction. The patient who developed TMD from full-mouth reconstruction said he previously could not occlude into maximum intercuspation, but now could and enjoyed continually clenching his teeth.

Occlusal therapy merely attempts to address one aspect of the multifactorial TMD problem. The TMD therapies provided in this book are comparatively much less expensive (in terms of price, time, adverse sequelae, etc.) and will provide greater symptom improvement than will occlusal therapy.

☾ FOCAL POINT
Occlusal therapy merely attempts to address one aspect of the multifactorial TMD problem.

◉ QUICK CONSULT
Using a Multidisciplinary Treatment Approach
The TMD therapies provided in this book are comparatively much less costly (in terms of price, time, adverse sequelae, etc.) and will provide greater symptom improvement than will occlusal therapy.

It is observed that many dentists prefer treating TMD by using the therapies they commonly provide, e.g., occlusal equilibration, restorative procedures, orthodontics, or orthognathic surgery. These treatments primarily attempt to increase occlusal stability, and using only one aspect of care will provide limited benefits. Dentists must keep in mind that there are many other professionals who can assist with other aspects of their TMD patient's care.

If a practitioner observes that orthodontics, orthognathic surgery, prosthodontics, or other dental procedures would improve a patient's occlusal stability, the procedure's perceived benefits must be compared with its costs, e.g., in terms of price, time, and adverse sequelae. When comparing the benefits with the costs, occlusal therapy is very rarely a worthwhile endeavor if provided only to reduce TMD symptoms. If a patient desires the procedure, the decision to proceed should be based on the anticipated non-TMD benefits, e.g., improving esthetics or chewing efficiency.[20,21]

In the future, I believe better guidelines will be developed for the integration of occlusal therapy and traditional TMD therapy. It has been observed, for instance, that TMD symptoms of several patients have been resolved by only the extraction of third molars. It appears to me that third molars erupting into a nonharmonious relationship decreases the occlusal stability and could cause patients to become symptomatic if the patients are prone to developing TMD symptoms. This could be why the removal of these teeth eliminated symptoms for those patients. It has been speculated that deep third-molar wear facets or other third-molar occlusal disharmonies may be predictors for third-molar removal providing significant TMD symptom benefit. It has also been observed that many TMD patients report that having their third molars removed provided no TMD symptom improvement. Further studies in this and in integrating occlusal therapy with TMD therapies are needed.

◉ QUICK CONSULT
Integrating Occlusal Therapy and Traditional TMD Therapy
In the future, I believe better guidelines will be developed for the integration of occlusal therapy and traditional TMD therapy.

OCCLUSAL EQUILIBRATION

For many years, occlusal equilibration has been recommended for treatment of TMD,[22-25] and it has been speculated that this therapy is still one of the most common procedures that dentists use to treat TMD.[26] Occlusal equilibration generally increases

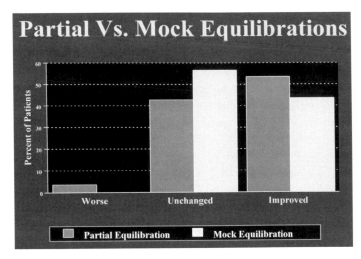

Figure 18-1. Partial equilibration provides only slightly better symptom improvement than does mock equilibration and causes some individual's symptoms to worsen.[28]

occlusal and orthopedic stability, thereby increasing the masticatory system's ability to tolerate excessive forces generated during parafunctional habits.[1-3]

Some practitioners provide only a partial equilibration by adjusting the most significant interferences. This has unpredictable results and may cause some TMD patients' symptoms to worsen (Figure 18-1).[27,28] For instance, a patient might have a prominent balancing interference on the second molar for which the patient has developed subconscious engrams to avoid contacting. The first molar may be positioned in such a way that, when the prominent second molar balancing interference is removed, the first molar's balancing interference comes into contact. Once the second molar's balancing interference is adjusted, the patient may start to play with the new first molar interference and the TMD symptoms worsen. If a partial equilibration is performed, I warn the patient to avoid playing with new contacts that will probably develop.

A complete full-mouth occlusal equilibration is more predictable than a partial equilibration for improving TMD symptoms and is typically performed in the studies evaluating TMD symptom change.[18,29,30] Some individuals in the studies experience worsening of their symptoms, and postoperative thermal sensitivity is common.[18,31]

Intuitively one can reason that stabilization appliances can generally provide a more "ideal" occlusion than can a full-mouth equilibration, because acrylic can be added to certain aspects of the splint to provide a more ideal occlusion; e.g., extra acrylic behind the maxillary anterior teeth might provide immediate disocclusion of the posterior teeth (coupling the anterior teeth). The closest study to comparing these is one in which the practitioner spent a median of four 1-hour appointments equilibrating the patient's dentition. The study compared the TMD symptom change with patients given stabilization appliances in combination with home exercises, which were shown to be more beneficial in treating TMD symptoms (see Figure 18-2).[18]

In the literature, a consensus has formed for three aspects of occlusal equilibrations:

1. Occlusal equilibration should not be provided as an initial therapy for TMD patients, except when symptoms are due to the placement of a nonharmonious restoration. Because of the increased tone in lateral

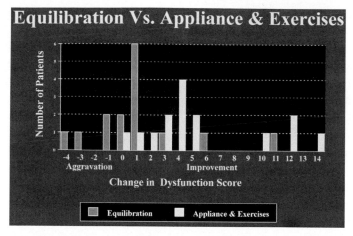

Figure 18-2. Stabilization appliances in conjunction with home exercises are more beneficial in reducing TMD symptoms than are 4-hour equilibrations.[18]

pterygoid muscles and/or TMJ inflammation, it is difficult to position a TMD patient's mandible in centric relation and/or obtain a reproducible closure position.[7,8] Disastrous consequences could occur if the dentition is equilibrated in an undesirable position. Prior to attending my TMD Fellowship, I had been taught and practiced using occlusal therapy as my primary treatment for TMD patients. Some became very occlusally obsessed, some would continually try to find minor remaining discrepancies and, if the adjustment was not perfect, it was virtually impossible to satisfy them.

2. Occlusal interferences do not cause bruxism, nor does removing them stop bruxism; therefore, an equilibration should not be performed with this objective.[3,16,32]

3. Occlusal equilibration should not be performed to prevent TMD signs or symptoms.[32-35]

If a full-mouth equilibration is performed, it must be done meticulously and has the potential to increase TMD symptoms.[18] An equilibration is time consuming, difficult to perform, and requires great precision.[27,36]

◉ **QUICK CONSULT**

Reducing TMD Symptoms through Full-mouth Equilibration

If a full-mouth equilibration is performed, it must be done meticulously and has the potential to increase TMD symptoms.

Contrary to what some practitioners are advocating, occlusal therapy is not needed to maintain a TMD patient's long-term symptom improvement.[9,14,37] This is discussed in "Long-term Management" in Chapter 19.

ORTHODONTIC–ORTHOGNATHIC THERAPY

Many clinical studies have examined the relationship between orthodontic treatment and TMD. Some longitudinal studies find a trend or statistically significant decrease in TMD signs and/or symptoms after orthodontic treatment.[38-41] This is probably due to an increase in occlusal stability, but orthodontics might decrease an individual's occlusal stability, thereby predisposing the patient to TMD.[2] There is no evidence that any particular type of orthodontic procedure or treatment approach (with or without tooth extraction) is associated with an increased risk of developing TMD.[42-44]

During the active orthodontic phase, patients tend to have fewer TMD signs and symptoms, even though there is a high prevalence of new occlusal interferences.[45,46] A proposed rationale is that teeth being orthodontically moved are so sensitive to percussion and opposing tooth contact that patients decrease their parafunctional habits.[45] This may be the reason some practitioners and patients develop the illusion that orthodontics provides clinically significant long-term TMD benefits. A survey of American Dental Association members found that 7 percent of the general dentists and 26 percent of the specialists (47 percent were orthodontists) use fixed orthodontics to treat TMD patients.[47]

Once patients are in the retention phase, their teeth are no longer sensitive, parafunctional habits return, and TMD signs and symptoms become more prevalent.[45,46,48] This can set the stage for the onset or return of TMD symptoms, causing some patients to believe orthodontics caused the TMD signs and/or symptoms. This tendency is compounded by the following: (a) children in their second and third decades of life tend to have an increase in frequency and severity of TMD signs and symptoms,[14] and (b) over the relatively lengthy course of orthodontic treatment, there is considerable opportunity for psychological distress, making patients more prone to developing TMD symptoms. In general, orthodontic treatment does not increase or decrease a patient's chance of developing TMD, even if the practitioner does not achieve a specific gnathologic ideal occlusion.[42-44]

✪ FOCAL POINT

In general, orthodontic treatment does not increase or decrease a patient's chance of developing TMD, even if the practitioner does not achieve a specific gnathologic ideal occlusion.

Occasionally, during the active orthodontic treatment phase, TMD symptoms occur to the point that TMD therapy is needed. Depending on severity of the symptoms, orthodontic treatment may need to be slowed or temporarily discontinued as TMD therapy is provided.[3,44] The therapy may involve TMD self-management therapies (i.e., the handout in Appendix 3), medications, adjunctive therapies, and/or occlusal appliance therapy.[3,46] If occlusal appliance therapy is deemed necessary, some practitioners may want to continue moving the teeth and use a partial coverage occlusal appliance, an occlusal appliance with springs or jack screws within it, or single "pods" of cement (e.g., glass ionomer) added to individual teeth to act as miniocclusal appliances.[3]

Practitioners performing orthodontic therapy should warn prospective orthodontic patients that TMD symptoms could develop or worsen and to be prepared to deal with their onset or exacerbation.[3,14] Because of the potential for TMD signs and symptoms during orthodontic treatment, it is imperative that a TMD screening examination be performed prior to orthodontic therapy.[44]

Even though TMD symptoms tend to diminish during active orthodontic treatment, I recommend delaying orthodontic therapy for the following patients until their symptoms reduce sufficiently:

1. TMD patients using an occlusal appliance who cannot tolerate being without it. It is recommended their TMD symptoms be further reduced through adjunctive TMD therapies prior to initiating orthodontics.

2. TMD patients with such significant TMD pain that they desire relatively immediate reduction of their symptoms. These patients should be treated with traditional TMD therapy to reduce their symptoms sufficiently.

3. Patients who have an intermittent acute TMJ disc displacement without reduction that occurs more often than once a week. It is feared that orthodontic therapy

could sufficiently aggravate their TMD symptoms so that they progress from intermittent to constant. This would be much more difficult to treat than the intermittent form. These patients should be treated with traditional TMD therapy to reduce the disorder sufficiently. Since these patients' TMD symptoms appear to have such a high potential of interrupting their active orthodontic treatment, it is recommended that TMD therapy be provided prior to initiation of orthodontic treatment. A controlled study observed that TMD symptoms eliminated prior to orthodontic treatment were not likely to recur during the subsequent orthodontic care.[46]

For the correction of skeletal malocclusions, orthognathic surgery may be considered in conjunction with orthodontic treatment.[47] TMD signs and symptoms tend to diminish following orthognathic surgery.[49-51] The results of one controlled study that followed the cases of patients with class II malocclusion after they received orthognathic surgery suggests that the correction does not cause a clinically significant increase or decrease in TMD signs or symptoms. The study also found that the amount of horizontal overlap corrected and the degree of TMD improvement were not related.[49]

Surgical treatment for skeletal asymmetries and growth anomalies with the specific intent of alleviating TMD symptoms is rarely indicated and should only follow careful evaluation and management of contributing factors.[13] However, in those TMD patients with severe skeletal malocclusion who desire improved esthetics, function, and/or occlusal stability, orthognathic treatment is often the method of choice.

Orthodontic and orthognathic therapy generally improve occlusal stability, thereby decreasing the negative impact that clenching and/or bruxing has on the masticatory system.[2-4] These procedures are costly and time consuming, and studies show that most patients do not obtain clinically significant TMD improvement.

PROSTHODONTIC THERAPY

Prosthodontic therapy can also increase an individual's occlusal stability by replacing missing teeth, restoring teeth where cusps do not contact the opposing teeth, and providing more ideal occlusal relationships for minor dental malalignments. Improving occlusal stability through prosthodontic therapy is very costly and time consuming, and periodically prosthodontic therapy needs to be replaced.

If a patient's primary problem is TMD pain, the therapies provided in this book are comparatively much less expensive (in terms of price, time, adverse sequelae, etc.) and will provide greater symptom improvement than will prosthodontic therapy. When comparing the benefits with the costs, prosthodontic therapy is very rarely a worthwhile endeavor if provided only to reduce TMD symptoms.[10,52] Additionally patients who have nocturnal parafunctional habits will often need to wear a stabilization appliance at night after extensive prosthodontic rehabilitation.[20]

⊙ **QUICK CONSULT**

Reducing TMD Symptoms through Prosthodontic Therapy

When comparing the benefits with the costs, prosthodontic therapy is very rarely a worthwhile endeavor if provided only to reduce TMD symptoms.

If a practitioner is contemplating a prosthodontic procedure, the decision should be based on the anticipated non-TMD benefits, e.g., restoring function and improving esthetics.[20,21] I once had a TMD patient with complete dentures for whom a maxillary acrylic stabilization appliance was provided that snapped onto her maxillary denture teeth. She wore the appliance 24 hours a day, including while eating (I do not recommend patients with natural teeth wear an occlusal appliance this often or eat with it) and obtained about 50 percent improvement in her TMD symptoms. She strongly believed her problem was caused by her dentures and, against my recommendations, had a new set made. The dentist took extraordinary measures to obtain the most accurate jaw position possible and made her a very nice set of dentures. As one would anticipate, the patient did not gain any additional TMD symptom improvement.

Prosthodontic therapy can enhance or worsen masticatory orthopedic stability and has caused or contributed to TMD symptoms.[13,52] I have been referred patients who received or were in the process of receiving fixed prosthetics, who developed TMD symptoms from tooth pain associated with the procedure, and masticatory muscle and TMJ pain from the long dental procedures.

TMD is a common disorder, so some patients desiring prosthodontic therapy will have TMD symptoms. Dentists need to proceed cautiously with these patients because they often have an increased tone in their lateral pterygoid muscles and/or TMJ inflammation, which make it difficult to position the mandible into centric relation and/or obtain a reproducible closure position.[7,53] Some TMD patients have a lateral pterygoid myospasm, which causes the condyle to be held in a partially translated position, and therefore temporarily have a distorted occlusion.

Practitioners with patients who have TMD symptoms and are in need of extensive prosthodontics or who will need to be restored in a position different than maximum intercuspation should first stabilize the TMD.[21,53-55] The better the TMD symptoms are controlled prior to prosthodontic treatment, the better the final occlusal results are.[56] If the TMD symptoms are significant and extensive prosthodontics is planned, the practitioner may desire to maintain the pa-

tient in this stable condition for 6 months prior to initiating prosthodontic therapy. Clinical judgment and a degree of compromise may be required for some patients.[52]

▼ TECHNICAL TIP
Stabilizing TMD Prior to Extensive Prosthodontics

Practitioners with patients who have TMD symptoms and are in need of extensive prosthodontics or who will need to be restored in a position different than maximum intercuspation should first stabilize the TMD.

Because there are less expensive (in terms of price, time, adverse sequelae, etc.) and more rapid treatments for TMD, prosthodontic rehabilitation should not be used as a TMD therapy and is not needed to prevent a recurrence.[53,55] Patients who have TMD and are in need of extensive prosthodontics should have the disorder stabilized prior to initiating prosthodontics.

TMJ SURGERY AND IMPLANTS

TMJ surgery is indicated for the treatment of a wide variety of pathological conditions. Among TMD patients, its purpose is to reduce their symptoms and dysfunction, not to make the TMJ disc-condyle relation "normal." The belief that a displaced disc is generally only a very minor contributor to TMD is supported by studies that show a large percentage of the general population has a displaced disc but not TMD symptoms.[57,58] Additionally a disc that is surgically moved to its "normal" position becomes displaced again in the majority of cases.[59,60]

When conservative TMD therapy is used, as described in this book, it is relatively rare for TMD patients to need TMJ surgery. One study that tracked over 2,000 TMD patients from many practices found that only 2.5 percent underwent TMJ surgery (1.4 percent arthrocentesis, 1.0 percent arthroscopy, and 0.1 percent open joint procedures).[61] TMD referral candidates are patients with specific diagnoses who have not received adequate benefit from conservative therapy, desire more rapid improvement than is traditional from conservative TMD therapy, or will not benefit from conservative TMD therapy.

TMJ surgery is significantly more expensive than conservative TMD therapy. Based on insurance records, the average cost of TMJ surgery (not including the hospitalization) is two to three times the cost of nonsurgical TMD therapy. The records also reflect a considerable gender bias for patients receiving TMJ surgery compared with conservative care. The male-to-female ratio was 1 to 10 for surgical care but 1 to 2 for nonsurgical therapy.[62]

TMJ surgery is not beneficial for all appropriately selected and treated patients. There is no scientifically determined protocol for determining which TMD patients should be referred to a surgeon.[63] To provide referral guidance, the following generalizations are based on the literature and my clinical experience. There are exceptions to these, so practitioners should proceed with caution.

Other than for the obvious reasons (e.g., infection, fracture, or neoplastic growth), there are primarily three TMD disorders for which practitioners may want to refer TMD patients to a surgeon: TMJ inflammation, acute TMJ disc displacement without reduction, and TMJ ankylosis.

FOCAL POINT

Other than for the obvious reasons (e.g., infection, fracture, or neoplastic growth), the primary TMD disorders for which practitioners may want to refer TMD patients to a surgeon are TMJ inflammation, acute TMJ disc displacement without reduction, and TMJ ankylosis.

TMJ inflammation is extremely common among TMD patients, is generally secondary to overloading of the TMJ from excessive parafunctional activity,[64,65] and generally resolves with conservative therapy.[66] Many invasive procedures can rapidly reduce TMJ inflammation and its associated symptoms. Trained practitioners may find that a corticosteroid injection into the TMJ adequately resolves the symptoms or may want to remove the inflammatory and pain mediators surgically. When the mediators are surgically removed, a corticosteroid is generally deposited at the end of the procedure to obtain its potent anti-inflammatory response.[67]

The choice of procedures will vary with a patient's history, signs, symptoms, and imaging findings, and the practitioner's clinical exam, training, and experience. If removal of the inflammatory and pain mediators is all that is thought necessary, arthrocentesis would most likely be the treatment choice. If surgical alterations within the TMJ are contemplated, arthroscopic or open joint surgery may be recommended. These surgical options are explained below.

Since TMJ inflammation is generally secondary to excessive parafunctional activity, that activity needs to be adequately reduced or the inflammatory and pain mediators will probably return after the invasive procedure. Therefore, prior to making a surgical referral for TMJ inflammation, the conservative therapies thought to be beneficial should be exhausted.

Consider referring the patient whose TMD symptoms are primarily due to TMJ inflammation when (a) the contributing factors are controlled as much as possible, (b) conservative therapy has not adequately resolved the pain, and (c) the pain from the TMJ is so significant that an invasive procedure is desired. Keep in mind that, if the perpetuating contributing factors are not adequately controlled, the inflammatory and pain mediators may return after the surgery.

Acute TMJ disc displacement without reduction can generally be treated by conservative therapies (see Chapter 10, "Acute TMJ

Disc Displacement without Reduction"). Invasive procedures are an option if a patient does not appear to be improving from the conservative therapy, is frustrated with the slow progress, or desires to obtain the rapid improvement generally achieved through arthrocentesis or arthroscopic surgery.[63] Studies show conservative therapy, arthrocentesis, and arthroscopic surgery provide a similar degree of improvement for this disorder.[68,69] Flushing the pain and inflammatory mediators out of the TMJ through arthrocentesis or arthroscopic surgery appears (a) to eliminate the TMJ pain caused by these mediators and (b) to enable patients to stretch the retrodiscal tissue rapidly, thereby enabling them to regain a normal opening. If the perpetuating contributing factors (parafunctional habits, etc.) are not adequately controlled prior to the procedure, the inflammatory and pain mediators may return after the surgery, and the contributing factors will need be addressed to resolve the new symptoms.[70,71]

When it becomes evident that conservative therapy will not be successful, referral for these surgical procedures should not be delayed, for the longer the patient has this disorder, the less likely he or she is to receive as much benefit from arthrocentesis and the more likely the patient may need arthroscopic surgery (which is more expensive and invasive).[72] TMJ injections with anesthetic, steroid, and/or sodium hyaluronate (not yet approved by the FDA for use in the TMJ) have also been recommended and are reasonable considerations for treating this disorder.[73,74]

Consider referring patients whose TMD symptoms are due to this disorder when patients (a) do not appear to be improving from the conservative therapy, (b) are frustrated with the slow progress and desire more rapid results through surgical intervention, or (c) desire to obtain the rapid improvement generally achieved through arthrocentesis or arthroscopic surgery. My

most common referral to oral surgeons are patients with this disorder who do not adequately improve from conservative therapy. Keep in mind that, if the perpetuating contributing factors are not adequately controlled, the inflammatory and pain mediators may return after the surgery.

TMJ ankylosis can be due to fibrous or osseous union within the TMJ, causing a firm restriction of the condyle, which is generally not associated with pain. Digital palpation of the ankylosed TMJ during maximal movements will demonstrate no or very limited translation of the condyle.[14,75,76] The patient's limited opening due to ankylosis will not be improved by conservative TMD therapy.

Treatment for fibrous ankylosis depends on the degree of dysfunction and discomfort. If a patient has adequate function and minimal discomfort, no treatment is indicated. If a patient desires to have the disc-condyle assembly released, TMJ surgery (e.g., arthroscopy or open joint surgery) will be needed.[75] Bony ankylosis is rare, and treatment involves open joint surgery to resect and recontour the osseous structures and any additional interventions that may be necessary.[14,75] Consider referring patients with an ankylosed TMJ when the degree of dysfunction and discomfort are such that the patients desire surgical intervention.

Arthrocentesis, arthroscopy, and open joint procedures are traditionally used to treat TMD, but a modified condylotomy and joint replacement may be considered.

Arthrocentesis is historically performed by placing a needle, connected to a syringe with saline, into the TMJ and then injecting the saline into the joint. The mandible is generally manipulated to allow the fluid into the recesses of the TMJ, and the syringe plunger is pulled back, sucking the mixture from the TMJ. The syringe is removed from the needle, replaced by more fresh saline, and the procedure is repeated multiple times to irrigate the inflammatory and pain mediators from the TMJ. More recently many practitioners use two ports so a continuous flow of saline flushes the TMJ, and the mandible is similarly manipulated to allow the saline access to the recesses of the TMJ.[77] Steroid is often placed in the joint space at the end of the procedure.

Arthroscopy uses two ports to provide constant flushing of the TMJ with saline. Additionally a scope is inserted through one port and small instruments are inserted through the other. This enables the surgeon to view the TMJ, remove adhesions, and provide other minor surgical procedures.

The success rate for arthroscopic surgery ranges from 60 to 93 percent, and a retrospective study of 450 arthroscopic surgeries provides a sense of its effectiveness. Patients reported an average pain reduction of 66 percent (mean, 0 to 10 visual analog scale score dropped from 8.8 to 3.2), patients had statistically significant improvement in opening and excursive movements, and 22 percent of the patients required another surgery within 1 year.[78]

Open joint surgery provides surgeons with better visibility and access than can be obtained with arthroscopy. Surgeons will require this type of access when treating a bony ankylosis, removing a previously placed alloplastic disc, removing a neoplasm, etc.

Modified condylotomy benefits patients primarily by decreasing the ability to load the TMJ. This is accomplished by the surgeon providing a sagittal split of the ramus, wiring the teeth together, and allowing the condyle to obtain an unloaded position within the TMJ. One study reported that 78 percent of the patients receiving this procedure found it was tremendously helpful, 15 percent reported it was somewhat helpful, and 7 percent found it had no effect.[79] It is believed that similar unloading of the TMJ can be achieved with a stabilization appliance that is adjusted using the *neutral jaw posture* described in "Mandibular Positions and Bite Registration" in Chapter 12. Additionally,

minimal loading of the TMJ can be achieved throughout the day if the patient learns to keep the masticatory muscles relaxed.

Joint replacement can be partial replacement (i.e., limited to the condyle) or total replacement of the TMJ. A surgeon can replace portions of the joint with tissues from a patient's body (i.e., a rib to replace the condyle) or with different alloplastic prostheses available. If a patient had this procedure, the case is not being followed, and the patient's general dentist is unsure of the patient's replacement type or management, it is recommended the practitioner refer the patient to, or work in conjunction with, someone who has greater expertise in this area.

Alloplastic disc implants composed of Teflon-Proplast and Silastic have been used as prosthetic replacements for discs. They have a history of fragmenting, stimulating a foreign-body response that can cause a progressive degeneration of the condyle and glenoid fossa. A specific protocol has been recommended for these implants and total joint prostheses.[80] If the practitioner is unsure of the disc implant type or management, it is recommended the practitioner refer the patient to, or work in conjunction with, someone who has greater expertise in this area.

Postsurgical exercises are a very important component of the surgery's success.[81] If a physical therapist will be involved in a patient's follow-up, it is appropriate for the patient to be referred to a physical therapist prior to surgery. This enables the patient to learn about the postsurgical exercises, possibly start them, and schedule the recommended postsurgical appointments. Patients who receive physical therapy after TMJ surgery have better results.[82,83] The immediate postsurgical use of stabilization appliances is controversial.

REFERENCES

1. Pertes RA. Occlusal appliance therapy. In: Pertes RA, Gross SG (eds). Clinical Management of

Temporomandibular Disorders and Orofacial Pain. Chicago: Quintessence, 1995:197–210.

2. Okeson JP. Management of Temporomandibular Disorders and Occlusion, 5th edition. St Louis: CV Mosby, 2003:98, 218, 507, 555.

3. Morrish RB Jr, Stround LP. Long-term management of the TMD patient. In: Pertes RA, Gross SG (eds). Clinical Management of Temporomandibular Disorders and Orofacial Pain. Chicago: Quintessence, 1995:273–95.

4. Tarantola GJ, Becker IM, Gremillion H, Pink F. The effectiveness of equilibration in the improvement of signs and symptoms in the stomatognathic system. Int J Periodontics Restorative Dent 1998;18(6):594–603.

5. Okeson JP (ed), for the American Academy of Orofacial Pain. Orofacial Pain: Guidelines for Assessment, Diagnosis and Management. Chicago: Quintessence, 1996:150–3.

6. Pertes RA. Occlusal appliance therapy. In: Pertes RA, Gross SG (eds). Clinical Management of Temporomandibular Disorders and Orofacial Pain. Chicago: Quintessence, 1995:197–210.

7. Obrez A, Turp JC. The effect of musculoskeletal facial pain on registration of maxillomandibular relationships and treatment planning: a synthesis of the literature. J Prosthet Dent 1998;79(4): 439–45.

8. Dawson PE. New definition for relating occlusion to varying conditions of the temporomandibular joint. J Prosthet Dent 1995;74:619–27.

9. McNeill C. Management of temporomandibular disorders: concepts and controversies. J Prosthet Dent 1997;77:510–22.

10. Dental Practice Parameters Committee. American Dental Association's dental practice parameters: temporomandibular (craniomandibular) disorders. J Am Dent Assoc Suppl 1997;128:29–32–S.

11. Ash MM. Occlusal adjustment: quo vadis? Cranio 2003;21(1):1–4.

12. Obrez A, Turp JC. The effect of musculoskeletal facial pain on registration of maxillomandibular relationships and treatment planning: a synthesis of the literature. J Prosthet Dent 1998;79(4): 439–45.

13. Goldstein BH. Temporomandibular disorders: a review of current understanding. Oral Surg Oral Med Oral Pathol Oral Radiol Endod 1999;88: 379–85.

14. American Academy of Orofacial Pain, with Okeson JP (ed). Orofacial Pain: Guidelines for Assessment, Diagnosis and Management. Chicago: Quintessence, 1996:117, 137, 141–58.

15. Tsukiyama Y, Baba K, Clark GT. An evidence-based assessment of occlusal adjustment as a treatment for temporomandibular disorders. J Prosthet Dent 2001;86:57–66.

16. Clark GT, Tsukiyama Y, Baba K, Watanabe T. Sixty-eight years of experimental occlusal interference studies: what have we learned? J Prosthet Dent 1999;2:704–13.

17. Forssell H, Kalso E, Koskela P, Vehmanen R, Puukka P, Alanen P. Occlusal treatments in temporomandibular disorders: a qualitative systematic review of randomized controlled trials. Pain 1999;83(3):549–60.

18. Wenneberg B, Nystrom T, Carlsson GE. Occlusal equilibration and other stomatognathic treatment in patients with mandibular dysfunction and headache. J Prosthet Dent 1988;59(4):478 83.

19. Yatani H, Minakuchi H, Matsuka Y, Fujisawa T, Yamashita A. The long-term effects of occlusal therapy on self-administered treatment outcomes of TMD. J Orofac Pain 1998;12(1):75–88.

20. Hilsen KL (ed), for the American College of Prosthodontics. Temporomandibular disorder prosthodontics: treatment and management goals. J Prosthodontics 1995;4:58–64.

21. De Boever JA, Carlsson GE, Klineberg IJ. Need for occlusal therapy and prosthodontic treatment in the management of temporomandibular disorders. Part II: Tooth loss and prosthodontic treatment. J Oral Rehabil 2000;27(8):647–59.

22. Kirveskari P. The role of occlusal adjustment in the management of temporomandibular disorders. Oral Surg Oral Med Oral Pathol Oral Radiol Endod 1997;83:87–90.

23. Tarantola GJ, Becker IM, Gremillion H, Pink F. The effectiveness of equilibration in the improvement of signs and symptoms in the stomatognathic system. Int J Periodontics Restorative Dent 1998;18(6):594–603.

24. Forssell H, Kirveskari P, Kangasniemi P. Effect of occlusal adjustment on mandibular dysfunction: a double-blind study. Acta Odontol Scand 1986;44(2):63–9.

25. Nassif NJ. Perceived malocclusion and other teeth-associated signs and symptoms in temporomandibular disorders. Compend Contin Educ Dent 2001;22(7):577–85.

26. Syrop SB. Initial management of temporomandibular disorders. Dent Today 2002;21(8):52–7.

27. Dawson PE, for the American Equilibration Society. Position paper regarding diagnosis, management, and treatment of temporomandibular disorders. J Prosthet Dent 1999;81(2):174–8.

28. Tsolka P, Morris RW, Preiskel HW. Occlusal adjustment therapy for craniomandibular disorders: a clinical assessment by a double-blind method. J Prosthet Dent 1992;68(6):957–64.

29. Jeffery RW, McGuire MT, French SA. Prevalence and correlates of large weight gains and losses. Int J Obes Relat Metab Disord 2002;26(7):969–72.

30. Dahlstrom L. Conservative treatment of mandibular dysfunction: clinical, experimental and electromyographic studies of biofeedback and occlusal appliances. Swed Dent J Suppl 1984;24:1–45.

31. Kirveskari P, Jamsa T, Alanen P. Occlusal adjustment and the incidence of demand for temporomandibular disorder treatment. J Prosthet Dent 1998;79:433–8.

32. Clark GT, Tsukiyama Y, Baba K, Simmons M. The validity and utility of disease detection methods and of occlusal therapy for temporomandibular disorders. Oral Surg Oral Med Oral Pathol Oral Radiol Endod 1997;83:101–6.

33. De Boever JA, Carlsson GE, Klineberg IJ. Need for occlusal therapy and prosthodontic treatment in the management of temporomandibular disorders. Part I: Occlusal interferences and occlusal adjustment. J Oral Rehabil 2000;27(5):367–79.

34. Conti PCR, Ferreira PM, Pegoraro LF, Conti JV, Salvador MCG. A cross-sectional study of prevalence and etiology of signs and symptoms of temporomandibular disorders in high school and university students. J Orofac Pain 1996;10(3):254–62.

35. Pullinger AG, Seligman DA, Gornbein JA. A multiple logistic regression analysis of the risk and relative odds of temporomandibular disorders as a function of common occlusal features. J Dent Res 1993;72(6):968–79

36. McHorris WH. Occlusal adjustment via selective cutting of natural teeth. Part II: Int J Periodontics Restorative Dent 1985;5(6):8–29.

37. Yatani H, Minakuchi H, Matsuka Y, Fujisawa T, Yamashita A. The long-term effect of occlusal therapy on self-administered treatment outcomes of TMD. J Orofac Pain 1998;12(1):75–88.

38. Lagerstrom L, Egermark I, Carlsson G. Signs and symptoms for temporomandibular disorders in 19-year-old individuals who have undergone or-

thodontic treatment. Swed Dent J 1998;22:177–86.

39. Henrikson T. Temporomandibular disorders and mandibular function in relation to class II malocclusion and orthodontic treatment: a controlled, prospective and longitudinal study. Swed Dent J Suppl 1999;134:1–144.

40. Egermark I, Thilander B. Craniomandibular disorders with special reference to orthodontic treatment: an evaluation from childhood to adulthood. Am J Orthod Dentofac Orthop 1992;101(1):28–34.

41. Henrikson T, Nilner M, Kurol J. Signs of temporomandibular disorders in girls receiving orthodontic treatment: a prospective and longitudinal comparison with untreated class II malocclusions and normal occlusion subjects. Eur J Orthod 2000;22(3):271–81.

42. Kim MR, Graber TM, Viana MA. Orthodontics and temporomandibular disorder: a meta-analysis. Am J Orthod Dentofac Orthop 2002;121(5):438–46.

43. McNamara JA. Orthodontic treatment and temporomandibular disorders. Oral Surg Oral Med Oral Pathol Oral Radiol Endod 1997;83:107–17.

44. Turp JC, McNamara JA Jr. Orthodontic treatment and temporomandibular disorder: is there a relationship? Part 2: Clinical implications. J Orofac Orthop 1997;58(3):136–43.

45. Egermark I, Ronnerman A. Temporomandibular disorders in the active phase of orthodontic treatment. J Oral Rehabil 1995;22(8):613–8.

46. Imai T, Okamoto T, Kaneko T, Umeda K, Yamamoto T, Nakamura S. Long-term follow-up of clinical symptoms in TMD patients who underwent occlusal reconstruction by orthodontic treatment. Eur J Orthod 2000;22(1):61–7.

47. Glass EG, Glaros AG, McGlynn FD. Myofascial pain dysfunction: treatments used by ADA members. Cranio 1993;11(1):25–9.

48. Greene CS. Orthodontics and temporomandibular disorders. Dent Clin North Am 1988;32(3):529–38.

49. Rodrigues-Garcia RCM, Sakai S, Rugh JD, Hatch JP, Tiner BD, van Sickels JE, Clark GM, Nemeth DZ, Bays RA. Effects of major class II occlusal corrections on temporomandibular signs and symptoms. J Orofac Pain 1998;12(3):185–92.

50. Dervis E, Tuncer E. Long-term evaluations of temporomandibular disorders in patients undergoing orthognathic surgery compared with a con-

trol group. Oral Surg Oral Med Oral Pathol Oral Radiol Endod 2002;94(5):554–60.

51. White CS, Dolwick MF. Prevalence and variance of temporomandibular dysfunction in orthognathic surgery patients. Int J Adult Orthod Orthognath Surg 1992;7(1):7–14.

52. Tanenbaum D. Prosthodontic therapy. In: Kaplan AS, Assael LA (eds). Temporomandibular Disorders: Diagnosis and Treatment. Philadelphia: WB Saunders, 1991:559–75.

53. Obrez A, Turp JC. The effect of musculoskeletal facial pain on registration of maxillomandibular relationships and treatment planning: a synthesis of the literature. J Prosthet Dent 1998;79(4): 439–45.

54. Pullinger AG, Seligman DA. Quantification and validation of predictive values of occlusal variables in temporomandibular disorders using a multifactorial analysis. J Prosthet Dent 2000;83(1): 66–75.

55. Litvak H, Malament KA. Prosthodontic management of temporomandibular disorders and orofacial pain. J Prosthet Dent 1993;69(1): 77–84.

56. Ettala-Ylitalo UM, Markanen H, Syrjanen S. Functional disturbances of the masticatory system and the effect of prosthetic treatment in patients treated with fixed prosthesis four years earlier. Cranio 1987;5(1):43–9.

57. Schiffman EL. Recent advances: diagnosis and management of TMJ disorders. In: Hardin JF (ed). Clark's Clinical Dentistry, volume 2. Philadelphia: JB Lippincott, 1998:1–5.

58. Ribeiro RF, Tallents RH, Katzberg RW, Murphy WC, Moss ME, Magalhaes AC, Tavano O. The prevalence of disc displacement in symptomatic and asymptomatic volunteers aged 6 to 25 years. J Orofac Pain 1997;11(1):37–47.

59. Montgomery MT, Gordon SM, van Sickels JE, Harms SE. Changes in signs and symptoms following temporomandibular joint disc repositioning surgery. J Oral Maxillofac Surg 1992;50(4):320–8.

60. Lieberman JM, Bradrick JP, Indresano AT, Smith AS, Bellon EM. Dermal grafts of the temporomandibular joint: postoperative appearance on MR images. Radiology 1990;176(1):199–203.

61. Brown DT, Gaudet EL Jr. Temporomandibular disorder treatment outcomes: second report of a large-scale prospective clinical study. Cranio 2002;20(4):244–53.

62. Marbach JJ, Ballard GT, Frankel MR, Raphael KG. Patterns of TMJ surgery: evidence of sex differences. J Am Dent Assoc 1997;128:609–14.

63. Reston JT, Turkelson CM. Meta-analysis of surgical treatments for temporomandibular articular disorders. J Oral Maxillofac Surg 2003;61(1): 3–10.

64. Stegenga B. Osteoarthritis of the temporomandibular joint organ and its relationship to disc displacement. J Orofac Pain 2001;15(3):193–205.

65. American Society of Temporomandibular Joint Surgeons. Guidelines for diagnosis and management of disorders involving the temporomandibular joint and related musculoskeletal structures [White paper]. Cranio 2003;21(1):68–76.

66. Wexler GB, McKinney MW. Temporomandibular treatment outcomes within five diagnostic categories. Cranio 1999;17(1):30–7.

67. Ganzberg S, Quek SYP. Pharmacotherapy. In: Pertes RA, Gross SG (eds). Clinical Management of Temporomandibular Disorders and Orofacial Pain. Chicago: Quintessence, 1995:211–26.

68. Schiffman E, Look J, Fricton J, Swift J, Wikes C, Templeton B, Anderson Q. TMJ disk displacement without reduction: a randomized clinical trial [abstract 3004]. J Dent Res (Special Issue) 1997;76:389.

69. Murakami K, Hosaka H, Moriya Y, Segami N, Iizuka T. Short-term treatment outcome study for the management of temporomandibular joint closed lock: a comparison of arthrocentesis to nonsurgical therapy and arthroscopic lysis and lavage. Oral Surg Oral Med Oral Pathol Oral Radiol Endod 1995;80(3):253–7.

70. Schiffman E. Five-year followup of RCT comparing surgical and non-surgical TMJ acute locks. In: 26th Scientific Meeting on Orofacial Pain and Temporomandibular Disorders, March 23–25, 2001, Washington DC. Mt Royal, NJ: American Academy of Orofacial Pain, 2001.

71. Dimitroulis G. A review of 56 cases of chronic closed lock treated with temporomandibular joint arthroscopy. J Oral Maxillofac Surg 2002;60(5): 519–24.

72. Sakamoto I, Yoda T, Tsukahara H, Imai H, Enomoto S. Comparison of the effectiveness of arthrocentesis in acute and chronic closed lock: analysis of clinical and arthroscopic findings. Cranio 2000;18(4):264–71.

73. Sato S, Sakamoto M, Kawamura H, Motegi K. Disc position and morphology in patients with

nonreducing disc displacement treated by injection of sodium hyaluronate. Int J Oral Maxillofac Surg 1999;28(4):253–7.

74. Suarez OF, Ourique SAM. An alternate technique for management of acute closed locks. Cranio 2000;18(3):168–73.

75. Pertes RA, Gross SG. Disorders of the temporomandibular joint. In: Pertes RA, Gross SG (eds). Clinical Management of Temporomandibular Disorders and Orofacial Pain. Chicago: Quintessence, 1995:85–6.

76. Manganello-Souza LC, Mariani PB. Temporomandibular joint ankylosis: report of 14 cases. Int J Oral Maxillofac Surg 2003;32(1):24–9.

77. Nitzan DW. Arthrocentesis for management of severe close lock of the temporomandibular joint. Oral Maxillofac Surg Clin North Am 1994;6:245–57.

78. Abd-Ul-Salam H, Weinberg S, Kryshtalskyj B. The incidence of reoperation after temporomandibular joint arthroscopic surgery: a retrospective study of 450 consecutive joints. Oral Surg Oral Med Oral Pathol Oral Radiol Endod 2002;93(4):408–11.

79. McKenna SJ, Cornella F, Gibbs SJ. Long-term follow-up of modified condylotomy for internal derangement of the temporomandibular joint. Oral Surg Oral Med Oral Pathol Oral Radiol Endod 1996;81(5):509–15.

80. American Association of Oral and Maxillofacial Surgeons. Recommendations for management of patients with temporomandibular joint implants. Temporomandibular Joint Implant Surgery Workshop. J Oral Maxillofac Surg 1993;51(10): 1164–72.

81. American Society of Temporomandibular Joint Surgeons. Guidelines for diagnosis and management of disorders involving the temporomandibular joint and related musculoskeletal structures [White paper]. Cranio 2003;21(1):68–76.

82. Kuwahara T, Bessette RW, Maruyama T. The influence of postoperative treatment on the results of TMJ meniscectomy. Part II: Comparison of chewing movement. Cranio 1996;14(2):121–31.

83. Austin BD, Shupe SM. The role of physical therapy in recovery after temporomandibular joint surgery. J Oral Maxillofac Surg 1993;51:495–8.

Chapter 19

Integrating Multidisciplinary Therapies

Practitioners from many disciplines find providing their disciplines' therapies to patients with TMD symptoms tends to improve these symptoms. Prosthodontists, orthodontists, and oral surgeons (providing orthognathic surgery) may observe this as they improve a patient's occlusal stability. Psychologists and psychiatrists may observe this as they treat patients for stress, anxiety, aggression, depression, etc. Additionally, physical therapists, massage therapists, and chiropractors may observe this as they treat patients for neck dysfunction.

Practitioners from many disciplines can target their therapies to treat patients' TMD disorders. Oral surgeons remove the inflammatory and pain mediators from the TMJ. Psychologists teach patients to break their daytime parafunctional habits and continually maintain their masticatory muscles in a relaxed state. Physical therapists, physicians, and massage therapists treat the masticatory muscles and TMJ as they would most other muscles or joints in the body. Acupuncturists balance the acupuncture meridian corresponding to TMD symptoms. Dentists fabricate occlusal appliances and prescribe medications.

With practitioners from so many various disciplines able to help relieve TMD patients' symptoms, the goal in developing a treatment plan is to identify which practitioners and therapies would provide each patient with the greatest benefits with the least costs, e.g., in terms of price, time, and adverse sequelae. This will vary with each patient, and awareness of a patient's perpetuating contributing factors, which are identified during the initial evaluation, will help develop the patient's best personal course of treatment.

☯ FOCAL POINT

With practitioners from so many various disciplines able to help relieve TMD patients' symptoms, the goal in developing a treatment plan is to identify which practitioners and therapies would provide each patient with the greatest benefits with the least costs, e.g., in terms of price, time, and adverse sequelae.

TREATMENT SUMMARIES AND CLINICAL IMPLICATIONS

There is no scientifically determined protocol for treating TMD patients, but the following treatment summaries and clinical implications are based on the literature and my clinical experience.

Occlusal Appliances

These generally provide a beneficial effect for masticatory muscle pain, TMJ pain, TMJ noise, and jaw mobility.[1] Wearing an occlusal appliance at night generally reduces morning TMD symptoms, is very easy for patients to do, and causes little interruption in their daily lives.[2] There are many different types of appliances, but no one appliance appears to be significantly superior to another.[3]

⊙ QUICK CONSULT
Using an Occlusal Appliance at Night
Wearing an occlusal appliance at night generally reduces morning TMD symptoms, is very easy for patients to do, and causes little interruption to their daily lives.

Self-management Therapy

This has been reported to help 60 to 90 percent of TMD patients. These instructions are easy for patients to implement, and this should be the first treatment provided to the majority of people diagnosed with TMD. Patients are asked to read the "TMD Self-management Therapies" handout (Appendix 3) during their initial evaluation appointment. The handout is then reviewed with them to emphasize its importance and answer any questions. Additionally some contributing factors are identified during this discussion, e.g., excessive caffeine consumption and stomach sleeping. A trained staff member can effectively review these instructions with patients.[4]

Closure Muscle-stretching Exercise

This is designed to decrease the masseter, temporalis, and medial pterygoid muscle pain and increase range of motion.[5] Patients should be able to optimize the benefits derived from this exercise by warming the painful area(s) before stretching the muscles.[6] This exercise is easy and not time-consuming. This exercise is not recommended to patients who have significant TMJ or lateral pterygoid muscle pain, because it may aggravate those structures.

Ask appropriate TMD patients to read the "Jaw Muscle-stretching Exercise" handout (Appendix 5) during the initial evaluation appointment. Then review it with them and answer any questions. A trained staff member can effectively review these instructions with patients.[7]

Posture Exercises

"Posture Improvement Exercises," Appendix 6, provided a mean TMD and neck symptom reduction of 42 and 38 percent among TMD patients whose pain was primarily of muscle origin.[8] Typically, TMD patients with neck symptoms do not derive as much improvement from conservative TMD therapies as do other patients.[9] Therefore, attempt to reduce cervical symptoms among TMD patients who have them. Well-motivated patients with neck pain may find the posture exercise handout beneficial. Additionally the study found TMD patients with a further forward head posture obtained greater TMD symptom benefit from these exercises.[8]

▼ TECHNICAL TIP
Observing Cervical Symptoms
Typically, TMD patients with neck symptoms do not derive as much improvement from conservative TMD therapies as do other patients. Therefore, attempt to reduce cervical symptoms among TMD patients who have them.

Massage and Trigger-point Compression

These are effective techniques to temporarily increase the muscle's vasodilation, inactivate trigger points, and thereby decrease the muscle pain and associated symptoms. These techniques are not in the "TMD Self-management Therapies" handout, but can easily be taught to patients who are motivated to perform additional self-management therapies. These techniques can be applied to the masticatory and/or cervical regions. Some TMD patients prefer having a massage therapist provide these, but this is not cost effective. Keep in mind that the contributing factors perpetuating the irritable trigger points must also be addressed and controlled, or the trigger points will tend to reactivate.

Trigger-point Injections

These can be administered for persistent trigger points and may provide an immediate decrease in trigger-point pain and its associated symptoms. It may be helpful to follow the injection with spray and stretch, hot packs, and have the patient actively move the injected muscle through its full range of motion. Generally, over days or weeks, the pain gradually returns, but not to the initial intensity. Administering repeated trigger-point injections may provide a stair-step lowering of pain and its associated symptoms. Trigger-point injections are recommended only after traditional conservative managements in addition to exercises and other physical therapy modalities have failed to provide a lasting effect.

Physical Therapy

This can be an effective adjunct that is generally beneficial for masticatory and/or concomitant neck pain. For TMD patients who have neck pain to the degree that they desire to be referred to a physical therapist, this is generally done at their initial evaluation appointment. By using the other conservative TMD therapies, I can generally resolve patients' TMD symptoms satisfactorily. For patients whose TMD symptoms are refractory to therapy, I consider referring them for a physical therapist's assistance in treating the masticatory structures.

Practitioners may desire to refer TMD patients to physical therapy for stretching exercises, physical therapy modalities, posture and posture biomechanics training, education on changing or correcting sleep posture, education on diaphragmatic breathing, and treatment of concomitant neck pain. Two examples of physical therapist referrals are provided in Appendix 9, "Examples of Physical Therapy Consultations."

Acupuncture

This has been reported to be as effective as occlusal appliance therapy in relieving TMD symptoms, but appears to lose its effectiveness over time. A study also found that TMD patients who did not improve with occlusal appliance therapy usually did not improve with acupuncture.[10] Treatment with acupuncture typically involves multiple treatments with periodic follow-up treatments to maintain its effectiveness. I do not refer TMD patients for acupuncture because I prefer using other conservative therapies rather than subjecting patients to long-term continual acupuncture treatments.

▼ TECHNICAL TIP
Referring Patients for Acupuncture

I do not refer TMD patients for acupuncture because I prefer using other conservative therapies rather than subjecting patients to long-term continual acupuncture treatments.

Chiropractics

This has been shown to be beneficial in treating neck pain and cervicogenic headaches.[11,12] Concomitant neck pain negatively impacts TMD, and the patients with such pain do not respond as well to conservative TMD therapy.[9] Chiropractics is one of many avenues that can be used to treat cervical pain. It is felt that this has been an effective treatment approach when a patient's neck pain is resolved and the improvement is maintained after two or three chiropractic treatments. On the other hand, if a patient cannot obtain adequate relief or maintain the improvement after two or three chiro- practic treatments, I recommend traditional medical interventions rather than further chiropractic therapy.

Some chiropractors also directly treat the masticatory system. These treatments vary with the chiropractor, but it is speculated that traditional TMD therapies are probably more effective. I currently do not refer pa- tients to chiropractors, but they are a reason- able alternative for treatment of coexisting neck pain.

Magnetic Therapy

This has been shown to be beneficial for per- sistent neck pain, headache, and other mus- cle or arthritis-like pains.[13-15] Clinically it has been observed that some patients find magnetic therapy beneficial in treating their TMD pain, whereas a few others find that the coldness of the magnet aggravates their pain. It would be reasonable for TMD pa- tients with refractory neck or TMD pain to try magnetic therapy. Esthetic considerations limit the application of magnetic therapy for the masticatory region primarily to the evening and night.

Breaking Daytime Parafunctional, Muscle-tightening, or Fatiguing Habits

This appears to be a very beneficial therapy for treating daytime TMD symptoms, but not the symptoms with which a patient awakes. Practitioners may desire to refer pa- tients to a psychologist for this treatment. Psychologists will often include relaxation and stress management in conjunction with these instructions and, if this does not ade- quately resolve the daytime pain, they can escalate therapy by providing biofeedback with relaxation.

Relaxation

This has been shown to reduce TMD symp- toms[16-18] and is traditionally provided in conjunction with habit-reversal and biofeed- back therapies.[19-21] Generally patients find that relaxation not only reduces their TMD pain temporarily, but also helps them be- come aware of what tense and relaxed masti- catory muscles feel like and develop the capability to relax these muscles rapidly whenever they notice the muscles are tight.

Clinically it has been observed that few TMD patients who are just handed an au- diotape program have the motivation to lis- ten to the tape and practice the therapy con- sistently.[22] Most appear to need a trained relaxation instructor to motivate them to practice and assist them with problems they may encounter.

Patients who are motivated to practice this therapy on their own can be given the options of using a relaxation tape or compact disk purchased from a bookstore, quietly lis- tening to soothing music, taking a warm re- laxing shower or bath, quietly sitting and taking slow deep breaths, etc. Some patients may prefer to practice the therapy while using a heating pad. They should be encour- aged to use the therapy form that provides them the greatest degree of relaxation and enjoyment. The more pleasurable the experi- ence is, the greater is the probability for long-term compliance.

Once patients become aware of what re- laxed muscles feel like and develop the abil- ity to reestablish this relaxed state whenever they choose, they must identify when they are tensing their masticatory muscles or performing parafunctional habits, and consciously stop these habits and bring forth the relaxed state they learned.

This enables patients to obtain long-term daytime symptom relief. If this therapy is used just prior to sleep, it often leads to more peaceful sleep and a decrease in nocturnal parafunctional habits.[23]

Hypnotherapy

Hypnotherapy, or hypnosis, assists patients to attain a deep level of relaxation and is beneficial in treating TMD symptoms.[24,25] Throughout the hypnotic session, patients maintain control of their thoughts and can leave the relaxed state whenever they desire.[24] Patients are generally given an audiocassette or compact disk of one of the hypnotic sessions that they repeatedly listen to at home, which enables them to practice attaining the relaxed state and deal with any residual or future stress or anxiety.[24,26] This provides a similar effect as relaxation therapy to improve daytime symptoms. Listening to the tape just prior to sleep often leads to more peaceful sleep and a decrease in nocturnal parafunctional habits.[27]

Biofeedback with Relaxation

This is an effective adjunctive therapy to treat a TMD patient's daytime symptoms, but not the symptoms with which he or she awakes. It is time-consuming therapy, the patient must be taught to transfer its effect from the therapist's office into everyday life, and the patient must be motivated to practice it. The relaxation portion appears to be the more beneficial component of this combined therapy.[28] My experience with patients who are first taught habit-reversal and relaxation techniques is that those who find they continue to have daytime symptoms and relate they can relax their entire body except their masticatory muscles often find biofeedback exceptionally beneficial.

Stress Management

This teaches coping skills to deal with stressful situations in life. Such situations typically exacerbate the tendency for patients to perform parafunctional habits and hold more tension in their muscles. One study found that stress management combined with biofeedback, relaxation, and occlusal appliance therapy increased a TMD patient's rate of improvement and decreased the relapse that may occur with occlusal appliance therapy alone.[29] This therapy is time consuming, and patients tend be less compliant with counseling than with occlusal appliance therapy.[30] Therefore, patients being referred for this therapy should be interested in receiving it and motivated to practice it.

Pharmacological Management

This can generally reduce TMD pain and sometimes speed recovery. I avoid prescribing muscle relaxants to patients with chronic TMD symptoms, unless they have an acute exacerbation. If a patient with chronic symptoms desires a prescription, medications that can be used long term are typically prescribed, i.e., nonsteroid anti-inflammatory drugs (NSAIDs) on an as-needed basis and/or tricyclic antidepressants. Patients with chronic TMD symptoms typically need to change their perpetuating factors to obtain long-term control of their symptoms. If possible, it is preferable to control a patient's chronic TMD symptoms through nonpharmaceutical management, e.g., self-management therapies, occlusal appliance therapy, or habit-breaking techniques.

▼ **TECHNICAL TIP**
Controlling Chronic TMD Symptoms
It is preferable to control a patient's chronic TMD symptoms through nonpharmaceutical management, e.g., self-management therapies,

occlusal appliance therapy, or habit-breaking techniques.

TMD pharmacological management most commonly involves over-the-counter analgesics (including NSAIDs), prescription anti-inflammatory drugs, muscle relaxants, low-dose tricyclic antidepressants, nutritional supplements, and topical analgesic cream. The "TMD Self-management Therapies" handout (Appendix 3) recommends over-the-counter medications for patients who desire to try one. Practitioners must weigh the medication's potential benefits against its side-effect risks, along with their competence in managing patients taking the medication.[31]

Occlusal Therapy

This generally improves occlusal stability, thereby decreasing the negative impact that clenching or bruxing has on the masticatory system.[32-34] Occlusal therapy addresses only one aspect of the multifactorial TMD problem. The TMD therapies provided in this book are comparatively much less expensive (regarding price, time, adverse sequelae, etc.) and provide greater symptom improvement than occlusal therapy. Dentists must keep in mind there are many practitioners outside of the dental profession who can assist with the other aspects of their TMD patient's care.

Most TMD patients have increased tone in their lateral pterygoid muscles and/or TMJ inflammation, making it difficult to position the mandible in centric relation and/or obtain a reproducible closure position.[35,36] Providing occlusal therapy for these patients without first resolving these problems may have a disastrous outcome. For these reasons and others, most practitioners recommend that TMD patients not be initially treated through occlusal therapy.[37-41]

TMD patients with constant chronic symptoms (a) will be given a stabilization appliance that is worn at night, which should provide the patient with an "ideal" occlusion, and (b) will be taught not to touch their teeth together during the day, except momentarily for swallowing and the occasional bumping while eating. Using these two therapies, the teeth almost never touch. If the teeth rarely touch, the occlusion is not a significant factor in any residual TMD symptoms, and it is speculated that any occlusal therapy will provide minimal to no benefit.

Patients with intermittent pain are generally provided the treatment that addresses the contributing factors related to their pain; i.e., patients who awake with pain are given a stabilization appliance that is worn at night, and those with daytime pain are taught not to touch their teeth together during the day. Therefore, it is similarly speculated that any occlusal therapy would have minimal impact on residual TMD symptoms.

Contrary to what some practitioners advocate, occlusal therapy is not needed to maintain a TMD patient's long-term symptom improvement.[37,42,43] Long-term management is discussed in its section later in this chapter.

It is recommended that a patient's occlusion be adjusted at the initial visit only if the TMD symptoms developed as a result of the placement of a restoration that is not in harmony with the rest of the dentition.[32,33,39] In this situation, it is generally much more cost effective to refine the restoration's occlusion than to provide traditional TMD therapy. This typically resolves the TMD symptoms, but the practitioner must keep in mind that there are other potential reasons TMD symptoms develop after the placement of a restoration (see Chapter 8, "TMD Secondary to Dental Treatment").

TMJ Surgery

This is indicated for the treatment of a wide variety of pathological conditions. Among

TMD patients, its purpose is to reduce their symptoms and dysfunction, not to make the TMJ disc-condyle relation "normal." Using conservative TMD therapy, as described in this book, it is relatively rare for TMD patients to need TMJ surgery. One study that tracked over 2,000 TMD patients from many practices found that only 2.5 percent received TMJ surgery (1.4 percent arthrocentesis, 1.0 percent arthroscopy, and 0.1 percent open joint procedures).[44]

TMJ surgery is significantly more expensive than conservative TMD therapy. Based on insurance records, the average cost of TMJ surgery (not including the hospitalization) is two to three times the cost of nonsurgical TMD therapy.[45] Other than for the obvious reasons (e.g., infection, fracture, or neoplastic growth), there are primarily three TMD disorders for which TMD patients might be referred to a surgeon: TMJ inflammation, acute TMJ disc displacement without reduction, and TMJ ankylosis. The referral recommendations for these disorders are discussed in "TMJ Surgery and Implants" in Chapter 18.

A specific protocol has been recommended for patients who have received a TMJ implant or prosthesis.[46] If a practitioner is unsure of a patient's implant type or management, it is recommended the practitioner refer the patient to, or work in conjunction with, someone who has greater expertise in this area.

INTEGRATING CONSERVATIVE THERAPIES

A multidisciplinary treatment approach is generally more effective than any single TMD therapy.[47,48] The most common referrals I initially make are to a physical therapist for treatment of the neck and to a psychologist for training to help patients in breaking daytime habits, relaxation, biofeedback, etc.

▼ **TECHNICAL TIP**

Referring Patients for Adjunctive Treatments

The most common referrals I initially make are to a physical therapist for treatment of the neck and to a psychologist for training to help patients in breaking their daytime habits, relaxation, biofeedback, etc.

Not every TMD patient needs a multidisciplinary treatment approach, and I do not mean to imply this because of the amount of material spent on this concept in this book. Practitioners generally find that patients with minimal symptoms or specific symptom characteristics (e.g., symptoms that primarily occur on awaking) do well with just TMD self-management therapies and an occlusal appliance worn at night. These TMD therapies are traditionally provided by dental practitioners and generally cannot provide satisfactory symptom improvement for patients with more significant daytime symptoms or in need of other therapies. One of the goals of this book is to help readers understand the wide choice of TMD therapies available and how to decide most effectively which would be the most beneficial for the majority of patients the readers evaluate.

During the initial patient evaluation, practitioners will generally identify non-TMD disorders (e.g., neck pain, widespread pain, rheumatic disorders, poor sleep, or depression) that may negatively impact a patient's TMD, decrease the probability that the practitioner will achieve satisfactory TMD symptom improvement, and are part of a patient's list of perpetuating contributing factors.[9,49,50] Patients should be informed about the impact these disorders may have on their TMD symptoms and asked whether they would like a referral.

I may refer patients to a physician for shoulder and/or back pain (dentists can directly refer to physical therapy for head and/or neck pain), a rheumatologist or internist for unexplained generalized muscle and/or joint pain, a neurologist or internist for migraine headaches, an otolaryngologist or physician for ear and/or sinus pain, and a psychologist and/or psychiatrist (whichever the patient prefers, after the different treatment approaches are discussed) for depression or other psychological disorders. Practitioners should not be reluctant to seek additional providers' expertise for other contributing ailments.

Parafunctional and muscle-tensing habits are probably the most significant contributing factors for the majority of TMD patients and can occur during the day and/or at night. It has been suggested that diurnal and nocturnal parafunctional habits are different in their character and origin.[32,51]

◉ QUICK CONSULT

Understanding the Most Significant Contributing Factors

Parafunctional and muscle-tensing habits are probably the most significant contributing factors for the majority of TMD patients.

Diurnal parafunctional habits may include, but are not limited to, teeth clenching or grinding, cheek or tongue biting or chewing, fingernail or cuticle biting and chewing, unusual jaw posture habits, and a wide range of habits related to occupation. Additionally a diurnal habit of tensing or holding tension in the jaw or neck muscles may contribute to the TMD symptoms. TMD symptoms related to diurnal habits have been closely related to increased emotional stress.[32]

Conversely, nocturnal parafunctional habits are generally limited to teeth clenching or grinding. These have been reported to be closely tied to emotional stress, physical exhaustion during waking hours, and sleep patterns.[32,52]

A patient's daily TMD symptom pattern may help identify whether the habits that contribute to the symptoms are diurnal and/or nocturnal. Patients whose nocturnal habits contribute to their symptoms will awake with symptoms, whereas those with contributing diurnal habits will exhibit daytime symptoms.[2,53,54]

The efficacy of some treatments will differ for patients whose habits are diurnal or nocturnal. Studies indicate that relaxation and biofeedback are more effective for patients with diurnal habits, whereas nighttime wear of a stabilization appliance is more effective for patients with nocturnal habits.[55-57]

Clinically patients can learn to break their diurnal parafunctional and muscle-tension habits. They may need a psychologist's help to use external and internal cues and learn how to relax their tight muscles (or drain the tension held in these muscles) (see "Breaking Daytime Habits" in Chapter 16). Patients cannot control their nocturnal parafunctional activity so they need to wear an occlusal appliance at night if these habits are contributing to their TMD symptoms.

Intuitively it makes sense that certain therapies would be more beneficial for patients with specific daily symptom patterns; e.g., breaking a stomach-sleeping habit would probably be more beneficial for a patient who awakes with TMD symptoms rather than a patient who awakes symptom free.

In light of these clinical findings as well as empirical observations, I primarily consider the following therapies *for patients who awake with TMD symptoms*: improvement in sleeping positions, nighttime wear of a stabilization appliance, administration of medications that decrease nocturnal electromyelographic (EMG) activity (e.g., amitriptyline, nortriptyline, or diazepam), and relaxation prior to sleep.[23]

I primarily consider the following therapies for *patients with daytime symptoms*: breaking daytime parafunctional and muscle-tensing habits,[58] relaxation, stress management, biofeedback, daytime wear of a stabilization appliance (as a temporary crutch until diurnal habits are broken or to encourage cognitive awareness to facilitate breaking diurnal habits), and administration of a tri-cyclic antidepressant that can be taken during the day (e.g., desipramine).

Clinically some residual treatment effects appear to carry over to the other portion of the day, so a patient who only has minimal daytime pain may find that nocturnal use of the occlusal appliance provides satisfactory improvement of that pain.

Therapies that appear beneficial for both categories of patients include physiotherapy (heat, ice, ultrasound, iontophoresis, etc.), jaw-stretching exercises, head and neck posture improvement exercises (based on unpublished data), and administration of oral NSAIDs and/or steroids.

Some patients fall into both categories, having symptoms throughout the day, but often a more predominant category can be identified. For these, consider all the aforementioned therapy categories, keeping in mind the more predominant category.

It is recommended that these therapies be modulated with the symptom severity, anticipated compliance, abilities of adjunctive personnel (physical therapist, psychologist, etc.), impact on a patient's lifestyle (for both symptoms and treatment), and costs (in terms of price, time, adverse sequelae, etc.).

Some TMD therapies have not been discussed here because I do not routinely use them or have not developed a good clinical sense for their effect on the daily symptom patterns. It is recommended that the least invasive procedures be used first and, if this adequately resolves the pain, no other treatment is needed.[37,38,42,59]

TMD Refractory to Initial Therapy

Despite the documented success of the various forms of conservative care, some TMD patients do not improve. The reasons vary: the pain's primary etiology may be an unidentified disorder (i.e., referred pain from an acute pulpalgia[60-62]) that mimics TMD; relevant contributing factors may not have

been adequately addressed or even recognized;[63] and patients who have greater TMD pain, nonadaptive coping skills, more psychosocial tendencies, anxiety, depression, widespread pain complaints, and nonspecific symptoms tend not to improve.[64-68]

⊙ **QUICK CONSULT**

Failing with Therapy

A patient's TMD symptoms may not improve because the pain's primary etiology is an unidentified disorder (i.e., referred pain from an acute pulpalgia) that mimics TMD, the relevant contributing factors are not adequately addressed or even recognized, or the patient has a characteristic of patients who tend not to do as well from TMD therapy; i.e., they have greater TMD pain, nonadaptive coping skills, more psychosocial tendencies, anxiety, depression, widespread pain complaints, and nonspecific symptoms.

There is no scientifically determined protocol for proceeding with patients whose TMD symptoms are refractory to initial therapy. If a patient has acute TMJ disc displacement without reduction, it is recommended the practitioner follow the guidance provided in Chapter 10, "Acute TMJ Disc Displacement without Reduction," rather than the related recommendations that follow.

If a patient has not obtained satisfactory improvement in TMD symptoms by using the recommended therapies, the following are recommended in the order listed:

1. Evaluate the patient's compliance with the therapies provided, such as TMD self-management therapies, any additional instructions (e.g., stretching exercises or massage), relaxation exercises, or implementation of biofeedback training into stressful times of the patient's life. The patient may be missing important facets of therapy and need a better understanding of or motivation to perform the procedures.

It is important to document the instructions that patients are given and periodically inquire about them. This reinforces the importance of the instructions and increases the probability of patients' performing them.

2. Reevaluate the patient for non-TMD. The patient's chief complaint may be due to a non-TMD condition, and/or non-TMD contributors (neck pain, fibromyalgia, etc.) may have been missed during the evaluation. If a panoramic radiograph was not previously taken, it is recommended one be taken at this time. Recommend appropriate evaluations for non-TMD conditions and contributors.

3. Review the list of the patient's perpetuating contributing factors and ensure they have been addressed to the degree possible. Some patients may have declined referrals for different components, or some of the components [e.g., fibromyalgia or posttraumatic stress disorder (PTSD)] may not be able to be treated adequately. Patients who previously declined referrals may change their mind at this time.

4. Consider whether the patient appears to have a significant psychosocial component to his or her contributing factors. By this time, the practitioner should have a feel for this and may have heard remarks suggestive of psychosocial stress; e.g., "I hate my job" or "I hate my boss."

Once, a patient with constant 6 out of a possible 10 bilateral jaw, preauricular, and temple pain did not improve from traditional conservative therapy. At her reevaluation appointment, she was questioned about many possible contributing factors, including depression. She admitted she was constantly depressed and had checked "Never" on her initial patient questionnaire because she had previously been treated by a psychologist, the sessions had not helped, and she was afraid of being referred to a psychologist if she marked "Always." Upon discussing the treatments for depression, she was open to trying antidepressant medications. After a psychiatrist placed her on an antidepressant, her TMD pain dropped to a 2 to 3 out of 10.

If your patient appears to have a significant psychosocial component, refer him or her for a psychological evaluation.

5. Ask if the patient tried a tricyclic antidepressant medication? If not, it is recommended the practitioner review the different tricyclic antidepressants ("Tricyclic Antidepressants" in Chapter 17) to determine which might be the most appropriate and ask whether the patient would be interested in trying this therapy.

6. If the patient has not gone to physical therapy for treatment of the masticatory structures, I recommend the practitioner refer the patient at this time. The physical therapist can evaluate the patient for other contributors (e.g., neck pain, or body mechanics at the patient's workstation) and implement local modality therapies. Physical therapists can also teach other therapies within their realm that they believe would be beneficial, e.g., diaphragmatic breathing or posture exercises.

7. If the patient still has not obtained satisfactory TMD improvement and wears a stabilization appliance, at this time consider altering the appliance to an anterior positioning. Does the patient meet the criteria (provided in Chapter 13, "Anterior Positioning Appliance") for this appliance? If the patient does not, it is speculated that this appliance has a low probability of helping the patient.

8. If the patient's parafunctional habits and other contributing factors have been controlled to the extent possible through conservative therapies and the patient has moderate to severe pain primarily from the TMJ, at this time consider referring the patient for a surgical evaluation.

LONG-TERM MANAGEMENT

Through conservative TMD therapies, attempt to satisfactorily reduce patients' symptoms so they need to wear their occlusal appliance only at night. I plan for the great majority of patients to wear their appliance at night for many years.

After patients have obtained and can maintain satisfactory symptom improvement, I like them to test periodically whether the therapies are still needed. Patients naturally do this by periodically forgetting to perform certain therapies, enabling them to discover how beneficial each is. Once they determine which are no longer needed, they can separately discontinue each to observe whether they can maintain their symptom improvement without them.

As symptoms improve, most patients on their own will (a) resume their normal diet and desired caffeine intake; (b) decrease or stop thermotherapy, jaw and posture exercises, and relaxation; and (c) occasionally forget to wear their occlusal appliance or take their medications, unintentionally testing whether they need to continue these.

Even as patients improve and decrease some therapies they were provided, hopefully they will continue (a) to maintain the new tongue and jaw postures they have learned, (b) to keep their muscles relaxed through internal cues, (c) to use the improved daytime and sleep postures they have learned, (d) to reduce their daytime parafunctional habits, and (e) to use the learned coping skills.

TMD tends to be a cyclic disorder that is often related to situations in a patient's life.[47] If the TMD symptoms recur, patients can implement the treatments that they discontinued.

◉ **QUICK CONSULT**

Treating Recurrence of Symptoms

If the TMD symptoms recur, patients can implement the treatments that they discontinued.

Since patients may periodically have some degree of TMD symptom exacerbation, it is recommended that they continue wearing their occlusal appliance at night even though they find it is no longer needed, for, if they stop wearing their occlusal appliance, their teeth may shift and the appliance may no longer fit when they need it. It is also recommended that patients periodically return to their practitioner to ensure the appliance is appropriately adjusted. If patients find they have not needed their appliance and it needs to be replaced, this is probably an appropriate time to discontinue its use.

▼ **TECHNICAL TIP**

Wearing Occlusal Appliance Long Term

Since patients may periodically have some degree of TMD symptom exacerbation, it is recommended that they continue wearing their occlusal appliance at night even though they find it is no longer needed.

The majority of TMD patients are between the ages of 20 and 40.[32] As patients age beyond this range, their TMD has a propensity to resolve. Therefore, over time, most patients will generally be able to discontinue their TMD therapies. Conversely, elderly individuals who never previously had TMD symptoms occasionally seek treatment for TMD. Typically I find that their primary contributing factor is related to being a caregiver or fear related to a health issue.

REFERENCES

1. Bush FM, Abbott FM, Butler JH, Harrington WG. Oral orthotics: design, indications, efficacy and care. In: Hardin JF (ed). Clark's Clinical Dentistry, volume 2, chapter 39. Philadelphia: JB Lippincott, 1998:1–33.
2. Lobbezoo F, Lavigne GJ. Do bruxism and temporomandibular disorders have a cause-and-effect relationship? J Orofac Pain 1997;11(1):15–23.
3. Schiffman EL. Recent advances: diagnosis and management of TMJ disorders. In: Hardin JF (ed). Clark's Clinical Dentistry, volume 2. Philadelphia: JB Lippincott, 1998:1–5.

4. Dworkin SF, Huggins KH, Wilson L, Mancl L, Turner J, Massoth D, LeResche L, Truelove E. A randomized clinical trial using research diagnostic criteria for temporomandibular disorders-axis II to target clinic cases for a tailored self-care TMD treatment program. J Orofac Pain 2002;16(1): 48–63.

5. Dall Arancio D, Fricton J. Randomized controlled study of exercises for masticatory myofascial pain [abstract 76]. J Orofac Pain 1993;7(1): 117.

6. Lentell G, Hetherington T, Eagan J, Morgan M. The use of thermal agents to influence the effectiveness of a low-load prolong stretch. J Orthop Sports Phys Ther 1992;16(5):200–7.

7. Magnusson T, Syren M. Therapeutic jaw exercises and interocclusal therapy: a comparison between two common treatments of temporomandibular disorders. J Swed Dent 1999;22:23–37.

8. Wright EF, Domenech MA, Fischer JR Jr. Usefulness of posture training for TMD patients. J Am Dent Assoc 2000;131(2):202–10.

9. Raphael KG, Marbach JJ, Klausner J. Myofascial face pain: clinical characteristics of those with regional vs. widespread pain. J Am Dent Assoc 2000;131(2):161–71.

10. List T, Helkimo M. Acupuncture and occlusal splint therapy in the treatment of craniomandibular disorders. II: A 1-year follow-up study. Acta Odontol Scand 1992;50(6):375–85.

11. Nilsson N, Christensen HW, Hartvigsen J. The effect of spinal manipulation in the treatment of cervicogenic headache. J Manipulative Physiol Ther 1997;20:326–30.

12. Raphael KG, Marbach JJ. Widespread pain and the effectiveness of oral splints in myofascial face pain. J Am Dent Assoc 2001;132(3):305–16.

13. Foley-Nolan D, Barry C, Coughlan RJ, O'Connor P, Roden D. Pulsed high frequency (27 MHz) electromagnetic therapy for persistent neck pain: a double blind, placebo-controlled study of 20 patients. Orthopedics 1990;13(4): 445–51.

14. Sherman RA, Robson L, Marden LA. Initial exploration of pulsing electromagnetic fields for treatment of migraine. Headache 1998;38(3): 208–13.

15. Vallbona C, Hazlewood CF, Jurida G. Response of pain to static magnetic fields in postpolio patients: a double-blind pilot study. Arch Phys Med Rehabil 1997;78(11):1200–3.

16. Myers CD, White BA, Heft MW. A review of complementary and alternative medicine use for treating chronic facial pain. J Am Dent Assoc 2002;133(9):1189–96.

17. Winocur E, Gavish A, Emodi-Perlman A, Halachmi M, Eli I. Hypnorelaxation as treatment for myofascial pain disorder: a comparative study. Oral Surg Oral Med Oral Pathol Oral Radiol Endod 2002;93(4):429–34.

18. Carlson CR, Bertrand PM, Ehrlich AD, Maxwell AW, Burton RG. Physical self-regulation training for the management of temporomandibular disorders. J Orofac Pain 2001;15(1):47–55.

19. Townsen D, Nicholson RA, Buenaver L, Bush F, Gramling S. Use of a habit reversal treatment for temporomandibular pain in a minimal therapist contact format. J Behav Ther Exp Psychiatry 2001;32(4):221–39.

20. Gramling SE, Neblett J, Grayson R, Townsend D. Temporomandibular disorder: efficacy of an oral habit reversal treatment program. J Behav Ther Exp Psychiatry 1996;27(3):245–55.

21. Dahlstrom L. Conservative treatment of mandibular dysfunction: clinical, experimental and electromyographic studies of biofeedback and occlusal appliances. Swed Dent J Suppl 1984;24: 1–45.

22. Okeson JP, Moody PM, Kemper JT, Haley JV. Evaluation of occlusal splint therapy and relaxation procedures in patients with temporomandibular disorders. J Am Dent Assoc 1983;107(3): 420–4.

23. Lavigne GJ, Goulet J-P, Zucconi M, Morisson F, Lobbezoo F. Sleep disorders and the dental patient: an overview. Oral Surg Oral Med Oral Pathol Oral Radiol Endod 1999;88:257–72.

24. Loitman JE. Pain management: beyond pharmacology to acupuncture and hypnosis. J Am Med Assoc 2000;283(1):118–9.

25. Simon EP, Lewis DM. Medical hypnosis for temporomandibular disorders: treatment efficacy and medical utilization outcome. Oral Surg Oral Med Oral Pathol Oral Radiol Endod 2000;90(1): 54–63.

26. Dubin LL. The use of hypnosis for temporomandibular joint (TMJ). Psychiatr Med 1992;10(4):99–103.

27. Somer E. Hypnotherapy in the treatment of chronic nocturnal use of a dental splint prescribed for bruxism. Int J Clin Exp Hypn 1991;39(3):145–54.

28. Funch DP, Gale EN. Biofeedback and relaxation therapy for chronic temporomandibular joint pain: predicting successful outcome. J Consult Clin Psychol 1984;52(6):928–35.

29. Turk DC, Zaki HS, Rudy TE. Effects of intraoral appliance and biofeedback/stress management alone and in combination in treating pain and depression in patients with temporomandibular disorders. J Prosthet Dent 1993;70(2):158–64.

30. Kerschbaum TH, Wende KU. Compliance von Schmerz-Dysfunktions-Patienten [Compliance of CMD patients]. Dtsch Zahnarztl Z 2001;56:322–5.

31. [No authors listed.] Management of temporomandibular disorders. National Institutes of Health Technology Assessment Conference Statement. J Am Dent Assoc 1996;127(11):1595–606.

32. Okeson JP. Management of Temporomandibular Disorders and Occlusion, 5th edition. St Louis: CV Mosby, 2003:98, 153, 383–4, 417, 555.

33. Morrish RB Jr, Stround LP. Long-term management of the TMD patient. In: Pertes RA, Gross SG (eds). Clinical Management of Temporomandibular Disorders and Orofacial Pain. Chicago: Quintessence, 1995:273–95.

34. Tarantola GJ, Becker IM, Gremillion H, Pink F. The effectiveness of equilibration in the improvement of signs and symptoms in the stomatognathic system. Int J Periodontics Restorative Dent 1998;18(6):594–603.

35. Obrez A, Turp JC. The effect of musculoskeletal facial pain on registration of maxillomandibular relationships and treatment planning: a synthesis of the literature. J Prosthet Dent 1998;79(4):439–45.

36. Dawson PE. New definition for relating occlusion to varying conditions of the temporomandibular joint. J Prosthet Dent 1995;74:619–27.

37. McNeill C. Management of temporomandibular disorders: concepts and controversies. J Prosthet Dent 1997;77:510–22.

38. Dental Practice Parameters Committee. American Dental Association's dental practice parameters: temporomandibular (craniomandibular) disorders. J Am Dent Assoc Suppl 1997;128:29–32–S.

39. Ash MM. Occlusal adjustment: quo vadis? Cranio 2003;21(1):1–4.

40. Obrez A, Turp JC. The effect of musculoskeletal facial pain on registration of maxillomandibular relationships and treatment planning: a synthesis of the literature. J Prosthet Dent 1998;79(4):439–45.

41. Goldstein BH. Temporomandibular disorders: a review of current understanding. Oral Surg Oral Med Oral Pathol Oral Radiol Endod 1999;88:379–85.

42. Okeson JP (ed), for the American Academy of Orofacial Pain. Orofacial Pain: Guidelines for Assessment, Diagnosis and Management. Chicago: Quintessence, 1996:117, 137, 141–58.

43. Yatani H, Minakuchi H, Matsuka Y, Fujisawa T, Yamashita A. The long-term effect of occlusal therapy on self-administered treatment outcomes of TMD. J Orofac Pain 1998;12(1):75–88.

44. Brown DT, Gaudet EL Jr. Temporomandibular disorder treatment outcomes: second report of a large-scale prospective clinical study. Cranio 2002;20(4):244–53.

45. Marbach JJ, Ballard GT, Frankel MR, Raphael KG. Patterns of TMJ surgery: evidence of sex differences. J Am Dent Assoc 1997;128:609–14.

46. American Association of Oral and Maxillofacial Surgeons. Recommendations for management of patients with temporomandibular joint implants. Temporomandibular Joint Implant Surgery Workshop. J Oral Maxillofac Surg 1993;51(10):1164–72.

47. Vallon D, Milner M, Soderfeldt B. Treatment outcome in patients with craniomandibular disorders of muscular origin: a 7-year follow-up. J Orofac Pain 1998;12(3):210–8.

48. Gil IA, Barbosa CMR, Pedro VM, Silverio KCA, Goldfarb EP, Fusco V, Navarro CM. Multidisciplinary approach to chronic pain from myofascial pain dysfunction syndrome: a four-year experience at a Brazilian center. Cranio 1998;16(1):17–25.

49. Wright EF, Schiffman EL. Treatment alternatives for patients with masticatory myofascial pain. J Am Dent Assoc 1995;126(7):1030–9.

50. Garofalo JP, Gatchel RJ, Wesley AL, Ellis III E. Predicting chronicity in acute temporomandibular joint disorders using the research diagnostic criteria. J Am Dent Assoc 1998;129(4):438–47.

51. Molina OF, dos Santos J Jr, Nelson SJ, Nowlin T. Profile of TMD and bruxer compared to TMD and nonbruxer patients regarding chief complaint, previous consultations, modes of therapy and chronicity. Cranio 2000;18(3):205–19.

52. Rugh JD, Robbins JW. Oral habits disorder. In: Ingersoll BD (ed). Behavioral Aspects of

Dentistry. Norwalk, CT: Appleton-Century-Crofts, 1982:179–202.

53. Dao TT, Lund JP, Lavigne GJ. Comparison of pain and quality of life in bruxers and patients with myofascial pain of the masticatory muscles. J Orofacial Pain 1994;8(4):350–6.

54. Van Grootel RJ, Van der Glas HW, Buchner R. Daily changes of pain variables for myogenous TMD patients [abstract 2965]. J Dent Res (Special Issue) 2000;79:514.

55. Pierce CJ, Gale EN. A comparison of different treatments for nocturnal bruxism. J Dent Res 1988;67:597–601.

56. Hijzen TH, Slangen JL, Van Houweligen HC. Subjective, clinical and EMG effects of biofeedback and splint treatment. J Oral Rehabil 1986;13:529–39.

57. Dahlstrom L, Carlsson SG. Treatment of mandibular dysfunction: the clinical usefulness of biofeedback in relation to splint therapy. J Oral Rehabil 1984;11:277–84.

58. Gramling SE, Neblett J, Grayson R, Townsend D. Temporomandibular disorder: efficacy of an oral habit reversal treatment program. J Behav Ther Exp Psychiatry 1996;27(3):245–55.

59. Greene CS. The etiology of temporomandibular disorders: implications for treatment. J Orofac Pain 2001;15(2):93–105.

60. Wright EF, Gullickson DC. Identifying acute pulpalgia as a factor in TMD pain. J Am Dent Assoc 1996;127:773–80.

61. Wright EF, Gullickson DC. Dental pulpalgia contributing to bilateral preauricular pain and tinnitus. J Orofacial Pain 1996;10:166–8.

62. Falace DA, Reid K, Rayens MK. The influence of deep (odontogenic) pain intensity, quality, and duration on the incidence and characteristics of referred orofacial pain. J Orofac Pain 1996;10(3):232–9.

63. Fricton JR. Etiology and management of masticatory myofascial pain. J Musculoske Pain 1999;7(1/2):143–60.

64. Epker J, Gatchel RJ, Ellis III E. A model for predicting chronic TMD: practical application in clinical settings. J Am Dent Assoc 1999;130:1470–5.

65. Garofalo JP, Gatchel RJ, Wesley AL, Ellis III E. Predicting chronicity in acute temporomandibular joint disorders using the research diagnostic criteria. J Am Dent Assoc 1998;129(4):438–47.

66. Krogstad BS, Jokstad A, Dahl BL, Vassend O. Relationship between risk factors and treatment outcome in a group of patients with temporomandibular disorder. J Orofac Pain 1996;10(1):48–53.

67. Almekinders LC. Tendinitis and other chronic tendinopathies. J Am Acad Orthop Surg 1998;6(3):157–64.

68. Raphael KG, Marbach JJ. Widespread pain and the effectiveness of oral splints in myofascial face pain. J Am Dent Assoc 2001;132(3):305–16.

Part V

Case Scenarios

FAQs

Q: What measurements would you consider to be minimum for normal opening and excursive movements?

A: I consider 40 mm to be the minimum for a normal opening and 7/7/6 mm to be the minimum for normal excursive movements.

Q: Do stabilization appliances stop patients from bruxing?

A: No. Patients with nocturnal bruxing habits usually continue to brux, even when they wear a stabilization appliance.

The following 18 cases are of patients who were referred to me because of TMD-like symptoms; not all had TMD. This section hopefully will help readers better identify patients with non-TMD symptoms and provide readers a better feel for how I integrate the various TMD therapies.

For the sake of expediency, most patients' identified perpetuating contributing factors (e.g., excessive caffeine consumption, stomach sleeping, neck pain, or poor sleep) are not reported. It is felt these factors were adequately discussed previously in this book and need not be revisited here. During my initial evaluation for TMD, I always document patients' perpetuating contributing factors and attempt to decrease them to the degree possible in order to reduce the TMD symptoms. Contributing factors that may not be changeable [e.g., widespread pain and posttraumatic stress disorder (PTSD) nightmares] are also important to document, because occasionally one needs to justify the reason a patient is not obtaining the symptom improvement that other patients typically do.

⊙ **QUICK CONSULTS**
Perpetuating Contributing Factors

Most patients' identified perpetuating contributing factors (e.g., excessive caffeine consumption, stomach sleeping, neck pain, or poor sleep) are not reported in the following cases.

Decreasing Perpetuating Factors

During my initial evaluation for TMD, I always document patients' perpetuating contributing factors and attempt to decrease them to the degree possible, in order to reduce the TMD symptoms.

The drawings provided with the cases depict the locations where patients drew their pain on the "Initial Patient Questionnaire" (Appendix 1), with the most significant locations indicated with a *yellow star*. The provided mandibular range-of-motion opening includes the overlap of the anterior teeth (I consider 40 mm to be the minimum for a normal opening). For simplicity, the excursive movements are designated with three numbers separated by slashes. These numbers are the millimeters for which these patients moved their mandible in right lateral, left lateral, and protrusive directions, respectively (I consider 7/7/6 mm to be the minimum for normal excursive movements).

The designation 5/10 is used to represent that the patient's average pain is a 5 on a 0 to 10 pain scale and similarly designate the other reported pain levels. For simplicity, TMJ noise or dysfunction is only reported if it is present or the patient has a history of it. Readers should assume a patient's complaints are chronic and not due to the placement of a restoration, unless noted otherwise.

The masticatory and cervical structures were palpated as recommended in "Palpation" in Chapter 3. As mentioned in that section, if a muscle is tender to palpation, the most probable diagnosis is myofascial pain. Ideally the practitioner would identify trigger points to arrive at this diagnosis, but they may be difficult to discern, even for practitioners experienced in palpating muscles.[1] From a clinically practical perspective, if the muscle is tender to palpation and no other muscle diagnosis in Chapter 5, "TMD Diagnostic Categories," better describes a patient's condition, I recommend the muscle tenderness be diagnosed as myofascial pain.

⊙ **QUICK CONSULT**
Diagnosing Myofascial Pain

If the muscle is tender to palpation and no other muscle diagnosis in Chapter 5, "TMD Diagnostic Categories," better describes a patient's condition, I recommend the muscle tenderness be diagnosed as myofascial pain.

For some patients, self-massage and/or trigger-point compression are provided as part of their self-management instructions. The decision to provide this is based on a patient's interest in additional self-management therapies, and the magnitude it is felt this therapy will benefit the patient. For simplicity, these therapies are not delineated in the case treatments.

⊙ **QUICK CONSULT**
Delineating Self-massage and/or Trigger-point Compression

The decision to provide these is based on a patient's interest in additional self-management therapies, and the magnitude it is felt this therapy will benefit the patient. For simplicity, these therapies are not delineated in the case treatments.

CASE 1: PULPAL PATHOSIS MIMICKING TMD SYMPTOMS

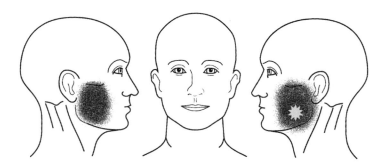

The patient related she had constant bilateral 2 to 3/10 dull/pressure pain (left worse than right) in the masseter muscle area. Every day, she had 8/10 throbbing pain in her left masseter muscle that could last minutes to hours and occur several times a day. Her pain was aggravated by yawning, lying down, and drinking cold beverages. Her range of motion was 36 mm opening and 7/7/6 (right lateral, left lateral, and protrusive). Palpation of the masticatory and cervical structures identified that her tenderness was limited to both masseter muscles, with the left masseter significantly more tender than the right. The masseter muscle palpation reproduced her complaint.

Is there anything that appears unusual about her symptoms? Are these symptoms typical for a patient with TMD? Do the aggravating symptoms suggest anything? Based on her symptoms, I would ask her why lying down aggravates her symptoms and determine whether there is a rational explanation relating the symptoms to TMD. The pain aggravation could be due to the patient lying on the tender masseter muscle, as when a patient with an acute pulpalgia lies down, etc.

It is often observed that TMD pain (not tooth pain) aggravated by drinking cold beverages is associated with a pulpal pathosis that is referring pain to masticatory structures (e.g., muscles or TMJ). Generally I ask patients with this aggravator which tooth the cold beverage touches to cause the aggrava-

tion. The answer gives me a feel for which area of the mouth is probably contributing to the pain. This patient related that, when cold liquid touched tooth 19 (mandibular left molar), her left masseter muscle pain was aggravated, and it often elicited the throbbing component. A panoramic radiograph that was taken showed a deep carious lesion in tooth 19.

◉ QUICK CONSULT

Observing for Drinking Cold Beverages Aggravating Symptoms

It is often noticed that TMD pain (not tooth pain) aggravated by drinking cold beverages is associated with a pulpal pathosis that is referring pain to masticatory structures (e.g., muscles or TMJ).

Next, I like to determine whether there is a connection between a patient's left masseter muscle pain and the tooth. The patient's mandibular left posterior teeth were percussed with the mouth-mirror handle, and the patient related that only tooth 19 was tender to percussion. It is not uncommon for a TMD patient to have many teeth tender to percussion from parafunctional habits. If a tooth is contributing to the pain, it should be significantly more tender than the other teeth.[2]

A very cold cotton pellet was then held to tooth 19 for approximately 5 seconds, and the patient related that this aggravated her left masseter muscle area pain and caused the throbbing. The TMD-like symptoms are not always reproduced when a patient has an acute pulpalgia referring pain to these areas. An acute pulpalgia is also suspected when the test produces lingering pain only within the tooth, as is commonly observed with an acute pulpalgia.

If this test suggests the tooth has an acute pulpalgia, I next administer a ligamentary injection along the tooth. This eliminates the patient's masseter muscle area pain. To obtain a positive response to this test, I like to see the pain reduced dramatically. If further understanding of this disorder or diagnostic technique is desired, several relevant articles are available.[2-4]

Both the cold and anesthetic tests being positive suggests the pulpal disorder is causing or contributing to the left masseter muscle area pain. The right masseter muscle pain or tenderness is probably independent of this finding. It was noted that, although the pain was eliminated by the anesthetic test, the patient continued to have a limited range of motion. The right masseter muscle pain and tenderness, and limited opening when tooth 19 was anesthetized, suggest an underlying TMD condition.

Since the pain on the left was related to the pulpal disorder, and the left masseter was significantly more tender than the right, my clinical impression was that the primary diagnosis for this complaint was pulpal pathosis of tooth 19, with a secondary diagnosis of myofascial pain.

The treatment provided was (a) recommending she return to her general dentist for treatment of tooth 19; (b) reviewing with her the "TMD Self-management Therapies" handout (Appendix 3), since she appeared to have a mild underlying TMD condition; (c) informing her that it was anticipated these therapies would adequately resolve her TMD symptoms, but, if they did not, she should return to my office for further evaluation and treatment. She never returned to my office, so it was assumed they adequately resolved her complaint.

Generally I find that patients who have an acute pulpalgia as the primary etiology for their TMD symptoms relate (if asked) that their TMD pain is aggravated by drinking hot or cold beverages, but several of these patients with acrylic crowns covering the offending tooth not having this symptom have been observed. Acrylic crowns appear to provide sufficient thermal protection so the pulp may not be aggravated by these thermal changes.

CASE 2: CHRONIC SINUSITIS

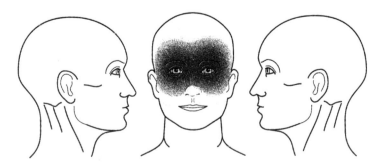

The patient related that every day she had 2/10 dull/pressure pain in the area marked on the drawing. Her pain occurred at variable times of the day, generally lasted 3 to 10 hours, and was aggravated by bending forward. Her range of motion was 40 mm opening and 7/7/6 (right lateral, left lateral, and protrusive). Palpation of her masticatory and cervical structures identified mild tenderness limited to bilateral masseter muscles and lateral pterygoid areas.

Are these symptoms typical for a patient with TMD? Bending forward can aggravate TMD symptoms, but this is also common among individuals who have sinus pain. Based on her symptom location and its aggravation when bending forward, it was suspected that her pain might be due to sinusitis. I asked her whether she had tried a decongestant for her symptoms, and she had not.

Her maxillary and frontal sinuses were then palpated, and she reported this aggravated her pain. Sinus palpation *cannot* rule out sinusitis, because many patients with sinusitis report this does not aggravate their pain. The patient was told that, since her pain could not be reproduced (or aggravated) through palpation of her masticatory or cervical structures, it was felt her pain was not related to these structures. My clinical impression was that her pain was probably due to chronic sinusitis. Sometimes I provide a trial with a decongestant to understand better the etiology of a patient's pain, but, since this was her only complaint and I planned for her to see her physician for this, a decongestant trial was not provided.

The patient's masseter muscle and lateral pterygoid area tenderness may have been independent of her sinus pain. Since its treatment would only have involved self-management instructions that I typically provide during my initial evaluation and would not have had a negative impact if it were not needed, I chose to assume the tenderness was independent of the sinus disorder. Therefore, she was given a secondary diagnosis of myofascial pain and told I would like to give her some recommendations for how she could reduce the mild tenderness noted in her masseter muscles and lateral pterygoid areas.

The treatment provided to this patient was recommending she see her primary medical provider to evaluate her for probable chronic sinusitis and reviewing with her the "TMD Self-management Therapies" handout (Appendix 3). She was told she could implement whichever of the self-management therapies she desired, and I informed her that, if the muscles became symptomatic in the future, she could increase the implementation of these recommendations and return to my office for further evaluation, if she desired.

CASE 3: CHRONIC FOREHEAD PAIN REFERRED FROM THE NECK

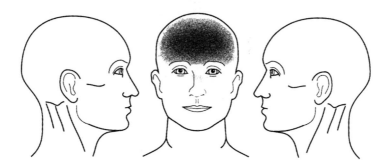

The patient related every morning she awoke with 2 to 3/10 dull/pressure pain in her forehead, which lasted approximately 2 to 3 hours. Approximately once a week, this was a 6/10 throbbing pain that lasted approximately 5 hours after she awoke. Her range of motion was 42 mm opening and 8/8/7 (right lateral, left lateral, and protrusive).

Palpation of her masticatory and cervical structures identified no tenderness among the masticatory structures, but did find tenderness of her cervical muscles. By holding pressure on the most tender firm nodules within her suboccipital muscles (cervical trigger points), her forehead pain could be reproduced; she felt that she would also develop the throbbing pain if pressure was maintained on these points, a common finding from greater aggravation of trigger points.

Does this patient have TMD? Since none of the masticatory structures were tender, and she did not have a history of TMJ noise, she did not have TMD. She has cervical muscle tenderness with trigger points, which I recommend practitioners diagnose as myofascial pain. This criteria does not rise to the definition of cervical myofascial pain, but the other features, such an associated taut band, are difficult even for practitioners experienced in palpating muscles to identify.

Since her forehead headache could be reproduced by holding pressure on her cervical trigger points, it was felt the aggravation of these trigger points was contributing to her headache. Her throbbing pain may have been due to greater aggravation of the trigger points. It is common for individuals to have forehead and/or periorbital pain referred from the neck.[5] Many of these individuals notice only the referred pain (the forehead pain for this patient) and do not notice pain at the source (the neck for this patient).

☯ FOCAL POINT

If a patient's forehead headache can be reproduced by holding pressure on his or her cervical trigger points, it is felt the aggravation of these trigger points is contributing to the headache.

◉ QUICK CONSULT

Observing Forehead and/or Periorbital Pain

It is common for individuals to have forehead and/or periorbital pain that is referred from the neck.

Assuming that her pain was primarily due to referred cervical pain, her daily symptom pattern suggested that something was aggravating her cervical myofascial pain at night, so I inquired about her sleep posture, identified some potential aggravations (e.g., intermittent stomach sleeping), and offered her suggestions to improve these. Many other treatments can be provided for a patient whose cervical myofascial pain is aggravated during the night, e.g., providing posture improvement exercises (Appendix 6), referral to a physical therapist or to a chiropractor, recommending the patient use relaxation or self-hypnosis just prior to or while going to sleep, prescribing a muscle relaxant or tricyclic antidepressant, and correcting poor sleep.

There are other potential causes for this chronic form of forehead pain: the throbbing pain could be a migraine headache, other less common conditions, or a combination of these. I prefer initially to treat headaches that can be reproduced or aggravated by palpating cervical tender nodules, without symptoms of a more serious disorder, with a nonpharmaceutical approach directed at the source of the referral pattern. Because of variabilities with combined etiologies and practitioners' skills, response to cervical treatment and referred pain varies. I generally find positive results with this therapeutic approach, but will escalate to pharmaceutical management if unsuccessful or if the patient desires this as a first line of therapy. Sometimes a neurologist's expertise is needed to manage these patients pharmaceutically.

The treatment provided to this patient was recommending improvements in her sleep posture and referring her to a physical therapist. She was told that, if she did not gain adequate improvement from this therapy, she should follow it up with her primary medical provider or return to my office.

CASE 4: MYOFASCIAL PAIN SECONDARY TO NOCTURNAL PARAFUNCTIONAL HABITS

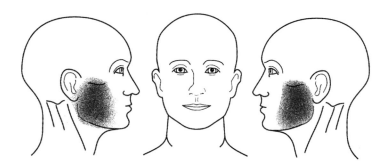

A 20-year-old patient related that every morning he awoke with 4/10 bilateral masseter muscle dull/pressure pain that lasted approximately 2 to 3 hours. His range of motion was 42 mm opening and 8/8/7 (right lateral, left lateral, and protrusive). Palpation of his masticatory and cervical structures identified approximately the same degree of tenderness limited to both masseter muscles. The masseter muscle palpation reproduced his pain.

Since the masseter muscle palpation reproduced his symptoms, and no other TMD muscle diagnosis better describes his condition, his complaint was diagnosed as myofascial pain. The patient's daily symptom pattern suggested nocturnal parafunctional habits as the primary contributing factor. Since this young healthy man had no additional perpetuating factors, it was felt he would probably obtain satisfactory improvement from following "TMD Self-management Therapies" handout (Appendix 3) and a maxillary stabilization appliance worn at night.

The patient would probably also find implementing the "Jaw Muscle-stretching Exercise" handout (Appendix 5) beneficial, but I believed he would not need the exercise, so he was not offered it as part of his initial therapy. If he did not derive satisfactory improvement from the initial therapies, this would be the first additional therapy I would consider.

Some practitioners would prescribe medication for this patient to use until they inserted a stabilization appliance. If he was prescribed 800 mg ibuprofen at bedtime, he would probably awake with minimal pain. This is a legitimate option, but I tend not to prescribe medications to patients with this relatively low degree of pain and who it is felt will obtain adequate relief from non-pharmaceutical management. This is because of the following: (a) I like these patients to work with the self-management procedures rather than rely on pain medication. (b) This patient had this pain for quite a while, and it was felt he would find adequate relief when he received his occlusal appliance in a week or two. (c) I find that most patients with this symptom severity are not interested in taking medications and would not fill the prescription. (d) The self-management instructions handout discusses using over-the-counter medications, and patients are informed they can use them if they desire. It is appropriate to write a prescription and, if a patient with this symptom severity of muscle origin requested an analgesic, I would prescribe 800 mg ibuprofen.

CASE 5: TOOTH ATTRITION—NO PAIN

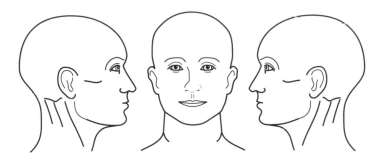

The patient had no pain, complained he was wearing down his teeth (Figure V-1), and said he would like to prevent further tooth wear. His range of motion was 55 mm opening and 9/9/7 (right lateral, left lateral, and protrusive). Palpation of his masticatory and cervical structures revealed no tenderness. Does this patient have TMD? Since none of the masticatory structures were tender, and he does not have a history of TMJ noise, he does not have TMD.

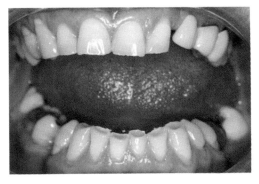

Figure V-1. Case 5: The patient complained of worn dentition.

The diagnosis for this patient's complaint is tooth attrition. The wear appears to be due to daytime and/or nighttime parafunctional habits that could be accelerated by certain foods or other items he puts in his mouth. The patient was not aware of any abrasive substances that could be contributing to the wear. The treatment provided this patient was (a) to discuss the potential that he may be performing parafunctional habits during the day and night, (b) to recommend he become aware of any daytime parafunctional habits and break them, and (c) to provide him with a maxillary acrylic stabilization appliance to wear at night.

Patients with nocturnal bruxing habits usually continue to brux, even though they wear a stabilization appliance. The maxillary appliance will protect his maxillary teeth from additional wear. As the mandibular teeth brux across the acrylic appliance, the acrylic will wear rather than his teeth. This is similar to acrylic denture teeth opposing natural teeth: the denture teeth wear rather than the natural teeth.

CASE 6: MYOFASCIAL PAIN SECONDARY TO DAYTIME PARAFUNCTIONAL HABITS

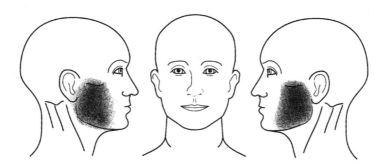

The patient related every morning he awoke pain free, but developed 4/10 bilateral masseter muscle dull/pressure pain later in the day that lasted into the evening. His range of motion was 42 mm opening and 8/8/7 (right lateral, left lateral, and protrusive). Palpation of his masticatory and cervical structures identified that approximately the same degree of tenderness was limited to both masseter muscles. Palpation of the masseter muscle reproduced his complaint.

The diagnosis was myofascial pain. The symptom pattern suggested that any nocturnal parafunctional habit had minimal impact on his symptoms, and that the daytime habits were the primary cause of his pain. Based on the limited information provided (no additional perpetuating factors, etc.), the patient was informed how his symptoms were affected by his daytime parafunctional habits, muscle tension, psychosocial stress, etc. At a minimum, I would initially treat such patients by offering them the "TMD Self-management Therapies" handout (Appendix 3) and the "Jaw Muscle-stretching Exercise" handout (Appendix 5), and observe whether the daytime symptoms were reduced satisfactorily.

There are many options if a patient cannot reduce daytime symptoms satisfactorily or desires to begin these additional therapies at the initial visit. These would be, for example, the temporary use of a daytime habit-breaking appliance, habit-reversal therapy (see "Breaking Daytime Habits" in Chapter 16), relaxation, or biofeedback. If the patient is interested, these options would be discussed and the patient could try to determine how he or she would like to proceed with escalating this therapy. I generally refer these patients to a psychologist who usually initially provides habit-reversal therapy and relaxation. If this does not adequately resolve the symptoms, the psychologist will escalate therapy in the direction that appears most appropriate, e.g., biofeedback or cognitive therapy.

CASE 7: TENSE, DEPRESSED, AND POOR SLEEP AS CONTRIBUTING FACTORS

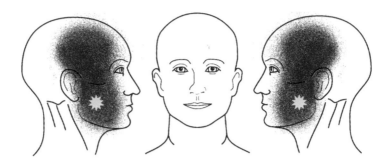

The patient related he had constant bilateral 6/10 preauricular and masseter muscle pain, and every morning he also had a 4/10 temporal headache. He related that his pain was worse when he awoke and again in the afternoon or evening. He also related that, during the usual day, he was tense all of the time, depressed half of the time, and could sleep only 4 to 6 hours because of insomnia. His range of motion was 34 mm opening and 6/6/5 (right lateral, left lateral, and protrusive). Palpation of his masticatory and cervical structures revealed generalized tenderness of these muscles; his TMJs were not tender. Palpation of multiple muscle sites reproduced his pain.

The diagnosis was myofascial pain. The symptom pattern suggested both daytime and nighttime habits negatively affected his pain, with the nighttime habits being the greater contributor. Other identified contributors were tension, depression, and insomnia.

It was first explained to the patient how these factors contributed to his pain. He was informed how a psychologist could help him reduce his tension and depression, in addition to teaching him habit reversal and relax-ation (other needed therapies may also be identified by the psychologist). The possibility of referring the patient to a psychiatrist for medical management of his depression and insomnia was also discussed. The possibility of referral to a physical therapist for treatment of the cervical myofascial pain was discussed. Such discussions help patients to realize the importance of these for adequately reducing pain and to make the cost (price, time, etc.)-benefit decision regarding which referrals they are open to receiving. Some patients initially decline certain referrals, but may be open to them later.

It is recommended initially providing patients with this presentation: (a) the "TMD Self-management Therapies" handout (Appendix 3), (b) "Jaw Muscle-stretching Exercise" handout (Appendix 5), (c) a stabilization appliance, and (d) whichever referrals patients are receptive to receiving. One of the more esthetic appliances could be fabricated and the patient asked to wear it temporarily for 24 hours a day, except when eating. The possibility of prescribing amitriptyline to help alleviate morning pain and improve insomnia should also be considered.

CASE 8: FIBROMYALGIA AS A CONTRIBUTING FACTOR

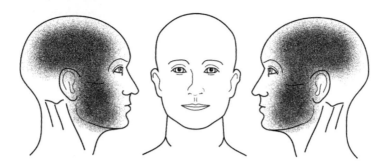

The patient related he had constant 8/10 bilateral preauricular, masseter, and temple muscle pain, which was worse when he awoke and again in evening. He related he had constant 6/10 generalized muscle tenderness throughout his body, restless sleep, and generalized muscle soreness when he awoke that felt like he just did 1,000 sit-ups. His range of motion was 45 mm opening and 8/8/7 (right lateral, left lateral, and protrusive). Palpation of his masticatory and cervical structures identified generalized tenderness of these structures, but no tenderness of his TMJs. Palpation of multiple muscle sites reproduced his pain.

He appeared to have a systemic disorder that was causing the constant 6/10 generalized muscle tenderness throughout his body. Since the masticatory symptoms were worse than his generalized body pain, local factors appeared to be making his masticatory symptoms more severe. Since his masticatory muscle palpation aggravated his pain, and no other TMD muscle diagnosis better described his condition, he was diagnosed as having myofascial pain. His generalized body symptoms were characteristic of fibromyalgia, and palpation of his fibromyalgia tender points revealed they were all tender, suggesting he had fibromyalgia.

◉ **QUICK CONSULT**

Deciding Whether Local Factors Are Contributing to Symptoms

If the masticatory symptoms are worse than the generalized body pain, local factors may be making the masticatory symptoms more severe.

The patient's masticatory symptom pattern suggested nocturnal and daytime habits were probably contributing to his pain. The patient was first informed that studies suggest patients with widespread pain do not generally obtain the degree of TMD symptom improvement as most other TMD patients. It was explained how these factors are probably contributing to his masticatory pain problem and that the best results I could hope for by treating his masticatory TMD symptoms would be to reduce them to the 6/10, as with the rest of his body. A referral to a physician to evaluate and manage his widespread pain and the possibility of him working with a psychologist to teach him habit reversal and relaxation was discussed.

⊗ **FOCAL POINT**

Patients with widespread pain are informed that studies suggest TMD patients with widespread pain do not generally obtain the degree of TMD symptom improvement as most other TMD patients.

It was recommended he initially be provided with (a) the "TMD Self-management

Therapies" handout (Appendix 3), (b) "Jaw Muscle-stretching Exercise" handout (Appendix 5), (c) a stabilization appliance, and (d) referral to a physician for probable fibromyalgia. If he did not obtain adequate improvement with his daytime symptoms, I would then consider referring him to a psychologist to learn habit reversal and relaxation.

CASE 9: TMJ DISC DISPLACEMENTS AND WHEN TO TREAT IT—NO PAIN

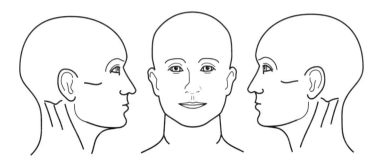

The patient related that, for the past year, he had a right TMJ click every time he opened and closed his mouth. He had noticed the noise was more prominent after eating tough foods or when stressed. His range of motion was 50 mm opening and 8/8/7 (right lateral, left lateral, and protrusive). Palpation of his masticatory and cervical structures revealed no tenderness there.

The diagnosis was right TMJ disc displacement with reduction. Should this patient be provided with any treatment? A nonpainful disc displacement with reduction does not need to be treated. The "TMJ Disc Displacements" diagram (Appendix 2) was discussed so he understood the cause of the noise. He was informed that, as with noises from other joints in the body, they do not need to be treated unless they cause discomfort. If discomfort occurred later, treatment would target the discomfort and may not have any effect on the noise. The patient was told he should return to my office for therapy if he developed discomfort (muscle or TMJ).

✪ FOCAL POINT

A nonpainful disc displacement with reduction does not require treatment.

If a patient's TMJ made a loud TMJ pop, should the patient be treated for this? Sometimes patients have such a loud pop that it can be heard across the room, which may embarrass the patient, spouse, or friends to the degree that the patient wants the noise decreased. Our TMD therapies are not always effective in decreasing TMJ noise, and patients should be aware of this possibility prior to treatment. If the noise is a serious problem, and conservative therapy cannot satisfactorily reduce it, surgical intervention may be required. Patients who do undergo surgical correction will probably continue to have some form of noise (crepitus, clicking, etc.) from the TMJ, but hopefully it will be less pronounced.

If a patient's noise is accompanied by intermittent locking (acute TMJ disc displacement without reduction), should the patient be treated for this? There is a concern that the patient's disorder may progress to a permanent lock, which is difficult to treat and the most common TMD disorder for which I refer patients to surgeons. For this reason, I recommend treating a patient who has intermittent locking even though it may not be a significant problem.

Recommending Treatment for Intermittent Lock

I recommend treating a patient who has intermittent locking even though it may not be a significant problem.

CASE 10: TMJ INFLAMMATION

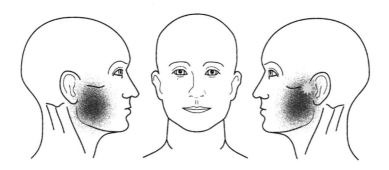

The patient related he had constant 3/10 bilateral preauricular and masseter dull/pressure pain that was worse when he awoke. He reported his left TMJ often clicked when he opened and closed his mouth. His range of motion was 36 mm opening and 6/6/5 (right lateral, left lateral, and protrusive). Palpation of his masticatory and cervical structures identified generalized tenderness of the masticatory muscles and TMJs (the left TMJ most readily reproduced his pain and was the most tender), whereas the cervical structures were not tender.

The problem had three diagnoses—i.e., primary, secondary, and tertiary diagnoses—that needed to be placed in the order of their contribution to the complaint. Since the primary complaint was pain, the structure that most readily reproduced it (the TMJ) was most likely the primary contributor to it. The diagnosis for TMJ palpation tenderness is TMJ inflammation, so this would be the patient's primary TMD diagnosis. The muscles were also tender (to a lesser degree), and the diagnosis for muscle palpation tenderness (when none of the other diagnoses better apply) is myofascial pain, so this would be

the secondary TMD diagnosis. The patient also had a left TMJ click, which generally contributes minimally to a patient's pain. The diagnosis for a TMJ click is most often disc displacement with reduction (unless a patient's history suggests another diagnosis; see Chapter 5, "TMD Diagnostic Categories"), so this patient's tertiary TMD diagnosis was left TMJ disc displacement with reduction.

▼ **TECHNICAL TIP**

Recording Diagnoses

It is helpful to list the diagnoses (primary, secondary, tertiary, etc.) in the order of their contribution to a patient's complaint.

Since this young healthy man had no additional perpetuating factors, it was felt he would probably obtain satisfactory improvement from following the "TMD Self-management Therapies" handout (Appendix 3) and a maxillary stabilization appliance worn at night. It was felt discussion of the self-management therapies and the carryover effect of the appliance worn at night would adequately resolve the daytime symptoms. If his daytime symptoms did not improve satisfactorily, then the therapies discussed in "Breaking Daytime Habits" in Chapter 16 would be implemented.

The patient had tender masticatory muscles, and the therapy presented in "Jaw Muscle-stretching Exercise" handout (Appendix 5) is normally beneficial for tender or painful masticatory muscles. The problem is that these stretching exercises tend to aggravate the TMJs and, since his TMJ was quite tender, I was afraid the exercise may further aggravate his TMJ. The patient's pain severity was relatively low, and his TMJs may have tolerated the exercise, but, out of this concern, these stretching exercises were not offered to him.

CASE 11: INTERMITTENT ACUTE TMJ DISC DISPLACEMENT WITHOUT REDUCTION

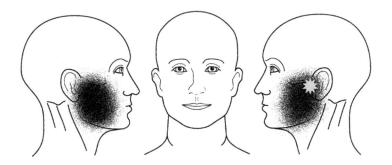

The patient related she had constant 5/10 bilateral preauricular and masseter dull/pressure pain that was worse in the evening. Her left TMJ continuously clicked when she opened and, two to three times a week, the disc blocked her from opening very wide (only approximately 23 mm). The locking never occurred when she first awoke. When asked, she related she also had constant 5/10 neck pain. Her range of motion was 34 mm opening and 6/6/5 (right lateral, left lateral, and protrusive). Palpation of her masticatory and cervical structures identified generalized tenderness of these structures, with the left TMJ most readily reproducing her pain and being the most tender.

The patient's problem had four diagnoses and, since the primary complaint was pain, the structure that most readily reproduced her pain (the TMJ) was the primary contributor to her complaint, so the primary diagnosis was TMJ inflammation. The masticatory and cervical muscles less readily reproduced her pain and were less tender, so the secondary diagnosis was myofascial pain (of the masticatory and cervical regions). The intermittent locking was of greater concern than the clicking, and its diagnosis (and the tertiary TMD diagnosis) was left intermittent acute TMJ disc displacement without reduction. Finally, the quaternary TMD diagnosis was left TMJ disc displacement with reduction.

That the patient's intermittent locking never occurred in the morning suggested her daytime parafunctional and/or muscle tightening habits were greater contributors than were her nocturnal habits. This was supported by her greater symptom severity later in the day.

◉ **QUICK CONSULT**
Observing an Intermittent Locking Pattern
The daytime pattern of a patient's intermittent locking suggests the time of day when the primary contributing factors are occurring.

The treatment provided to this patient was (a) using the "TMJ Disc Displacements" diagram (Appendix 2) to explain the mechanism for her TMJ click and intermittent lock, and how her parafunctional habits and muscle tension contributed to this problem; (b) reviewing with her the "TMD Self-management Therapies" handout; (c) fabricating and inserting a stabilization appliance (one of the more esthetic appliances could be fabricated and the patient asked to wear it temporarily 24 hours a day, except when eating); (d) referring her to a physical therapist for treatment of her constant neck pain; (e) referring her for habit-reversal and relaxation therapy (if that does not satisfactorily relieve the daytime symptoms, we can escalate therapy); and (f) offering to prescribe 500 mg naproxen taken twice a day.

CASE 12: ACUTE TMJ DISC DISPLACEMENT WITHOUT REDUCTION—UNLOCKED

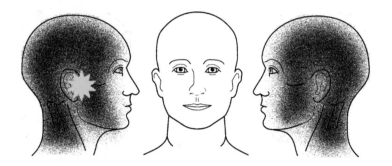

The patient related she had not worn her stabilization appliance the previous night, awoke with 4/10 right preauricular pain and, an hour ago, her right TMJ had locked (the disc blocks her from being able to open very wide) and would not unlock. She related she had constant 10/10 bilateral preauricular, masseter, temple, and neck pain. She also related that her right TMJ had not clicked or locked since it had been operated on for this problem a year ago.

Her range of motion was 19 mm opening and 5/1/3 (right lateral, left lateral, and protrusive). Palpation of her masticatory and cervical structures revealed their generalized tenderness, with exquisite tenderness of her right TMJ. These palpations aggravated her complaint, with the right TMJ reproducing the most intense portion of her pain.

What are the patient's diagnoses? Since the TMJ inflammation is due to acute TMJ disc displacement without reduction, the recommendations are acute TMJ disc displacement without reduction as the primary diagnosis, bilateral TMJ inflammation as the secondary diagnosis, and myofascial pain as the tertiary diagnosis.

Should one attempt to unlock her right TMJ? Since it locked only an hour ago, I would recommend trying to unlock it. Techniques to unlock the TMJ and a technique to fabricate an immediate anterior positioning appliance that would be used once it is unlocked are discussed in Chapter 10, "Acute TMJ Disc Displacement without Reduction."

Her condyle was reduced onto the disc (see Figures 10-1, 10-2, and 10-3), which was confirmed by observing that she regained a normal opening of 44 mm. Her mandible needed to be stabilized in this anterior position so the condyle would be maintained in the reduced disc-condyle position. If she were to retrude her mandible (i.e., close into maximum intercuspation), her condyle would move posterior off the disc and her TMJ would probably lock again. Therefore, to stabilize her mandible in this position, a temporary anterior positioning appliance was immediately fabricated from the putty used for crown and bridge impressions.

The patient related that her constant bilateral preauricular, masseter, temple, and neck pain had decreased from 10/10 to 9/10. She was instructed to wear the appliance 24 hours a day, including while eating, and was prescribed Medrol Dosepak, taken as directed on the package; Naproxen 500 mg, 1 tablet b.i.d., starting on day 4 of the Dosepak; and diazepam 5 mg, 1 to 2 tablets h.s. and 1/2 tablet in the morning and the afternoon, if that did not cause drowsiness.

After a week, she transitioned from wearing the anterior positioning appliance to wearing her stabilization appliance 24 hours a day, modulating this transition with the propensity for her TMJ to lock again. Similarly, over time, she slowly reduced the use of the stabilization appliance, again modulated by the propensity for her TMJ to lock.

She had been a patient of mine before and understood the mechanics of her TMJ disorder. She previously had an acute TMJ disc displacement without reduction, which I could not resolve through conservative therapies, so she was referred to an oral surgeon. With magnetic resonance imaging (MRI), the oral surgeon found condylar bony irregularities, so he elected to perform open TMJ surgery to smooth them. It appeared to the surgeon and myself that the patient had multiple psychosocial issues that were the primary contributor to her continued TMD symptoms. She was not interested in continuing therapy for these issues and felt her TMD symptoms were satisfactorily minimal. Once this acute flare-up was resolved, she did not want to escalate TMD therapy by working on these issues and continued to wear her appliance at night and occasionally for short periods during the day.

CASE 13: ACUTE TMJ DISC DISPLACEMENT WITHOUT REDUCTION—NOT UNLOCKED

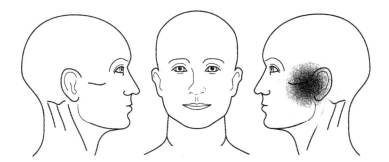

The patient related her left TMJ disc blocked her from opening wide. She had constant 4/10 left preauricular dull/pressure pain (worse later in the day) and momentary 5/10 left preauricular sharp pain when she tried to open wide. Her range of motion was 29 mm opening and 5/10/9 (right lateral, left lateral, and protrusive). Palpation of her masticatory and cervical structures revealed tenderness was limited to her left TMJ, masseter, and posterior digastric muscles. Palpation of the left TMJ was very tender and most readily reproduced her pain complaint, whereas her masseter and posterior digastric muscles were less tender. In an attempt to confirm the source of her restriction, her jaw was stretched open beyond this limited opening to aggravate the restriction.

She related this aggravation occurred within her left TMJ, suggesting that as the source of her restriction.

What were her TMD diagnoses? Since her primary complaint was that she could not open wide, the diagnosis was left acute TMJ disc displacement without reduction. Her secondary complaint was her pain, so left TMJ inflammation was the secondary diagnosis. She also had muscle tenderness, so the tertiary diagnosis was myofascial pain.

It is not uncommon to find the anterior and/or posterior digastric muscles painful among patients with an acute TMJ disc displacement without reduction. Patients with this disorder often repeatedly open the mouth and push against the disc in an attempt to free or stretch this restriction. These are small jaw-opening muscles not developed to provide repeated forceful contractions and generally become painful from repeatedly pushing against the restriction.

Should I have attempted to unlock her left TMJ? More information was needed to make that decision. She related that her left TMJ started intermittently locking 5 months ago and had been continuously locked for over 2 months. She also related she was not willing to wear an anterior positioning appliance 24 hours a day. Since her TMJ has been locked for over 2 months, it is unlikely that her TMJ would unlock even if tried. Since she refused to wear an anterior positioning appliance 24 hours a day even if her TMJ could be unlocked, it would probably just lock again soon afterward. Thus, I did not attempt to unlock her TMJ.

It has been shown that patients with this disorder do not need to have their TMJ unlocked to regain their opening and minimize their symptoms.[6] It is speculated that, over time, these patients stretch their retrodiscal tissues, moving the disc forward, enabling them to translate freely and regain their opening. With the disc out of the way, there is no longer the mechanical interference within the TMJ, and the TMJ inflammation reduces. If patients cannot stretch the retrodiscal tissue on their own, arthrocentesis or arthroscopics are generally very beneficial.

☻ FOCAL POINT

It has been shown that patients with a locked TMJ do not need to have it unlocked to regain their opening and minimize their symptoms.

The patient had a 29-mm opening, which was greater than I typically saw with patients who recently developed an acute TMJ disc displacement without reduction. Therefore, it was suspected that she had already partially stretched her retrodiscal tissue, but further stretching was needed.

My clinical experience with this disorder is based on the biased sample of individuals who come to me for help in regaining their opening and reducing their TMJ inflammation. It is observed that, as long as they have significant inflammation, they generally refuse to aggravate their TMJ more by stretching the retrodiscal tissue, so I first minimize the inflammation to the degree possible and then instruct them to perform stretching exercises, as shown in Figure 5-1, and anti-inflammatory medications are generally included in their initial conservative therapy.

▼ TECHNICAL TIP

Stretching Retrodiscal Tissue

If patients have significant TMJ inflammation, I first minimize the inflammation to the degree possible with anti-inflammatory medications and then instruct them to perform stretching exercises, as shown in Figure 5-1.

The patient had related that, during the intermittent locking phase, her TMJ locking always occurred later in the day, suggesting her daytime parafunctional and/or muscle-tightening habits were greater contributors to her locking than were her nocturnal habits. She also related that her current preauricular pain was worse later in the day, suggesting her daytime habits continued to be a more prominent problem for her than were the nocturnal habits.

She was provided the following treatment: (a) Using the "TMJ Disc Displacements" diagram (Appendix 2), I explained the mechanical interference that was occurring with her acute TMJ disc displacement without reduction, how I planned for the disc to move anteriorly so she would regain her opening, and how her parafunctional habits and muscle tension contributed to her complaint (see Chapter 10, "Acute TMJ Disc Displacement without Reduction"). (b) The "TMD Self-management Therapies" handout was reviewed with her. (c) It was discussed whether she preferred to try 500 mg naproxen taken twice a day alone or for me to prescribe the Medrol Dosepak-naproxen regimen discussed in "Anti-inflammatory Medications" in Chapter 17. (d) She was instructed to perform the stretching exercise as shown in Figure 5-1, hold the stretch 30 to 60 seconds, and sporadically perform this approxi-

mately six times daily. It was explained that she needed to balance the amount of force, length of time the stretch was held, and its number of times performed throughout the day so the resulting TMJ aggravation was within her pain tolerance. She was also told that heating the TMJ with a heating pad prior to performing the exercise usually allowed the retrodiscal tissue to stretch more. (e) She was informed that she should also receive a stabilization appliance to decrease the impact her clenching and/or bruxing was having on the masticatory system. One of the more esthetic appliances could be fabricated and the patient asked to wear it temporarily 24 hours a day, except when eating. (f) A physical therapy referral for treatment of her constant neck pain was discussed. (g) A referral for habit-reversal and relaxation therapy was discussed; if that did not relieve the daytime symptoms satisfactorily, therapy could be escalated.

CASE 14: OSTEITIS CAUSING INABILITY TO OPEN WIDE

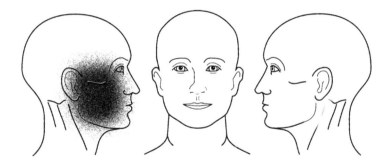

The patient related her right TMJ was locked, restricting her from fully opening her mouth. Tooth 1 (maxillary right third molar) had been extracted 5 days earlier, it was a difficult extraction, and "the surgeon put a lot of force on my jaw." She also related the pain from the extraction was completely gone, but she had constant 6 to 7/10 right preauricular and facial pain.

The findings on periapical radiography of

the extraction site were within normal limits (no root tips or fractured adjacent teeth were noted). Her range of motion was 25 mm opening and 3/5/3 (right lateral, left lateral, and protrusive). Palpation of her masticatory and cervical structures revealed tenderness limited primarily to her left masseter, medial pterygoid muscles, and lateral pterygoid areas. The muscle palpation aggravated her pain, and her right TMJ was minimally tender. In an attempt to confirm the source of her restriction, her jaw was stretched open beyond this limited opening, and this caused aggravation within the general area of these tender muscles. These findings suggested that her disorder was a primary muscle disorder (myositis, myospasm, or local myalgia) and not related to her right TMJ.

This patient was seen at the end of the day on a Friday in our emergency clinic. I had been called to this clinic to do a quick assessment and make recommendations. Since my assessment was that her problem was of muscle origin, the "TMD Self-management Therapies" handout (Appendix 3) was reviewed with her and it was recommended to the dentist that he prescribe her 800 mg ibuprofen, 1 tablet q.i.d.; and 5 mg diazepam, 1 to 2 tablets h.s. and 1/2 tablet in morning and afternoon, if that did not cause drowsiness. She made an appointment to see me first thing on Monday morning so I could perform a comprehensive TMD evaluation, observe for changes in her signs and symptoms, and recommend revisions in her therapy. After I left, the patient convinced the dentist that she also needed acetaminophen with codeine (Tylenol 3) for her pain, and he also prescribed that.

On Monday morning, the patient reported that her pain and her opening had not improved. She related the diazepam relaxed her, but it took the acetaminophen with codeine (Tylenol 3) to relieve her pain. This did not make sense to me, because, if her disorder was caused by the muscles, once they relaxed from the diazepam, her pain should have decreased and the opening should have increased. Once she completed

the "Initial Patient Questionnaire," it was discovered that cold beverages increased her pain, but she was not sure which tooth the cold liquid touched to cause the aggravation. While palpating her muscles and TMJs, it was observed that their tenderness had not changed and that none of the palpations reproduced her complaint.

My thoughts were that she may have an acute pulpalgia from a tooth in the area causing these symptoms. Bitewing radiographs revealed she had no large restorations or cavities on her right side. My next thought was of a possible osteitis in the extraction site, so her extraction site was irrigated, which reproduced her complaint. We packed the extraction site, and her pain was eliminated within 15 minutes. The next morning her opening was back to normal (46 mm).

Occasionally patients inadvertently lead practitioners into an erroneous thought process such as this. To arrive at the proper diagnosis, it is important to evaluate a patient's signs and symptoms (including those obtained from the "Initial Patient Questionnaire") and reproduce the chief complaint(s). When I palpated her muscles on Friday, the patient stated I was aggravating her pain, but when I inquired on Monday whether this was the same pain as her complaint, she said it was not.

⊙ **QUICK CONSULT**

Watching for Incorrect Assumptions

Occasionally patients inadvertently lead practitioners into an erroneous thought process.

CASE 15: LATERAL PTERYGOID MYOSPASM

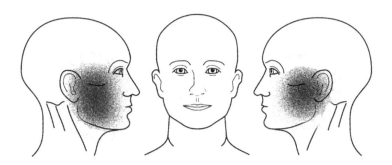

The patient related she could no longer interdigitate her right posterior teeth, could no longer open her mouth wide, and had constant 6/10 bilateral preauricular and masseter area dull/pressure pain (right much worse than left). Her pain was aggravated by trying to bite on her right posterior teeth, which caused a sustained 10/10 right preauricular sharp pain as long as she was biting. Her range of motion was 25 mm opening and 8/4/6 (right lateral, left lateral, and protrusive).

The patient was asked to lie back in the dental chair, relax her mandible with it slightly open, and close her teeth together slowly. It was observed that her left cuspids were repeatedly the first teeth to contact, even though her teeth appeared to have normal alignment.

Palpation of her masticatory and cervical structures revealed generalized tenderness of the masticatory structures, with the greatest tenderness in the right lateral pterygoid area, followed by the bilateral masseter, anterior region of the temporalis muscles, and left lateral pterygoid area, and followed by the TMJs. Masticatory palpations reproduced her pain. The right lateral pterygoid area was exquisitely tender, and the patient felt that its palpation exacerbated the most intense portion of her pain.

What were her TMD diagnoses? Many of these signs and symptoms are characteristic of a right lateral pterygoid myospasm, and that appeared to be the primary diagnosis.

To support this diagnosis, the patient was asked to bite on her right posterior teeth and remember the degree of pain that was created by this force. Next, three wooden tongue depressors (if she had less severe symptoms, I would use two tongue depressors) were placed over the occlusal surfaces of the posterior teeth, as shown in Figure 9-2, and she was asked to bite on the tongue depressors. She reported she had no pain when she bit on them. Based on her signs and symptoms, this test, and her right lateral pterygoid area most exquisitely reproducing her pain compared with her right TMJ, my clinical diagnoses for her were a primary diagnosis of right lateral pterygoid myospasm, a secondary diagnosis of myofascial pain, and a tertiary diagnosis of bilateral TMJ inflammation.

The lateral pterygoid myospasm is the most common disorder I see among the referred emergency TMD patients. Patients and their dentists are often frantic because it frequently develops relatively rapidly, and patients can no longer close their teeth into maximum intercuspation or open wide. Occasionally this occurs after dental treatment, creating quite a bit of anxiety for the dentist.

⊙ **QUICK CONSULT**

Observing for Lateral Pterygoid Myospasm

The lateral pterygoid myospasm is the most common disorder I see among the referred emergency TMD patients. Patients and their dentists are often frantic because it frequently develops relatively rapidly, and patients can no longer close their teeth into maximum intercuspation or open wide.

This patient was provided with the following treatment: (a) The drawing on the top left portion of the "TMJ Disc Displacements" diagram (Appendix 2) was used to explain the mechanics of her lateral pterygoid myospasm symptoms. (b) The "TMD Self-management Therapies" handout was reviewed with her. (c) An exercise to stretch the lateral pterygoid muscle, as depicted in Figure 9-3, was demonstrated to her, and she practiced the exercise to ensure she could properly perform it. She was asked to perform this stretch as a series of six stretches, six times a day, holding each stretch for 30 seconds. [Keep in mind the TMD stretching exercise handout (Appendix 5) is for closure muscles and will probably aggravate a lateral pterygoid myospasm.] (d) She was prescribed 5 mg diazepam, 1 to 2 tablets h.s., to relax the lateral pterygoid muscle and 500 mg naproxen, 1 tablet b.i.d., to alleviate the TMJ inflammation.

The great majority of my patients with a lateral pterygoid myospasm report this therapy resolves or controls their symptoms to the degree that they do not desire to escalate therapy. If these initial therapies do not resolve the myospasm or if the myospasm continues to recur, then traditional TMD therapies (e.g., occlusal appliance therapy, or identifying and changing contributing factors) should be implemented and have been shown to be beneficial.

For a more complete explanation of diagnosis and treatments for lateral pterygoid myospasm, please see Chapter 9, "Lateral Pterygoid Myospasm." Since the inability to close into maximum intercuspation is due to a temporary condition, it is important the practitioner does not adjust the occlusion at this transitory position.

Keep in mind that other, rarely observed, disorders may cause similar symptoms (and are beyond the scope of this book). I once observed an individual with an external ear infection that similarly caused the patient to be unable to close into maximum intercuspation. The patient clearly knew the ear was the source of his pain and inability to close into maximum intercuspation; additionally his opening was not restricted. If a patient does not respond to initial therapy adequately or there is cause for other concerns, the practitioner may desire to take a screening image of the TMJ with a plain (e.g., transcranial) radiograph or panoramic radiograph.

Case 16: Acute Exacerbation of TMD

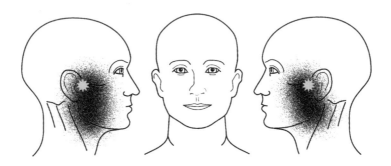

The patient related she was in town for a week-long continuing education course and for the past 4 days had severe exacerbation of her TMD symptoms. Her usual pain was 5/10 bilateral preauricular dull/pressure pain that occurred every day and was never present when she awoke. For the past 4 days, she had constant 7/10 bilateral preauricular and masseter dull/pressure pain without daily variation and momentary 8/10 bilateral preauricular sharp pain when she opened wide.

Her range of motion was 30 mm opening and 5/5/4 (right lateral, left lateral, and protrusive). Palpation of her masticatory and cervical structures revealed generalized tenderness of her masticatory muscles, with her TMJs being the most tender and her posterior digastric muscles being second most painful. Masticatory palpations reproduced her pain, and palpation of the TMJs most intensely reproduced her complaint. She had bilateral TMJ clicks on opening and closing.

What were her TMD diagnoses? The primary diagnosis was bilateral TMJ inflammation, the secondary diagnosis was myofascial pain, and the tertiary diagnosis was bilateral TMJ disc displacement with reduction.

The patient reported she had received the following treatments for her TMD symptoms: (a) A maxillary acrylic stabilization appliance that she wore only at night. She reported this was not beneficial and, since her usual symptoms were primarily caused by daytime habits, I would have expected her

not to obtain significant improvement from it. (b) She took 20 mg amitriptyline (a tricyclic antidepressant) at bedtime. She reported this was also not beneficial and, since her usual symptoms were primarily due to daytime habits, I would similarly have expected her not to obtain significant improvement from it. (c) Biofeedback (recommended for daytime symptoms), which she felt provided her minimal benefit. I was surprised that this did not provide her significant symptom improvement. In discussing her treatment, she related that she was taught to relax while in the therapist's quiet tranquil environment, but she had not been taught to transfer that ability into her normal environment. She was told that, since she could now relax in his office, her treatment was complete. Therefore, I understood the reason she did not have a better symptom response.

She was provided with the following treatment for the acute exacerbation: (a) The "TMJ Disc Displacements" diagram (Appendix 2) was used to explain visually the mechanism of her TMJ clicking and how her parafunctional habits and muscle tension contributed to the loading of her TMJs and their inflammation. (b) The "TMD Self-management Therapies" handout was reviewed with her. She was informed that the pain in her posterior digastric muscles suggested that she had a habit of repeatedly opening her mouth wide in an attempt to stretch or free her restricted opening. She was asked to observe for this and stop the habit, and her normal opening should return once she reduced her TMJ inflammation. (c) Since she had been taught to relax, she was asked to try to implement this training every 5 minutes. She was to try to obtain and continually maintain the relaxed state she achieved in her therapist's office. (d) She was advised that she could temporarily use her stabilization appliance more often than only at night. The maxillary appliance is unesthetic, so I was sure she would not wear it in public, but would wear it more often when she was in her hotel room. (e) She was prescribed the following medications for the acute exacerbation of her chronic pain: Medrol Dosepak, taken as directed on the package; 500 mg naproxen, 1 tablet b.i.d., starting on day 4 of the Dosepak; and 5 mg diazepam, 1 to 2 tablets h.s. and 1/2 tablet in morning and afternoon, if that did not cause drowsiness.

A few options were feasible if she wanted to escalate therapy once she returned home: (a) It was recommended that the treating dentist refer her to a psychologist to provide her with habit-reversal training and teach her to implement relaxation and biofeedback training into her daily life. If indicated, the psychologist may also desire to provide her with coping skills and other therapies. (b) The practitioner may want to provide her with a more esthetic appliance that she would wear temporarily 24 hours a day, except when eating. (c) If the practitioner felt comfortable in prescribing a tricyclic antidepressant, I recommended prescribing her 25 mg desipramine taken in the morning and afternoon, to determine whether this reduced her symptoms and had minimal side effects.

If these additions to her therapy did not improve her symptoms satisfactorily, I recommended considering the following therapies in the order presented: (a) referral to a physical therapist to evaluate her for other contributors (e.g., neck pain, or body mechanics at her workstation) and implementation of local modality therapies (e.g., iontophoresis to her TMJs); (b) alteration of her maxillary stabilization appliance to an anterior positioning appliance, if she met the criteria (provided in Chapter 13, "Anterior Positioning Appliance") for this appliance; or (c) referral for surgical evaluation, if she continued to have moderate to severe pain primarily from the TMJ and her parafunctional habits and other contributing factors had been controlled to the extent possible through conservative therapy.

CASE 17: MULTIPLE FORMS OF HEAD AND NECK PAIN AFTER CROWN INSERTION

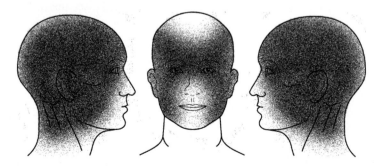

The patient related that, since crowns 18 and 19 (mandibular left first and second molars) were placed a year ago, she had multiple forms of head and neck pain, including (a) 10/10 eye pain, once a week, that started as tightness in back of her neck and progressed to throbbing pain in her right eye, associated with nausea and photophobia lasting 4 to 5 hours; (b) constant 6 to 7/10 bilateral temple dull/pressure pain that was worse in the evening; and (c) 3/10 bilateral maxillary and frontal sinus area pain two to three times a week.

Her range of motion was 51 mm opening and 9/9/7 (right lateral, left lateral, and protrusive). Palpation of her masticatory and cervical structures revealed generalized tenderness of these structures, and her muscles were more tender than her TMJs. These palpations did not reproduce her eye pain, but they revealed temporalis tenderness that reproduced her temple headache, and palpations of the sinuses revealed tenderness that reproduced her sinus area pain.

Evaluation of her occlusion revealed her occlusal contacts appeared evenly distributed on all of her posterior teeth in maximum intercuspation. Accufilm marks of her excursive movements revealed no contacts on crowns 18 and 19, except for a very slight centric relation to maximum intercuspation slide, with much heavier marks with this movement on other posterior teeth.

Do you believe the occlusion on crowns 18 and 19 is the cause of her symptoms? Do you believe that adjusting the very slight centric relation to maximum intercuspation slide on these crowns would alleviate the pain? Since she had fairly even posterior maximum intercuspation contacts, and the slides were heavier on other teeth, it was felt her occlusion was playing only a minor role in her TMD pain and that adjustment of the slide on these crowns would not change her symptoms.

It was felt the reason she associated her pain with the placement of the crowns could run along a continuum between the following: (a) She was very predisposed to TMD, and her masticatory system could not stand the normal strain needed for these procedures, which a normal patient has no problem tolerating. (b) She was not predisposed to TMD, and her masticatory system was subjected to unnecessary overstretching

and/or prolonged procedures. The pain could have also started at that time by coincidence; i.e., the dental procedure may have coincided with her starting a new job or with other stressors that were developing in her life.

Understandably, prior to performing dental treatment, it is prudent to inquire about TMD symptoms and perform a cursory TMD evaluation. Performing a cursory TMD evaluation on all dental patients by measuring their opening and checking for tenderness in the anterior region of the temporalis and masseter muscles, TMJs, and lateral pterygoid areas (Table 8-1) is recommended. Additionally palpations can be performed if further evaluation is indicated.

⊗ **FOCAL POINT**

Prior to performing dental treatment, it is prudent to inquire about TMD symptoms and perform a cursory TMD evaluation.

The patient was informed that, since her eye pain could not be reproduced, I did not know what its source or sources were. It could be created by a local problem, be migraine pain, be referred from a different area (e.g., the neck), be a more central problem (highly unlikely), or be a combination of these. She was informed that the tightness in back of her neck that occurred just prior to her eye pain could be a sign that her eye pain is coming from the neck, could indicate that the neck muscles are tightening in response to the beginning of the eye pain, or could be in response to a source that is behind both pains. She was given the choice of referral to a neurologist or first seeing what response she had from neck treatment by a physical therapist. Since she had chronic neck discomfort, she preferred to be referred to a physical therapist first and, if she did not improve satisfactorily, then be referred to a neurologist.

Palpation of the temporalis muscles reproduced her temporal headache. She was informed that this is due to TMD and could be treated with standard TMD therapies. Her TMD diagnoses were myofascial pain and bilateral TMJ inflammation.

For these TMD symptoms, she was provided with (a) the "TMD Self-management Therapies" handout (Appendix 3), (b) the "Jaw Muscle-stretching Exercise" handout (Appendix 5), (c) one of the more esthetic stabilization appliances that she would wear temporarily 24 hours a day, except when eating, (d) a referral for habit-reversal and relaxation therapy (if that did not relieve the daytime symptoms satisfactorily, we could escalate therapy); and (e) the choice of tak-

ing 800 mg ibuprofen, 1 tablet t.i.d. Patients tend to tighten their masticatory muscles in response to other pains, so relief of these other pains is also important.

The patient was informed that, since her maxillary and frontal sinus pain could be increased only by applying pressure over her sinuses, I believed this pain was due to chronic sinusitis. She related that she was aware this pain could be relieved with decongestants. We discussed her seeing her primary medical provider for this. She wanted to delay this and asked me to prescribe her a decongestant to be used when she had the pain, which I did.

CASE 18: APPLIANCE THAT POSITIONED CONDYLES INTO THEIR "PROPER POSITION"

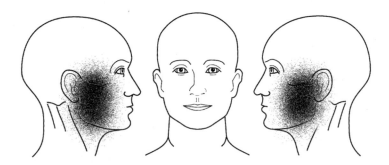

The patient related she needed to wear her appliance 24 hours a day, even when eating and when she had intolerable TMD pain. She had constant 3/10 bilateral preauricular and masseter dull/pressure pain even with continuous wear of her occlusal positioning appliance. When she removed her appliance and closed into maximum intercuspation, her pain increased greatly.

Her range of motion was 30 mm opening and 5/5/5 (right lateral, left lateral, and protrusive). Palpation of her masticatory and cervical structures revealed generalized tenderness of her masticatory muscles and, to a lesser degree, her TMJs; the palpations reproduced her pain.

She related that she had constant 6/10 bilateral preauricular and masseter pain 2 years

ago. Her dentist used sophisticated technology to determine the "proper positions" of her condyles and made her an occlusal appliance with occlusal indentations that positioned her mandible so the condyles were located in these positions. To reduce her TMD symptoms further, she needed orthognathic surgery and braces to align her teeth properly so they interdigitated at the position her condyles had been placed.

She was attempting to join the military, and I was responsible for screening recruits to identify those who had such significant TMD that they could not be deployed. I discussed with the recruit her desire to enter the service, how we are not equipped to repair or make occlusal appliances for deployed personnel who broke or lost their appliance, how the stress of the military would affect her TMD symptoms, and our ability to provide her desired treatment.

Despite this, she still wanted to enter the service. She was informed that she had to demonstrate she could tolerate not wearing her appliance. She was provided the "TMD Self-management Therapies" handout (Appendix 3) and "Jaw Muscle-stretching Exercise" handout (Appendix 5), which were reviewed with her, and it was suggested that she use these instructions. She left her appliance with me, worked with these instructions, and returned to my office 1 week later.

When she returned, she related that her symptoms had decreased and she could now occlude into maximum intercuspation without any symptom increase. I approved her for entering the service, returned her appliance, and asked her to wear it only at night. She was offered additional TMD therapies and joined our habit-reversal and relaxation therapy class.

She returned 2 weeks later stating her symptoms had continued to decrease, but now her appliance positioned her condyles so they were uncomfortable in that position. Her appliance was adjusted so it was the standard stabilization appliance. The patient applied the knowledge gained from our class, used her stabilization appliance at night, and was symptom free a few weeks later.

There are different groups that advocate using relatively expensive techniques to position the condyle into a specific location that each group believes is the best condylar position. One study compared appliances fabricated using a conventional jaw posture technique with appliances fabricated using the Myomonitor (to obtain the myocentric position). The results showed no significant electromyelographic (EMG) activity difference from clenching on the two appliances, and the appliance fabricated with the conven-

tional jaw posture had a more positive EMG activity result.[7]

I am not aware of a better method for positioning the mandible on appliances than what has been recommended in this book. Using one of these other systems appears to be a waste of time and money.

▼ **TECHNICAL TIP**
Positioning the Mandible
I am not aware of a better method for positioning the mandible on appliances than what has been recommended in this book.

REFERENCES

1. Sciotti VM, Mittak VL, DiMarco L, Ford LM, Plezbert J, Santipadri E, Wigglesworth J, Ball K. Clinical precision of myofascial trigger point location in the trapezius muscle. Pain 2001;93(3): 259–66.
2. Wright EF, Gullickson DC. Identifying acute pulpalgia as a factor in TMD pain. J Am Dent Assoc 1996;127:773–80.
3. Wright EF, Gullickson DC. Dental pulpalgia contributing to bilateral preauricular pain and tinnitus. J Orofac Pain 1996;10(2):166–8.
4. Falace DA, Reid K, Rayens MK. The influence of deep (odontogenic) pain intensity, quality, and duration on the incidence and characteristics of referred orofacial pain. J Orofac Pain 1996;10(3):232–9.
5. Wright EF, Domenech MA, Fischer JR Jr. Usefulness of posture training for TMD patients. J Am Dent Assoc 2000;131(2):202–10.
6. Sato S, Kawamura H, Nagasaka H, Motegi K. The natural course of anterior disc displacement without reduction in temporomandibular joint: follow-up at 6, 12, and 18 months. J Oral Maxillofac Surg 1997;55:234–8.
7. Carlson N, Moline D, Huber L, Jacobson J. Comparison of muscle activity between conventional and neuromuscular splints. J Prosthet Dent 1993;70:39–43.

Appendices

Appendices are available on-line at
www.dentistry.blackwellmunksgaard.com/wright

Appendix 1

Initial Patient Questionnaire

Name: _____ Date: _____

1. On the diagram, please shade the
   areas of your pain: Right ○ Left ○

Right   Left

2. When did your pain/problem begin? _____
   _____
   _____

3. What seemed to cause it to start? _____
   _____
   _____

4. What makes it feel worse? _____
   _____
   _____

5. What makes it feel better? _____
   _____
   _____

6. What treatments have you received? _____
   _____
   _____

7. When is your pain the worst? When first wake up ○   Later in the day ○
   No daily pattern ○   Other ○

8. What does the pain keep you from doing? _____

_____

_____

9. Is your pain (check as many as apply): Ache ○   Pressure ○   Dull ○   Sharp ○
   Throbbing ○   Burning ○   Other ○

10. Does your pain:
    Awake you at night? Yes ○   No ○
    Increase when you lie down? Yes ○   No ○
    Increase when you bend forward? Yes ○   No ○
    Increase when you drink hot or cold beverages? Yes ○   No ○

11. Please circle the number below to indicate your *present* pain level.
    (No pain) 0 - 1 - 2 - 3 - 4 - 5 - 6 - 7 - 8 - 9 - 10 (The worst pain imaginable)

12. Please circle your *average* pain level during the past 6 months.
    (No pain) 0 - 1 - 2 - 3 - 4 - 5 - 6 - 7 - 8 - 9 - 10 (The worst pain imaginable)

13. Is your pain always present? Yes ○   No ○   How often do you have it? _____

_____

_____

14. Please describe any symptoms other than pain that you associate with your problem.

_____

_____

_____

_____

15. Have you had:
    Head or neck surgery? Yes ○   No ○
    Whiplash or trauma to your head or neck? Yes ○   No ○
    Shingles on your head or neck? Yes ○   No ○

16. Do you have:
    A fever? Yes ○   No ○
    Nasal congestion or stuffiness? Yes ○   No ○
    Movement difficulties of your facial muscles, eyes, mouth or tongue? Yes ○   No ○
    Numbness or tingling? Yes ○   No ○
    Problems with your teeth? Yes ○   No ○
    Swelling over your jaw joint or in your mouth or throat? Yes ○   No ○
    A certain spot that triggers your pain? Yes ○   No ○
    Recurrent swelling or tenderness of joints other than in your jaw joint? Yes ○   No ○
    Morning stiffness in your body, other than with your jaw? Yes ○   No ○
    Muscle tenderness in your body (other than in your head or neck) for more than 50%
       of the time? Yes ○   No ○

17. Is your problem worse:
    When swallowing or turning your head? Yes ◯   No ◯
    After reading or straining your eyes? Yes ◯   No ◯

18. Do your jaw joints make noise? Yes ◯   No ◯   If yes, which: Right ◯   Left ◯

19. Have you ever been unable to open your mouth wide? Yes ◯   No ◯
    If yes, please explain: _____
    _____
    _____

20. Have you ever been unable to close your mouth? Yes ◯   No ◯   If yes, please explain:
    _____
    _____
    _____

21. Do you sleep well at night? Yes ◯   No ◯   Please explain: _____
    _____
    _____

22. How often are you tense, aggravated or frustrated during a usual day? Always ◯
    Half the time ◯   Seldom ◯   Never ◯

23. How often do you feel depressed during a usual day? Always ◯   Half the time ◯
    Seldom ◯   Never ◯

24. Do you have thoughts of hurting yourself or committing suicide? Yes ◯   No ◯

25. Do you play a musical instrument and/or sing more than 5 hours in a typical week?
    Yes ◯   No ◯

26. What percent of the day are your teeth touching? ____%

27. Are you aware of clenching or grinding your teeth: When sleeping? ◯
    While driving? ◯   When using a computer? ◯   Other times? ◯   Not aware? ◯

28. Are you aware of oral habits such as: Chewing your cheeks? ◯   Chewing objects? ◯
    Biting your nails or cuticles? ◯   Thrusting your jaw? ◯   Other habits? ◯
    Not aware? ◯

29. What treatment do you think is needed for your problem? _____
    _____
    _____

30. Is there anything else you think we should know about your problem? _____
    _____
    _____

31. If your age is 50 or older, please circle the correct response:
    Does your pain occur only when you eat? Yes ⭕   No ⭕
    Are you pain free when you open wide? Yes ⭕   No ⭕
    Do you have unexplainable scalp tenderness? Yes ⭕   No ⭕
    Are you experiencing unexplainable or unintentional weight loss? Yes ⭕   No ⭕
    Do you have significant morning stiffness lasting more than 1/2 hour? Yes ⭕   No ⭕
    Do you have visual symptoms or a visual loss? Yes ⭕   No ⭕

To the best of my knowledge, the above information is correct, and permission is granted for a written report to be sent to my referring and treating doctors and dentists.

Signature _____ Date _____

[Readers choosing to use this questionnaire agree to indemnify and hold the publisher and author harmless for all losses, liabilities, damages (including indirect, special, or consequential), and expenses (including attorneys' fees).]

Appendix 2

TMJ Disc Displacements

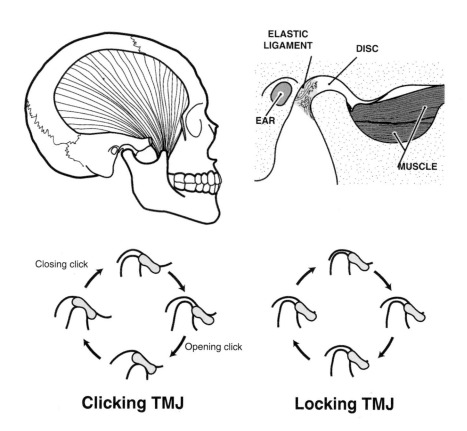

Clicking TMJ   **Locking TMJ**

Appendix 3

TMD Self-management Therapies

Your dentist determined you have a temporomandibular disorder that is often referred to as TMD. The "T" in TMD stands for the *temple*, "M" for the *mandible* or jaw, and "D" for a *disorder* within this complex. This disorder is usually due to an overuse of this system.

We use this system for many activities (talking, eating, yawning, laughing) and, when we are not engaged in these, we need to allow our jaw muscles and joints to relax. Many people have developed habits that do not permit their muscles or joints to relax for a sufficient amount of time. The following will help instruct you on how to reduce the TMD pain you are having:

1. Apply heat, ice, or a combination of heat and ice to the painful areas. Most patients prefer heat, but, if that increases your pain, use the combination or just the ice.
    a. Use heat for 20 minutes two or four times each day. Some patients prefer to use moist heat, whereas others find dry heat just as effective and less of a hassle. Moist heat can be obtained by wetting a thin washcloth with very warm water. The washcloth can then be kept warm by wrapping it around a hot-water bottle or placing it against a heating pad separated by a piece of plastic wrap.
    b. Use the combination of heat and ice two to four times each day. Apply heat to the painful area for approximately 5 minutes (less if it aggravates your pain). Then apply an ice cube wrapped in a thin washcloth.
    c. Apply ice wrapped in a thin washcloth until you first feel some numbness and then remove it (this usually takes about 10 minutes).
2. Eat soft foods like casseroles, canned fruits, soups, eggs, and yogurt. Do not chew gum or eat hard foods (e.g., raw carrots) or chewy foods (e.g., caramels, steak, and bagels). Cut other foods into small pieces, evenly divide the food on both sides of your mouth, and chew on both sides.
3. Avoid caffeine because it stimulates your muscles to contract and hold tension. Caffeine or caffeine-like drugs are found in coffee, tea, most sodas, and chocolate. Decaffeinated coffee also has some caffeine, whereas Sanka has none.
4. Your teeth should never touch except lightly when you swallow. Closely monitor yourself for a clenching or grinding habit. People often clench their teeth when they are irritated,

drive a car, use a computer, or concentrate. Learn to keep your jaw muscles relaxed, teeth separated, and tongue resting lightly on the roof of your mouth just behind your upper front teeth.

5. Observe for and avoid additional habits that put unnecessary strain on your jaw muscles and joints. Some habits include, but are not limited to, resting your teeth together; resting your jaw on your hand; biting your cheeks, lips, fingernails, cuticles, or any other objects you may put in your mouth; pushing your tongue against your teeth; and holding your jaw in an uncomfortable or tense position.

6. Posture appears to play a role in TMD symptoms. Try to maintain good head, neck, and shoulder posture. You may find that a small pillow or rolled towel supporting your lower back may be helpful. Ensure you maintain good posture when using a computer and avoid poor postural habits such as cradling the telephone against your shoulder.

7. Your sleep posture is also important. Avoid positions that strain your neck or jaw, such as stomach sleeping. If you sleep on your side, keep your neck and jaw aligned.

8. Set aside time once or twice a day to relax and drain the tension from your jaw and neck. Patients often benefit from simple relaxation techniques such as sitting in a quiet room while listening to soothing music, taking a warm shower or bath, and slow deep breathing.

9. Restrain from opening your mouth wide, such as yawning, yelling, or prolonged dental procedures.

10. Use anti-inflammatory and pain-reducing medications, such as Aleve, ibuprofen, Tylenol, aspirin, and Percogesic, to reduce joint and muscle pain. Avoid those with caffeine, e.g., Anacin, Excedrin, or Vanquish.

There is no cure for TMD, and you may need to follow these instructions for the rest of your life. Your dentist may suggest other therapies in addition to these instructions. No single therapy has been shown to be totally effective for TMD, and a percentage of patients receiving therapies report no symptom improvement (i.e., 10 to 20 percent of patients receiving occlusal appliances report no improvement). Based on your symptoms and identified contributing factors, an individualized treatment approach will be recommended that may be revised as your symptom response is observed.

Appendix 4

Occlusal Appliance Care Instructions

Your appliance is designed to protect and stabilize your jaw muscles and joints. It should help you feel more comfortable and allow healing to occur. It is adjusted to hit evenly on your back teeth. As your muscles relax and your TMJ inflammation resolves, it is common for your bite on the appliance to change so that your back teeth no longer hit evenly. Your appliance will need to be periodically adjusted for these changes. To maximize the benefits derived from your appliance, follow these recommendations:

1. Do not bite on your appliance. The appliance is a reminder to help you learn to keep your teeth apart and jaw muscles and tongue relaxed. Constantly monitor your jaw position and tension, and remember to keep your tongue up and teeth off of the appliance.

2. It is normal for the appliance to feel tight when you first put it in. If your appliance hurts your teeth or gums, leave it out and come back to have it adjusted. Occasionally the appliance may cause a temporary increase in jaw tension or joint noises, especially when you are first getting used to wearing it.

3. Never wear your appliance when you eat.

4. Clean the inside and outside of your appliance at least daily with your toothbrush and toothpaste. It can be soaked with baking soda or a denture-cleaner solution to help clean it.

5. When you are *not* wearing your appliance:
   a. Be careful where you place it, because it is very fragile.
   b. Do not let it lie around, because dogs and cats enjoy chewing on such items.
   c. Do not leave it in a warm place (e.g., inside your car on a warm day), because it may warp.
   d. If your appliance will be out of your mouth for more than 8 hours, store it in a moist environment. You can place it with a few drops of water in a ziplock bag or margarine tub.

6. Some patients find their appliance causes them to salivate, whereas others find it causes them to have a dry mouth. This is generally only a temporary situation.

7. When you take your appliance out, your jaw may take a few seconds to adjust back to the way your teeth normally fit together.

8. ALWAYS BRING YOUR APPLIANCE TO ALL DENTAL APPOINTMENTS. In the beginning, it will need to be adjusted for the changes that occur with your muscles and TMJs. Any dental work (restorations, sealants, etc.) may cause it not to fit and/or occlude properly, and it should be checked for changes.

Appendix 5

Jaw Muscle-stretching Exercise

People unconsciously stretch many of their muscles throughout the day. Patients who have jaw muscle stiffness or pain often find a significant improvement in their symptoms with this jaw-stretching exercise. Your dentist believes your symptoms will improve if you perform this simple jaw-stretching exercise 6 times a day, between 30 and 60 seconds each time, at the opening and duration you determine best for you.

It is best to warm your jaw muscles before you stretch by opening and closing them slowly about 10 times. You may also warm your muscles by applying heat to them (allow time for the heat to penetrate into your muscles). While stretching, you need to concentrate on relaxing your lips, facial muscles, and jaw. Do not bite on your fingers while stretching; they are only to give you a guide for the width you are stretching.

To determine what opening and duration are best for you, the first time you stretch, bend your index finger and place the middle knuckle between your upper and lower front teeth (see Figure 1). Hold this position for 30 seconds. If this does not aggravate your symptoms, the second time you stretch, increase the time to 45 seconds. If this does not aggravate your symptoms, the next time increase it to 60 seconds. If this does not aggravate your symptoms, increase your opening width to 2 fingertips (see Figure 2) and cut your time back to 30 seconds. Continue increasing your time and opening in this manner, but do not go beyond 3 fingertips. Find the largest opening and duration that does not cause even the slightest discomfort or aggravation of your symptoms and use this each time you stretch. If you experience any discomfort or aggravation, decrease your opening or time.

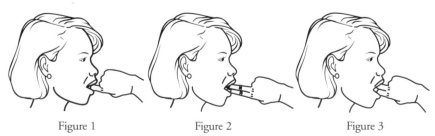

Figure 1   Figure 2   Figure 3

As your symptoms improve or if you have a flare-up, you will need to increase or decrease this opening and time. Be very careful not to cause yourself any aggravation with this exercise, because this may hurt your progress.

Patients report this exercise does not provide immediate symptom improvement, but takes about 1 to 2 weeks before benefits are noticed. Similarly, stopping does not cause immediate loss of these benefits, but also tends to take 1 to 2 weeks to be noticed. With the normal symptom fluctuation most TMD patients experience, it is often difficult for them to relate their symptom improvement or aggravation to the starting or stopping of this exercise.

Appendix 6

Posture Improvement Exercises

INSTRUCTIONS

Chin tucks	Tuck your chin back over the notch above your sternum, so that your ear is in line with the tip of your shoulder.
Chest stretch	Stand in a doorway or a the corner of a room. Lean forward, with your hands on the wall, until you feel significant stretch across the front of your chest. Do this exercise as requested in both positions.
Wall stretch	Stand with your back against the wall and your arms positioned as shown in the drawing. Straighten your upper back and flatten your lower back against the wall. Press your head back with your chin down and in, and pull your elbows back against the wall. Do this exercise as requested in both positions.
On-your-back chest stretch	Lie on your back with your hands clasped behind your head. As you exhale, slowly bring your elbows together touching in front of your face. As you inhale, slowly draw the elbows apart until they touch the floor.
Face-down arm lifts	Lie on your stomach as shown in the drawings (position 1 has the elbows at shoulder level and bent at 90°, whereas position 2 has elbows at ear level). Lift your arms, head, and chest off the floor and repeat until you can only move 50 percent through the range or to fatigue. Do this in both positions.

If these exercises cause any discomfort or aggravate your pain, discontinue them until you can discuss it with your provider.

Stretching should be done in a slow, gradual, easy, and painless manner. Move to the point of mild tension and hold. Do not bounce!

300

EXERCISES

Chin Tucks
Perform: 10 times on the hour
Hold: 5 seconds

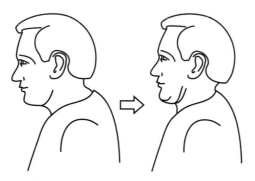

Chest Stretch
Perform: 3 times a day, 2 repetitions
Hold: 15 seconds

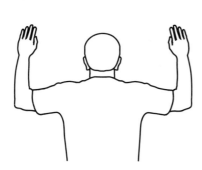
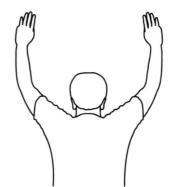

Wall Stretch
Perform: 3 times a day, 2 repetitions
Hold: 15 seconds

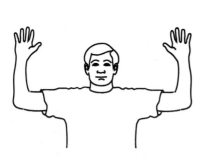
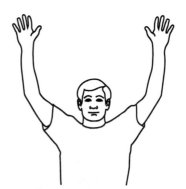

On-your-back Chest Stretch
Perform: before you retire, 10 repetitions

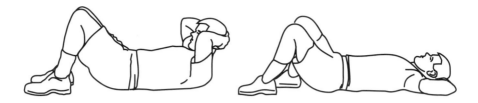

Face-down Arm Lifts
Perform: once a day, 5 days/week

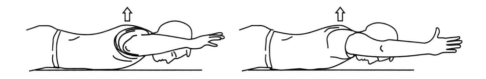

Appendix 7

Laboratory Occlusal Appliance Instructions

Please fabricate the occlusal appliance circled below. The patient is scheduled for insertion of this appliance on _____ .

MAXILLARY 0.15-INCH SOFT THERMOPLASTIC APPLIANCE AND MAXILLARY DUAL LAMINATE THERMOPLASTIC APPLIANCE

Please debubble cast(s), do not block out undercuts, carry the facial portion of the appliance only to the gingival margin and extend the lingual portion 5 mm along the gingiva.

For the dual laminate thermoplastic appliance, once the dual laminate material is on the articulator, adjust the incisal pin so the closest opposing tooth is 1 mm from the occlusal surface, enabling the thickness of the added acrylic to be 1 mm or more. Please add acrylic to the occlusal surface so the occlusal surface is flat without cuspal indentations, the nonsupporting posterior cusps are not in contact, the protrusive and canine guidances provide minimal posterior disocclusion (1/2 to 1 mm), and the occlusal line angles are rounded. Thank you.

MANDIBULAR 0.15-INCH SOFT THERMOPLASTIC APPLIANCE AND MANDIBULAR DUAL LAMINATE THERMOPLASTIC APPLIANCE

Please debubble cast(s), do not block out undercuts, carry the facial portion of the appliance only to the gingival margin and extend the lingual portion 10 mm below the gingival margin, keeping it short of lingual tori, vestibule, and frenum.

For the dual laminate thermoplastic appliance, once the dual laminate material is on the articulator, adjust the incisal pin so the closest opposing tooth is 1 mm from the occlusal surface, enabling the thickness of the added acrylic to be 1 mm or more. Please add acrylic to the occlusal surface so the occlusal surface is flat without cuspal indentations, the nonsupporting posterior cusps are not in contact, the protrusive and canine guidances provide minimal posterior disocclusion (1/2 to 1 mm), and the occlusal line angles are rounded. Thank you.

Maxillary 2-mm Hard Thermoplastic Appliance and Maxillary Acrylic Stabilization Appliance

Please:

1. Debubble the cast(s) and block out (a) deep grooves on and between the teeth and (b) all undercuts at 0°, with the exception of *no* blockout in the buccal embrasures of the posterior teeth.

2. Survey the cast and extend acrylic, so that (a) the buccal extent is carried 1/2 mm below the height of contour for the posterior teeth, (b) the labial extent is carried only 1 to 11/2 mm beyond the incisal edge of the anterior teeth, and (c) the lingual portion extends 5 mm along the gingiva.

3. For the acrylic stabilization appliance, adjust the incisal pin so the appliance's minimum occlusal thickness is 3 mm. Fabricate the occlusal surface so the surface is flat without cuspal indentations, the nonsupporting posterior cusps are not in contact, the protrusive and canine guidances provide minimal posterior disocclusion (1/2 to 1 mm), and the occlusal line angles are rounded. Please make the facial acrylic so it is 1 mm thick and flows with the contours of the teeth and make the lingual flange so it is only 1 mm thick.

Thank you.

Mandibular 2-mm Hard Thermoplastic Appliance and Mandibular Acrylic Stabilization Appliance

Please:

1. Debubble the cast(s) and block out (a) deep grooves on and between the teeth and (b) all undercuts at 0°, with the exception of *no* blockout in the buccal undercuts of the posterior teeth.

2. Survey the cast and extend acrylic, so that (a) the buccal extent is carried 1/2 mm below the height of contour for the posterior teeth, (b) the labial extent is carried only 1 to 11/2 mm beyond the incisal edge of the anterior teeth, and (c) the lingual extends 10 mm below the gingival margin, keeping it short of lingual tori, vestibule, and frenum.

3. For the acrylic stabilization appliance, adjust the incisal pin so the appliance's minimum occlusal thickness is 3 mm. Fabricate the occlusal surface so the surface is flat without cuspal indentations, the nonsupporting posterior cusps are not in contact, the protrusive and canine guidances provide minimal posterior disocclusion (1/2 to 1 mm), and the occlusal line angles are rounded. Please make the posterior facial acrylic so it is 1 mm thick and flows with the contours of the teeth and make the lingual surface so it is only 1 mm thick.

Thank you.

Appendix 8

Example of Dental Record Entries

INITIAL EXAM

S: Comprehensive TMD evaluation; CC: constant Rt preauricular dull/pressure pain, 4/10 upon awaking and 1/10 later in the day. Approximately once a week, she also awakes with 2/10 Rt temporal pain lasting approximately 2 hours. The pain began approximately 3 months ago after an increase in stress at work. The "Initial Patient Questionnaire" responses were reviewed with Pt.

O: Soft tissue and teeth were WNL. Palpation of selected masticatory and cervical structures revealed tenderness of her Rt and Lt masseter and Rt temporalis muscles, and Rt TMJ. The Rt masseter and Rt temporalis muscle palpations reproduced her pain complaints. A reciprocal click was present in her Rt TMJ. ROM: 38 mm opening, 6/6/5 (right lateral, left lateral, and protrusive).

A: Clinical TMD Dx: Myofascial pain, Rt TMJ inflammation, and Rt TMJ disc displacement with reduction. Nocturnal and daytime parafunctional habits (Pt relates her teeth are touching 30 percent of the day), tension, and caffeine consumption appear to be her major perpetuating contributing factors.

P: Explained to Pt the mechanics of her Rt TMJ reciprocal click. Written and oral TMD self-management instructions given; Pt agreed to decrease her caffeine consumption to 1 cup of coffee a day. Max and man alginate imp and bite registration taken for fab of a max acr stabilization appliance that Pt to wear at night. Pt reappt in 2 weeks for insertion of occlusal appliance.

INSERTION APPOINTMENT

Re: Myofascial pain, Rt TMJ inflammation, and Rt TMJ disc displacement with reduction. Pt reports slt improvement, which she attributes to implementing the TMD self-management instructions. Her Rt preauricular pain upon awaking is now 3/10, and she has only intermittent 1/10 daytime symptoms; she continues to have her weekly 2/10 Rt temporal pain. Ins max acr stabilization appliance for Pt to wear at night. Written and oral appliance care instr given and reviewed TMD self-management instructions. Pt reappt in 3 weeks for follow-up.

FOLLOW-UP

Re: Myofascial pain, Rt TMJ inflammation, and Rt TMJ disc displacement with reduction. Pt reports significant symptom improvement and has only 1/10 preauricular morning pain approximately once a week. Adj stabilization appliance and Pt reappt in 2 months for follow-up or to RTC sooner if improvement does not continue.

FOLLOW-UP

Re: Myofascial pain, Rt TMJ inflammation, and Rt TMJ disc displacement with reduction. Pt reports as long as she wears her appliance at night she has no TMD discomfort. ROM: 48 mm opening, palpation of selected masticatory structures revealed minimal tenderness, and reciprocal click is still present in Rt TMJ. Adj stabilization appliance and Pt to wear appliance nightly. Pt to RTC annually for follow-up or sooner if symptoms return, appliance needs adj, or another problem develops.

Appendix 9

Examples of Physical Therapy Consultations

Dentists commonly refer TMD patients to physical therapists to improve TMD pain, TMJ function, range of motion, daytime or sleeping postures, and/or neck symptoms. In addition to improving a patient's symptoms, a goal in physical therapy is to teach the patient to maintain this improvement. It has been demonstrated that physical therapy performed in conjunction with occlusal appliance therapy attains better improvement in TMD symptoms.

Two examples are presented below: the first is a patient whose TMD symptoms are limited to the masticatory system, and the second is a patient who has concomitant neck pain and the physical therapist is requested to treat just the cervical myofascial pain.

These referrals can be made on a prescription pad. Many third-party payers require also that the requested frequency and duration of treatment be documented; two to three times a week for a month is a reasonable request, and some third-party payers will allow practitioners to request "as therapist recommends." Inform the physical therapist of any precautions he or she should be aware of (e.g., previous surgery, tumor, screws, or wires in the region) and medical disorders that could complicate therapy (e.g., angioedema).

CC: Constant 6/10 Rt preauricular pain.

Dx: Rt TMJ inflammation, myofascial pain, and Rt TMJ disc displacement with reduction.

Please evaluate and treat. Pt also relates she intermittently sleeps on her stomach and cannot stop. Would you please help Pt break this habit? Thank you.

Precautions: None.

Pt was given an occlusal appliance and TMD self-management instructions.

CC: Constant 5/10 bilateral preauricular and masseter pain, and constant 5/10 neck pain.

Dx: Masticatory and cervical myofascial pain.

Please evaluate and treat Pt's cervical disorder. Palpation of her cervical muscles reproduced her masticatory pain. It is believed that the local component of her masticatory symptoms can be adequately relieved through TMD therapy, but need treatment of her neck pain to relieve the cervical component.

Precautions: None.

Pt was given TMD self-management instructions and will be give an occlusal appliance at her next appointment.

Clinical experience suggests referring TMD patients to physical therapy for any of the following:

1. The patient has neck pain. TMD patients with neck pain do not respond to TMD therapy as well as those without neck pain. Some TMD symptoms primarily come from the neck, and it has been observed that some TMD patients who have their cervical trigger points inactivated report a substantial decrease in their pain.

2. The patient has cervicogenic headaches, which are headaches that originate in the neck, and clinically it appears TMD patients tend to hold more tension in their masticatory muscles when they have a headache. Therefore, TMD patients with cervicogenic headaches who have their neck treated should have fewer headaches and may also obtain substantial TMD symptom improvement.

3. The patient has moderate to severe forward head posture. These patients have been shown to be most likely to derive significant TMD symptom improvement from posture exercises in combination with TMD self-management instructions.

4. The patient's TMD symptoms increase with abnormal postural activities. Instructing these patients in body mechanics (teaching patients how to perform tasks without straining the body) should help them maintain good posture, thereby improving their TMD symptoms.

5. The patient desires help in changing poor sleep posture. Stomach sleeping perpetuates TMD and neck symptoms and, if a patient cannot stop sleeping on his or her stomach, physical therapists are trained to help patients change their sleep position.

6. The patient did not derive adequate TMD symptom relief from other therapies. Physical therapists are trained to treat musculoskeletal disorders throughout the body and can apply their skills to the masticatory system.

7. The patient is to have TMJ surgery. It has been shown that patients who receive physical therapy following TMJ surgery have better results. It is appropriate for these patients to be given a physical therapy referral prior to surgery in order that they may learn about and possibly start the postsurgical exercises, and schedule the recommended postsurgical appointments.

Appendix 10

Examples of Psychology Consultations

It is well recognized that daytime parafunctional habits, tension, stress, anxiety, anger, depression, catastrophizing (thinking the worst of situations), pain-related beliefs, not coping well with "life's stuff," etc., negatively impact patients' TMD symptoms and their ability to improve with conservative TMD therapy. Cognitive-behavioral interventions are adjunctive TMD therapies that attempt to help patients reduce their daytime parafunctional habits and psychosocial contributing factors.

Patients with significant persistent daytime habits and/or psychosocial contributors often need additional help from a practitioner trained in cognitive-behavioral interventions. These interventions primarily encompass habit reversal, relaxation, hypnosis, biofeedback, stress management, and cognitive therapy (focuses on changing patients' distorted thoughts).

It has been observed that some psychologists desire to perform psychological testing prior to the cognitive-behavioral intervention to identify which therapies may be most beneficial for the patient. Other psychologists may provide a standard brief cognitive-behavioral intervention and may test only those patients who do not sufficiently improve.

Referring patients to a psychologist can be as easy as giving patients the psychologist's name and asking them to make an appointment. At the initial visit, the patient would tell the psychologist the problem, and the psychologist would assess the patient's condition.

It is my preference to write a note (as the examples below) to help the psychologist better understand my concerns. In the first example, the psychologist will probably primarily use habit-reversal therapy and, in the second example, primarily use stress management therapy:

Mrs. Jones has long-standing 6/10 daytime TMD symptoms that are primarily due to overloading her masticatory system from daytime oral habits. She has unsuccessfully attempted to break these habits on her own, and she is aware she touches her teeth together approximately 90 percent of the day and unconsciously squeezes them together when she becomes busy, frustrated, or deep in thought. Mrs. Jones would like your assistance to help her break her daytime oral parafunctional habits. She has an occlusal appliance that she wears for her nocturnal oral parafunctional habits. Thank you.

Miss Smith complains of 6/10 bilateral jaw pain, which was diagnosed as myofascial pain. Her primary contributing factor appears to be work-related stress. Her pain started 4 months ago, right after she started a new job that she finds very busy, hectic, and stressful. She would like to learn stress management and coping skills to better deal with her work situation. Would you please evaluate and treat as you feel is most appropriate? Thank you.

Appendix 11

Working with Insurance Companies

States that have laws that mandate medical insurance companies cover certain aspects of TMD therapy are Arkansas, California, Florida, Georgia, Illinois, Kentucky, Minnesota, Mississippi, Nebraska, Nevada, New Mexico, North Carolina, North Dakota, Texas, Vermont, Virginia, Washington, West Virginia, and Wisconsin. Small private insurance companies may be exempt from the law and may avoid covering these state-mandated procedures.

The Patient Advocacy Group listed in "Sources For Additional TMD Information" (Appendix 12) should be able to provide you with a copy of the portion of your state law that covers TMD mandated procedures. Additionally the American Academy of Orofacial Pain (also listed in Appendix 12) has an Access to Care Committee that should be able to provide you with answers to many of your insurance questions.

Electronic filing and proper coding tend to speed payment reimbursement and decrease the number of "misplaced" claim forms. Coding manuals and software are offered by one of the businesses listed in Appendix 12.

Medical TMD Diagnosis Codes
ICD-9

TMJ Disorders

524.60	Temporomandibular joint disorders, unspecified
524.61	TMJ adhesion and ankylosis (bony or fibrous)
524.62	TMJ arthralgia (TMJ inflammation, as used in this book)
524.63	Articular disc disorder (with or without reduction)
524.69	Other specified temporomandibular joint disorders
830.1	TMJ dislocation
848.1	TMJ sprain or strain

Muscular Disorders

728.85	Spasm of muscle (myospasm)
729.1	Myalgia and myositis (also use for myofascial pain)

Dental and medical TMD procedure codes

CDT-4   CPT

Initial Visit

D0150		Comprehensive oral evaluation [for normal TMD evaluation]
D0160		Detailed and extensive oral evaluation [for complex TMD evaluation]
D9310		Consultation
D9920		Behavioral management, by report [for each 15-minute increment]

Occlusal Appliance Insertion

D7880	21110	Occlusal orthotic device, by report
D9920		Behavioral management, by report [for each 15-minute increment]

Follow-up

D9920		Behavioral management, by report [for each 15-minute increment]
D9430		Office visit for observation [no other services provided]

Other Codes

D0330	70355	Panoramic film
D0321	70328	Radiological examination, TMJ, open and closed mouth, unilateral
D0321	70330	Radiological examination, TMJ, open and closed mouth, bilateral
D0321	76101	Radiological examination, TMJ tomogram, unilateral
D0321	76102	Radiological examination, TMJ tomogram, bilateral
D0460		Pulp vitality tests
D7899		Orthotic repair, by report
D7899		Chairside orthotic reline, by report
D9110		Palliative (emergency) treatment of pain
D9210		Local anesthesia not in conjunction with operative or surgical procedure
D9610		Therapeutic drug injection, by report
D9940		Occlusal guard, by report [for bruxism, if for TMD use D7880]

CPT Codes for Office Visit and Consultation

99201 to 99205	New patient office visit
99211 to 99215	Established patient office visit
99241 to 99245	Office consultation [for new or established patient]

Sources:

ICD-9: *Hospital & Payer ICD-9-CM*, 6th edition. Salt Lake City: Medicode, 2000.

CDT-4: *Current Dental Terminology*, 4th edition. Chicago: American Dental Association, 2002.

CPT: *Current Procedural Terminology 2003*. Chicago: AMA, 2002.

Appendix 12

Sources for Additional TMD Information

PATIENT BROCHURES

Among the many pamphlets about TMD available from various sources, the following pamphlets are preferred:

1. Temporomandibular Disorders (TMD), brochure OP-23. This is my favorite brochure and it is sponsored by the National Institute of Dental Research. It states that orthodontics, crowns, bridges, and occlusal adjustments are of little value. The brochure is free and can be ordered from the National Oral Health Information Clearinghouse on line (up to 50 copies) at www.nohic.nidcr.nih.gov or via telephone (301-402-7364).

2. The American Academy of Orofacial Pain (AAOP) has a good patient brochure that can be viewed on their Web site (www.aaop.org/AAOP) and ordered through their central office (856-423-3629).

PATIENT ADVOCACY GROUP

The TMJ and Orofacial Pain Society of America is a nonprofit organization that provides help with patient issues, publishes quarterly newsletters, and should be able to provide you with the mandated law insurance information for your state. Visit their Web site (www.tmjsociety.org) or telephone them (916-444-1985).

BOOKS FOR PATIENTS

During your interaction with patients, you may feel one enjoys reading, is self-motivated, and would benefit from reading one or more of the following books:

1. *Taking Control of TMJ* (1999), by Robert O. Uppgaard $13.95, gives patients more information about their TMD condition, self-management therapies, neck exercises, stress management, and many other suggestions.

2. *Feeling Good: The New Mood Therapy* (1999), by David D. Burns, $7.99, helps patients understand how our thoughts affect our moods and how to improve them.

3. *No More Sleepless Nights* (1996), by Peter Hauri, Shirley Linde, and Philip Westbrook, $16.95, helps patients with a sleep disorder better understand their problem and use techniques to attempt to improve their sleep.

TMD Practice Management Businesses

1. TMData Resources offers practice development consultations and a full line of services exclusively for TMD and snoring practices. They write and distribute TMD-related and snoring-related educational materials for doctor education, patient education, and physician referrals. They support TMJ patients with information and a national list of doctors who treat TMD. You can view their products and services (www.tmdataresources.com) or telephone them (800-533-5121).

2. Nierman Practice Management offers manuals and software for diagnostic and procedural codes, narrative reports, and other correspondence for collecting medical and dental insurance benefits for treatment of TMD. They also offer services for orthodontics, implants, general and esthetic dentistry, and sleep disorders. You can view their products and services (www.rosenierman.com) or telephone them (800-879-6468).

Professional TMD Organizations

There are two primary TMD professional organizations. They provide educational meetings, offer staff training at their meetings, worked with the American Dental Association to make TMD a recognized specialty, have diplomate certification boards, and each publishes one of the two journals listed below and provides other beneficial activities:

1. American Academy of Orofacial Pain (AAOP). Their Web site can be viewed at www.aaop.org. The AAOP Central Office telephone number is 856-423-3629.

2. American Academy of Craniofacial Pain (AACFP). Their Web site can be viewed at www.aacfp.org. The AACP Central Office telephone number is 800-322-8651.

Textbooks

The two outstanding TMD books are:

1. Okeson JP. *Management of Temporomandibular Disorders and Occlusion*, 5th edition. St Louis: CV Mosby, 2003. Telephone 800-621-0387.

2. American Academy of Orofacial Pain, with Okeson JP (ed). *Orofacial Pain: Guidelines for Assessment, Diagnosis and Management*. Chicago: Quintessence, 1996. Telephone 800-621-0387.

TMD Studies

TMD studies can be found in most dental and medical journals. The first two names below are journals that are dedicated primarily to TMD, and the third is a 16-page publication, printed 6 times a year, entailing recent TMD articles and their summaries:

1. *Journal of Orofacial Pain*. Quintessence. Telephone 800-621-0387.
2. *Cranio: The Journal of Craniomandibular Practice*. Chroma. Telephone 800-624-4141.
3. *TMJ Update*. Anadem. Telephone 800-633-0055.

Glossary

The words listed in the glossary are in bold print throughout the text.

Anterior positioning occlusal appliance holds the mandible in an anterior location, typically where the condyle is reduced onto the disc. It is primarily used for patients who have a disc displacement with reduction, and this position holds the condyle in the reduced position so the disc-condyle mechanical disturbances are temporarily eliminated and any forces loading the condyle are transmitted through the disc's intermediate zone rather than the retrodiscal tissue.

Centric relation (CR) is the maxillomandibular relationship in which the condyles are seated in their most anterior-superior location against the disc's intermediate zone (the thinnest avascular portion of the disc) and the posterior slopes of the articular eminences. This is a very reproducible position and appears to be the most musculoskeletally stable position for the mandible.

Cervical dysfunction is neck pain, tightness, or decreased range of motion. It is moderately prevalent among TMD patients and may not only directly affect the masticatory system and its ability to respond to therapy, but may also cause referred pain to the masticatory structures, which can add to a patient's TMD symptoms or be the sole cause for the symptoms.

Cognitive behavioral interventions primarily encompass habit reversal, relaxation, hypnosis, biofeedback, stress management, and cognitive therapy (focuses on changing patients' distorted thoughts). They are adjunctive TMD therapies that attempt to help patients reduce their daytime parafunctional habits and psychosocial contributing factors.

Contributing factors are the elements that directly or indirectly contribute to the TMD symptoms, impacting both muscle and TMJ pain. They can be subcategorized into *predisposing, initiating,* and *perpetuating* contributing factors. The perpetuating contributing factors are a TMD patient's contributing factors that perpetuate the disorder (not allowing it to resolve), e.g., nighttime parafunctional habits, gum chewing, daytime clenching, stress, and poor posture.

Direct trauma is a physical blow to the masticatory system (macrotrauma), thus differing from *indirect trauma* or *microtrauma*.

External cues are external stimuli that TMD patients use to remind themselves to check for oral habits or masticatory muscle tension. Examples of external cues are an unusually placed yellow Post-it note that will alert the patient, or a timer that rings every 5 minutes. Over time, they tend to blend into the background and need to be changed. Some patients prefer to work first with external cues and progress later to internal cues.

Fibromyalgia is characterized by widespread muscle pain, multiple tender points over the body, poor sleep, stiffness, and generalized fatigue. It is moderately prevalent among TMD patients, can add to the patient's TMD symptoms, and can decrease a patient's ability to respond to TMD therapy.

Indirect trauma is a nonimpact jolt to the jaw analogous to cervical whiplash, which can result in TMD symptoms from damage to the muscle or TMJ.

Initiating contributing factor is the event that caused the TMD symptoms, e.g., trauma to the jaw or the placement of a crown.

Internal cues are bodily features that TMD patients use to alert themselves when they are performing oral habits or have excessive masticatory muscle tension. The patient becomes very attuned to observing the chosen internal cue, so, when it occurs, the patient notices it despite other mental activity. The most common internal cues that TMD patients use are the teeth touching the opposing teeth or an occlusal appliance, their pain intensity, and muscle tension. Clinically, patients appear to have the best long-term success with breaking daytime oral habits if they have learned to use internal cues to maintain their desired behaviors or postures. Some patients prefer to work first with external cues and progress later to internal cues.

Lateral pterygoid myospasm is a condition in which the inferior lateral pterygoid muscle is in constant involuntary contraction at a partially shortened position. This is a common cause for patients reporting an inability to put the ipsilateral posterior teeth together without excruciating pain.

Maximum intercuspation (MI) is a maxillary to mandibular relation determined by the teeth, in which they are maximally intercuspating (occluding).

Microtrauma is chronic irritation to the masticatory structures, usually from chronic parafunctional habits. It generally predisposes or causes individuals to develop TMD, and makes it more difficult to resolve the manifested symptoms.

Neutral position is an unrestrained condylar position that approaches CR, but does not encroach upon inflamed retrodiscal tissue nor firmly seat the condyles.

Parafunctional habits are unproductive movement habits; in relation to TMD, these would be oral habits, e.g., lip biting, cheek biting, grinding teeth, clenching teeth, and pursing lips.

Perpetuating contributing factors are the elements that directly or indirectly aggravate the masticatory system and prevent the TMD symptoms from resolving, e.g., night-time parafunctional habits, gum chewing, daytime clenching, stress, and poor posture.

Predisposing contributing factors are the elements that make an individual more susceptible to developing TMD, e.g., fingernail biting, clenching, and biting on objects. Individuals who are very predisposed to developing TMD may be those who develop TMD from a slight occlusal change, e.g., from the placement of a pit and fissure sealant.

Primary diagnosis is the diagnosis for the disorder most responsible for a patient's chief complaint. This diagnosis can be of TMD origin (e.g., myofascial pain, TMJ inflammation, or acute TMJ disc displacement without reduction) or from a different source (e.g., pulpal pathosis, sinusitis, or cervicogenic headache).

Referred pain is pain perceived at a location different than its source. This is similar to how a patient suffering from a heart attack may perceive pain only in the left arm, whereas the source is the heart. Masticatory muscles, TMJs, tooth pulps, and cervical muscles and cervical spine commonly cause referred pain to each other. The true source must be identified and treatment directed toward the source, not the site where the pain is felt.

Secondary diagnosis is another TMD diagnosis that contributes to the primary diagnosis. Typically, the primary diagnosis will be of TMD origin (e.g., myofascial pain) and the secondary and tertiary diagnoses will be other TMD diagnoses (e.g., TMJ inflammation and TMJ disc displacement with reduction) that contribute to a patient's chief complaint. They are ordered by the degree they contribute to the patient's chief complaint.

Secondary gain is a situation in which a patient is rewarded for having TMD; e.g., a patient receives disability payments or is excused from undesirable chores or work. Clinically, I do not commonly observe this situation, but, if it is present, the patient may not relate improvement from any therapy.

Stabilization occlusal appliances have a flat surface occluding with the opposing dentition, which provides a gnathologically stable occlusal environment. It allows patients to move freely from maximum intercuspation and is most commonly used for those with tooth attrition or TMD symptoms.

Stress management is a cognitive approach to deal with the stresses, irritations, or frustrations that patients encounter. Some studies suggest the average TMD patient does not cope as well with stress as do non-TMD patients. TMD patients tend to tighten their masticatory muscles in these situations, and stress management teaches coping skills to help them better manage these situations and their thoughts about them.

Symptom patterns include the period of the day in which the symptoms occur or are most intense (e.g., worse upon awakening) and the location pattern (e.g., begins in the neck and then moves to the jaw).

Tertiary diagnosis is another TMD diagnosis that contributes to the primary diagnosis. Typically, the primary diagnosis will be of TMD origin (e.g., myofascial pain), and the secondary and tertiary diagnoses will be other TMD diagnoses (e.g., TMJ inflammation and TMJ disc displacement with reduction) that contribute to a patient's chief complaint. They are ordered by the degree they contribute to the patient's chief complaint.

TMJ click or pop is a very prevalent noise among TMD patients and non-TMD patients, are most commonly related to a patient having a disc displacement with reduction, and by themselves do not suggest the need for a patient to receive TMD therapy.

TMJ crepitus is a grating or crackling noise similar to the sound that is created when one walks over gravel. It is often subdivided into course and fine crepitus. *Course crepitus* is most commonly related to a patient having a chronic disc displacement without reduction, whereas *fine crepitus* does not appear to be highly related to any single articular diagnosis.

TMJ dislocation (also known as *subluxation*) occurs when the condyle catches or locks in front of the articular eminence, causing a patient difficulty or inability of retruding the condyle. This generally occurs at a jaw opening of 45 mm or wider.

Index